METHODS IN MOLECULAR BIOLOGY

For further volumes:
http://www.springer.com/series/7651

For over 35 years, biological scientists have come to rely on the research protocols and methodologies in the critically acclaimed *Methods in Molecular Biology* series. The series was the first to introduce the step-by-step protocols approach that has become the standard in all biomedical protocol publishing. Each protocol is provided in readily-reproducible step-by-step fashion, opening with an introductory overview, a list of the materials and reagents needed to complete the experiment, and followed by a detailed procedure that is supported with a helpful notes section offering tips and tricks of the trade as well as troubleshooting advice. These hallmark features were introduced by series editor Dr. John Walker and constitute the key ingredient in each and every volume of the *Methods in Molecular Biology* series. Tested and trusted, comprehensive and reliable, all protocols from the series are indexed in PubMed.

Oligonucleotide-Based Therapies

Methods and Protocols

Edited by

Olof Gissberg, Rula Zain, and Karin E. Lundin

Center for Advanced Therapies, Department of Laboratory Medicine, Karolinska Institutet, Stockholm, Sweden

Humana Press

Editors
Olof Gissberg
Center for Advanced Therapies
Department of Laboratory Medicine
Karolinska Institutet
Stockholm, Sweden

Rula Zain
Center for Advanced Therapies
Department of Laboratory Medicine
Karolinska Institutet
Stockholm, Sweden

Karin E. Lundin
Center for Advanced Therapies
Department of Laboratory Medicine
Karolinska Institutet
Stockholm, Sweden

ISSN 1064-3745 ISSN 1940-6029 (electronic)
Methods in Molecular Biology
ISBN 978-1-4939-9669-8 ISBN 978-1-4939-9670-4 (eBook)
https://doi.org/10.1007/978-1-4939-9670-4

This Humana imprint is published by the registered company Springer Science+Business Media, LLC part of Springer Nature.
The registered company address is: 233 Spring Street, New York, NY 10013, U.S.A.

Preface

The study of oligonucleotide (ON)-based therapies is a fast-growing field, targeting various biological processes like immune stimulation, translation, transcription, RNA splicing, and specific RNA regulation. The number of chemical modifications used in synthetic nucleic acid chemistry has grown extensively since the 1960s and can be applied to the backbone, the phosphate group, the sugar moiety, and also to the heterocyclic nucleobases.

Most of the existing therapeutic ONs are acting as antisense ONs to influence the splicing pattern of specific pre-mRNAs or to induce degradation of specific RNAs, as small interfering RNA (siRNA), through the RISC complex or as gapmers to induce degradation by RNase H. Other RNA-targeting ONs act as antagomirs to block cellular microRNAs or as microRNA mimics.

The aptamer field has provided ONs that interact with proteins like cellular receptors and can be used to enhance tissue-specific cell uptake, but can also act as protein mimics. New nucleic acid chemistries and the completion of DNA sequencing of the human genome have also allowed the use of anti-gene ONs to directly target DNA to modulate gene expression in cells, and extensive research to enhance the anti-gene field is ongoing.

Oligonucleotide-Based Therapies, part of the *Methods in Molecular Biology* series, provides a collection of comprehensive, up-to-date, and broadly applicable guides to the research and development fields of ON therapeutics. The aim of the book is to cover a wide-ranging and useful spectrum of methods and protocols needed to take full advantage of therapeutic applications involving ONs.

The two first chapters of the book present reviews of existing chemical modifications and ON delivery, including the hurdles of reaching the intended targets and the strategies to overcome these challenges. In the second part of the book, detailed protocols for the study of antisense as well as anti-gene effects are outlined. Methods to formulate or directly conjugate ONs with peptides and how to study in vivo delivery, physiochemical properties, targeting strategies, and toxicological effects are described. Elaborative chapters covering in silico protocols and bioinformatics to find suitable targets and reduce off-target effects are also provided. In addition, the book includes protocols placing the oligonucleotides in the context of drug discovery and development, introducing strategies for studying ONs PK/PD parameters and ADME properties.

We hope that the reader will find the background information and protocols provided in this book to be useful in the laboratory and as a reference guide when designing antisense and anti-gene oligonucleotides for therapeutic applications.

Stockholm, Sweden

Olof Gissberg
Rula Zain
Karin E. Lundin

Contents

Contributors

FRANK ABENDROTH • *Laboratory of Molecular Biology, Medical Research Council, Cambridge, UK; Institute of Pharmacy and Biochemistry, Johannes Gutenberg-University of Mainz, Mainz, Germany*

CHRISTINE AHLSTRÖM • *DMPK, Research and Early Development Cardiovascular, Renal and Metabolism, BioPharmaceuticals R&D, AstraZeneca, Gothenburg, Sweden*

ISABEL F. AMARAL • *i3S—Instituto de Investigação e Inovação em Saúde, Universidade do Porto, Porto, Portugal; INEB—Instituto de Engenharia Biomédica, Universidade do Porto, Porto, Portugal*

PIRET ARUKUUSK • *Institute of Technology, University of Tartu, Tartu, Estonia*

PAULA J. BATES • *Department of Medicine, University of Louisville, Louisville, KY, USA; Department of Biochemistry, University of Louisville, Louisville, KY, USA; Experimental Therapeutics Program of the James Graham Brown Cancer Center, University of Louisville, Louisville, KY, USA*

FRANZISKA BOESS • *Roche Pharma Research and Early Development, Pharmaceutical Sciences (PS), Roche Innovation Center Basel, Basel, Switzerland*

ANDREAS BRINK • *Roche Pharma Research and Early Development, Roche Innovation Center Basel, F. Hoffmann-La Roche Ltd., Basel, Switzerland*

STEVEN EVANS • *Immunology and Inflammation Research, Worldwide Research and Development, Pfizer Inc., Cambridge, MA, USA*

MICHAEL FAULER • *Institute of General Physiology, University of Ulm, Ulm, Germany*

MANFRED FRICK • *Institute of General Physiology, University of Ulm, Ulm, Germany*

MICHAEL J. GAIT • *Laboratory of Molecular Biology, Medical Research Council, Cambridge, UK*

PETER GENNEMARK • *DMPK, Research and Early Development Cardiovascular, Renal and Metabolism, BioPharmaceuticals R&D, AstraZeneca, Gothenburg, Sweden*

OLOF GISSBERG • *Center for Advanced Therapies, Department of Laboratory Medicine, Karolinska Institutet, Stockholm, Sweden*

OKSANA GOROSHCHUK • *Department of Laboratory Medicine, Clinical Research Center, Karolinska Institutet, Huddinge, Sweden*

HELEN GRAVES • *CamPhos Therapeutics, Cambridge, UK*

PETER H. HAGEDORN • *Therapeutic Modalities, Roche Pharma Research and Early Development, Roche Innovation Center Copenhagen, Hørsholm, Denmark*

SUZAN M. HAMMOND • *Department of Paediatrics, University of Oxford, Oxford, UK*

DMYTRO HONCHARENKO • *Department of Biosciences and Nutrition, Karolinska Institutet, Huddinge, Sweden*

MALGORZATA HONCHARENKO • *Department of Biosciences and Nutrition, Karolinska Institutet, Huddinge, Sweden*

CHRISTOPHE HUSSER • *Roche Pharma Research and Early Development, Roche Innovation Center Basel, F. Hoffmann-La Roche Ltd., Basel, Switzerland*

RASMUS JANSSON-LÖFMARK • *DMPK, Research and Early Development Cardiovascular, Renal and Metabolism, BioPharmaceuticals R&D, AstraZeneca, Gothenburg, Sweden*

PHILIPP MICHAEL KLEIN • *Pharmaceutical Biotechnology, Center for System-Based Drug Research, Ludwig-Maximilians-Universität München, Munich, Germany*

TROELS KOCH • *Therapeutic Modalities, Roche Pharma Research and Early Development, Roche Innovation Center Copenhagen, Hørsholm, Denmark*
ERICH KOLLER • *Roche Pharma Research and Early Development, Roche Innovation Center Basel, F. Hoffmann-La Roche Ltd., Basel, Switzerland*
IRYNA KOLOSENKO • *Department of Laboratory Medicine, Clinical Research Center, Karolinska Institutet, Huddinge, Sweden*
KARIN E. LUNDIN • *Center for Advanced Therapies, Department of Laboratory Medicine, Karolinska Institutet, Stockholm, Sweden*
TANJA MINZ • *Roche Pharma Research and Early Development, Pharmaceutical Sciences (PS), Roche Innovation Center Basel, Basel, Switzerland*
PEDRO M. D. MORENO • *i3S—Instituto de Investigação e Inovação em Saúde, Universidade do Porto, Porto, Portugal; INEB—Instituto de Engenharia Biomédica, Universidade do Porto, Porto, Portugal*
STERGHIOS A. MOSCHOS • *Department of Applied Sciences, Faculty of Health and Life Sciences, Northumbria University, Newcastle Upon Tyne, UK*
NEGIN MOZAFARI • *Department of Laboratory Medicine, Center for Advanced Therapies, Karolinska University Hospital Huddinge, Karolinska Institutet, Stockholm, Sweden*
LENNART NILSSON • *Department of Biosciences and Nutrition, Karolinska Institutet, Huddinge, Sweden*
KÄRT PADARI • *Institute of Molecular and Cell Biology, University of Tartu, Tartu, Estonia*
CAROLINE PALM-APERGI • *Department of Laboratory Medicine, Clinical Research Center, Karolinska Institutet, Huddinge, Sweden*
LYKKE PEDERSEN • *Therapeutic Modalities, Roche Pharma Research and Early Development, Roche Innovation Center Copenhagen, Hørsholm, Denmark*
ANA P. PÊGO • *i3S—Instituto de Investigação e Inovação em Saúde, Universidade do Porto, Porto, Portugal; INEB—Instituto de Engenharia Biomédica, Universidade do Porto, Porto, Portugal; Faculdade de Engenharia da Universidade do Porto, Porto, Portugal; Instituto de Ciências Biomédicas Abel Salazar (ICBAS), Universidade do Porto, Porto, Portugal*
NICOLETTE POLLOCK • *Department of Molecular and Cellular Biology, Beckman Research Institute, City of Hope, Duarte, CA, USA*
MARGUS POOGA • *Institute of Molecular and Cell Biology, University of Tartu, Tartu, Estonia; Institute of Technology, University of Tartu, Tartu, Estonia*
LY POROSK • *Institute of Technology, University of Tartu, Tartu, Estonia*
ELSA M. REYES-REYES • *Division of Pulmonary, Allergy, Critical Care, and Sleep Medicine, University of Arizona College of Medicine, Tucson, AZ, USA; Department of Cellular and Molecular Medicine, University of Arizona Cancer Center, Tucson, AZ, USA*
CRISTINA S. J. ROCHA • *Clinical Pharmacology & Safety Sciences, BioPharmaceuticals R&D, AstraZeneca, Gothenburg, Sweden*
TERESA RODRIGUES • *i3S—Instituto de Investigação e Inovação em Saúde, Universidade do Porto, Porto, Portugal; INEB—Instituto de Engenharia Biomédica, Universidade do Porto, Porto, Portugal*
JOHN ROSSI • *Department of Molecular and Cellular Biology, Beckman Research Institute, City of Hope, Duarte, CA, USA*
SIMONE SCHADT • *Roche Pharma Research and Early Development, Roche Innovation Center Basel, F. Hoffmann-La Roche Ltd., Basel, Switzerland*
SABINE SEWING • *Roche Pharma Research and Early Development, Pharmaceutical Sciences (PS), Roche Innovation Center Basel, Basel, Switzerland*

C. I. Edvard Smith • *Department of Laboratory Medicine, Center for Advanced Therapies, Karolinska University Hospital Huddinge, Karolinska Institutet, Stockholm, Sweden*
Roger Strömberg • *Department of Biosciences and Nutrition, Karolinska Institutet, Huddinge, Sweden*
Pantazis I. Theotokis • *National Heart and Lung Institute, Imperial College, London, UK; Cardiovascular Research Centre, Royal Brompton and Harefield NHS Foundation Trust, Imperial College London, London, UK*
Marília Torrado • *i3S—Instituto de Investigação e Inovação em Saúde, Universidade do Porto, Porto, Portugal; INEB—Instituto de Engenharia Biomédica, Universidade do Porto, Porto, Portugal*
Tea Umek • *Department of Laboratory Medicine, Center for Advanced Therapies, Karolinska Institutet, Karolinska University Hospital Huddinge, Stockholm, Sweden*
Louise Usher • *School of Life Sciences, University of Westminster, London, UK*
Linda Vidarsdottir • *Department of Laboratory Medicine, Clinical Research Center, Karolinska Institutet, Huddinge, Sweden*
Alessandra Villa • *Department of Biosciences and Nutrition, Karolinska Institutet, Huddinge, Sweden*
Ernst Wagner • *Pharmaceutical Biotechnology, Center for System-based Drug Research, Ludwig-Maximilians-Universität München, Munich, Germany; Nanosystems Initiative Munich, Munich, Germany*
Matthew J. A. Wood • *Department of Paediatrics, University of Oxford, Oxford, UK*
Xin Xia • *Department of Molecular and Cellular Biology, Beckman Research Institute, City of Hope, Duarte, CA, USA*
Rula Zain • *Center for Advanced Therapies, Department of Laboratory Medicine, Karolinska Institutet, Stockholm, Sweden; Department of Clinical Genetics, Center for Rare Diseases, Karolinska University Hospital, Stockholm, Sweden*
Margherita Zamboni • *Jonas Frisén Lab, Department of Cell and Molecular Biology, Karolinska Institute, Stockholm, Sweden*
Jiehua Zhou • *Department of Molecular and Cellular Biology, Beckman Research Institute, City of Hope, Duarte, CA, USA*

Part I

Reviews

Chapter 1

Chemical Development of Therapeutic Oligonucleotides

Karin E. Lundin, Olof Gissberg, C. I. Edvard Smith, and Rula Zain

Abstract

The development of several different chemical modifications of nucleic acids, with improved base-pairing affinity and specificity as well as increased resistance against nucleases, has been described. These new chemistries have allowed the synthesis of different types of therapeutic oligonucleotides. Here we discuss selected chemistries used in antisense oligonucleotide (ASO) applications (e.g., small interfering RNA (siRNA), RNase H activation, translational block, splice-switching, and also as aptamers). Recently approved oligonucleotide-based drugs are also presented briefly.

Key words Base analogs, Ribose modifications, Phosphodiester linkage, Phosphorodiamidate morpholino (PMO), Locked nucleic acid (LNA), Peptide nucleic acid (PNA), Tricyclo-DNA

1 Introduction

Oligonucleotide (ON) based therapies is a fast-growing field, where efforts are made to target various biological processes like immune-stimulation, transcription, RNA splicing, translation and RNA stability. An important biological property of endogenous nucleic acids is that they are degraded once outside their natural environment, if not properly protected. In particular, single strand (ss) nucleic acids are hydrolyzed by specific endonucleases and exonucleases. This is an important step within gene regulation, and DNA repair, as well as a defence mechanism against virus infections. Nucleic acid degradation also takes place outside the cell in the extracellular compartments. During the last third of the twentieth century a number of new chemically modified nucleic acid analogs were described. The possibility to synthesize modified ONs with increased resistance against nucleases facilitates the development of ON-based therapies.

One advantage of ONs as therapeutics, in comparison to small molecule medicines, is the possibility to design, in a sequence-specific manner, the mode of action and define the biomolecule to be targeted (e.g., mRNA, noncoding RNA, DNA, or even

Olof Gissberg et al. (eds.), *Oligonucleotide-Based Therapies: Methods and Protocols*, Methods in Molecular Biology, vol. 2036, https://doi.org/10.1007/978-1-4939-9670-4_1,

protein). ONs interact with nucleic acids via a sequence specific Watson–Crick base pairing between Guanine and Cytosine and between Adenine and Thymine or Uracil; or as triplex forming ONs binding to the polypurine strand in a DNA duplex via Hoogsteen or reverse Hoogsteen interactions. A drawback compared to small molecule drugs is the relatively large size of ONs, which renders their intracellular delivery a challenge. Spontaneous uptake into the target cell is highly dependent on the chemistry of the ONs. Different approaches to solve the delivery issue are addressed in the review by Xia, Zhou and Rossi, found in Chapter 2.

Beside the delivery issue, there are three major features to carefully address in order to design a biologically active ON: (1) the nuclease stability, (2) the binding strength to the target site and (3) the specificity (the risk for off-target binding). Methods to study the effects of ONs on cellular base, methods to influence cellular uptake and specific tissue delivery, and some strategies to reduce the off-target effects are described in different chapters of this volume. There are numerous chemical modifications of nucleic acids published so far, including heterocyclic nucleobase, sugar, phosphodiester linkage, and more extensive backbone modifications, and many of these have been incorporated in ONs and tested for DNA and RNA interactions using in vitro and in vivo models.

2 The History of Nucleic Acid Chemical Modifications

Since the mid 1960s when the 2′-Fluoro (2′-F) substitution in the ribose moiety of nucleic acids [1, 2] and the phosphorothioate (PS) [3] modification of the phosphodiester backbone in synthetic ONs were first reported, a plethora of different modifications has been described. The chemical structures of selected nucleic acid modifications can be seen in Fig. 1, given in a chronological order according to their initial incorporation in ON synthesis.

The 2′ position of the ribose ring was found to tolerate numerous modifications in addition to 2′-F, without hampering the ability of base-pairing, and many different substitutions were reported during the 1960s. Today two frequently used modifications in ON therapeutics are the 2′-*O*-Methyl (2′-*O*-Me) [4] and the 2′-*O*-Methoxyethyl (2′-*O*-MOE) [5] substitutions.

In the end of 1989, the phosphorodiamidate morpholino (PMO) chemistry was developed. PMO oligomers have a morpholino-phosphoroamidate backbone and thus are charge-neutral. Still, PMOs display good water solubility and in contrast to a PS ON, PMOs have also higher affinity toward an RNA target than the corresponding unmodified DNA [6]. In 1991 an additional nucleic acid analog, the peptide nucleic acid (PNA), was first presented [7]. PNA is based on an *N*-(2-aminoethyl)-glycine

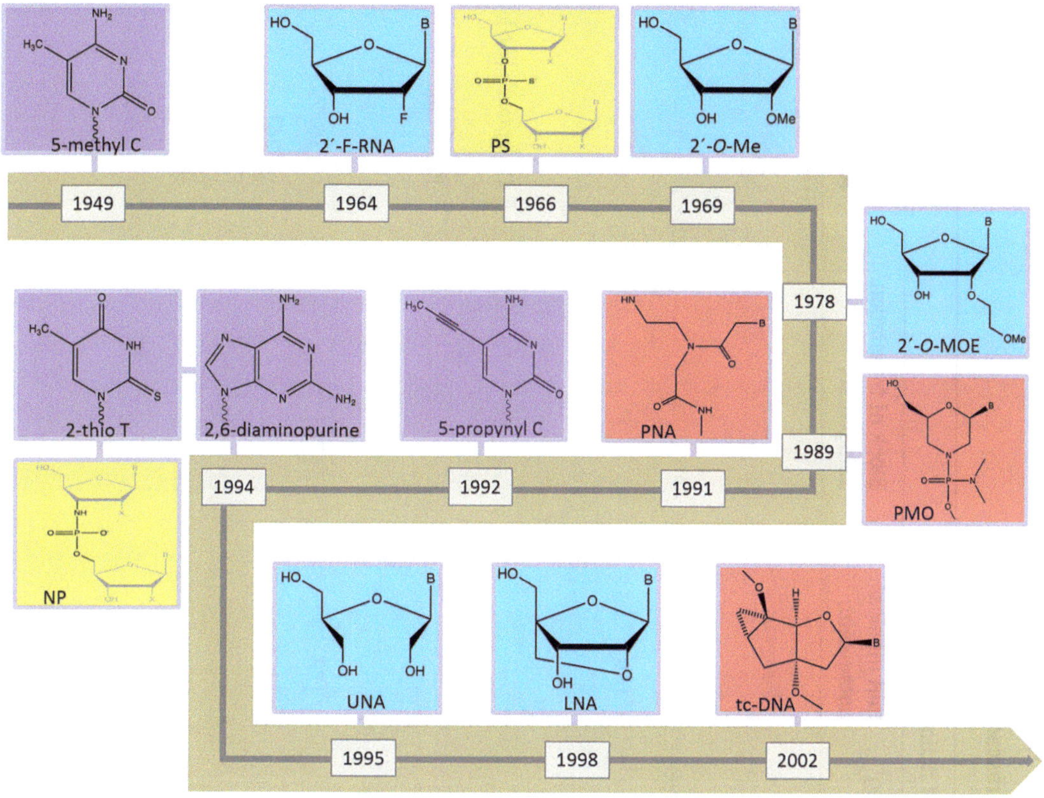

Fig. 1 Time axis of the development of selected chemistries used in synthetic oligonucleotides. *X* = H (DNA) or OH (RNA). Modifications of base (purple boxes), sugar (blue boxes), phosphodiester (yellow boxes), and other backbone (red boxes). Abbreviations: 2′-F, 2′-fluoro; 2′-*O*-Me, 2′-*O*-methyl; 2′-*O*-MOE, 2′-*O*-methoxyethyl; B, heterocyclic nucleobase; LNA locked nucleic acid; NP, N3-phosphoramidate; PS, phosphorothioate; *tc-DNA*, tricyclo-DNA; UNA, unlocked nucleic acid

backbone and binds with much higher affinity toward both RNA and DNA than previously described nucleic acid oligomers do.

In 1995 a new nucleoside analog with a flexible open ribose structure was synthesized and incorporated into an ON [8]. This nucleoside analog, which is designated unlocked nucleic acid (UNA), was shown to stabilize against 3′-exonucleases when placed at the 3′ end but destabilized the duplex formation when several modifications were introduced inside the ON. Later this modification has been incorporated in several types of therapeutic ONs (*see* Table 1). At the end of the 1990s two different groups independently synthesized an RNA analog with a modified ribose, where the nucleosides contain a methylene bridge between the 2′-oxygen and the 4′-carbon in the ribose, creating a locked nucleic acid (LNA) [9, 10]. This modification locks the ribose in a north conformation and increases the melting temperature (*T*m) of an LNA-containing ON forming a duplex with DNA and even more in a duplex with RNA. Various LNA analogs, or bridged nucleic acids

Table 1
Selected chemically modified nucleic acids used in therapeutic oligonucleotide research

Chemical modifications	Chemically modified oligonucleotides' mechanisms of action					
	siRNA	RNase-H-dependent ASOs	Changed splicing pattern	miR mimics/ antagomirs	Block of translation/ antagonists	Aptamers
Base modifications						
5-methyl C[#]	√	√	√	√	√	√
5-propynyl C		√ [67, 68]				
2-thio T		√ [16]				
2,6-diaminopurine				√ [69]		
Sugar modifications						
2′-F-RNA#	√	√[a]	√	√		√ Pegaptanib [56]
2′-*O*-Me-RNA #	√ Patisiran [61]	√[a] [70]	√ Drisapersen [71]	√	√	√ Pegaptanib [56]
2′-*O*-MOE-RNA		√[a] Mipomersen [19]	√ Nusinersen [20]			
LNA	√ [24, 25]	√[a] [21]	√ [41, 72]	√ [73, 74]	√ [75]	√ [76, 77]
UNA	√ [25]			√ [27]		√ [26]
Linkage modifications						
Phosphorothioate (PS)	√	√ Fomivirsen[b] [55] Mipomersen [19]	√ Nusinersen [20]	√	√	√ [78]

N3′-5′ phosphoramidate (NP)				√ [79]
N3′-P5′ thio phosphoramidate				√ [80] GRN163L (Imetelstat) [29, 66]
Additional backbone modifications				
PMO		√ [39, 42] Eteplirsen [40]		√ [39]
PNA		√ [48, 81] ISIS 208529 [82]	√ [48]	√ [48, 75, 83]
Tricyclo-DNA	√[a] [53]	√ [50, 53]		√ [51, 53]

2′-F, 2′-fluoro; 2′-*O*-Me, 2′-*O*-methyl; 2′-*O*-MOE, 2′-*O*-methoxyethyl; LNA, locked nucleic acid; UNA, unlocked nucleic acid; PNA, peptide nucleic acid; PMO, phosphorodiamidate morpholino

[#]These modifications are common in oligonucleotides within all groups of actions, mostly in combination with modifications in other parts of the nucleotides

[a]The chemical modification is used in the flanking region of the "gapmer" ONs

[b]Fomivirsen is an all DNA PS modified ON, the ASO mechanism of action is not clear, the drug is no longer available from the manufacturer

(BNAs), with constrained conformation have the ability to improve ON performance, such as 2,4-constrained ethyl (cEt)-BNA [11]. In 2002, Tricyclo-DNA, which also belongs to the family of conformationally restricted oligodeoxynucleotide analogs, was developed [12]. It differs structurally from DNA by an additional ethylene bridge to which a cyclopropane unit is fused (Fig. 1). The tricyclo-DNA modification imposes an increased rigidity on the modified ON, with increased *Tm* toward both DNA and RNA targets.

3 Selected Chemistries Used in Experimental ON Therapeutics

The choice of chemical modification(s) to be used in a therapeutic ON depends on the desired mechanism of action. ONs have, for example, been used to degrade specific RNAs (siRNA and gapmer antisense ONs (ASOs)), to influence splicing of pre-mRNA, to block translation by preventing required protein–RNA interaction, and to modulate transcription by binding to DNA [13]. ONs have also been used as aptamers, where the base-pairing property within the ON itself creates a three-dimensional structure interacting with diverse biological molecules, and they may also act as adjuvants. A summary over selected nucleic acid chemical modifications that have been applied in several ON targeting mechanisms is shown in Table 1. Antigene ONs targeting double strand DNA (dsDNA), through triplex forming or dsDNA invasion mechanisms, have not been included since these have not yet reached clinical trials. Neither has the use of ONs as immunological adjuvants been addressed. For a more detailed review including these mechanisms, *see* [14].

Nucleic acid modifications can be introduced in the heterocyclic nucleobase, the ribose and deoxyribose, the phosphodiester linkage or as larger backbone modifications. Biologically active ONs frequently include a combination of chemical modifications.

3.1 Nucleobase Modifications

A frequently used base modification is the addition of a methyl group in position 5 of the cytosine. This base modification is also naturally occurring. The methyl group increases the binding affinity toward the complementary RNA and has been used in many types of ONs, mostly in combination with sugar or linkage modifications. The introduction of a propynyl group in the same position further increases the *Tm* as compared to the methyl substitution. The propynyl group has been demonstrated to be effective in antisense applications, but seems to be detrimental when incorporated in siRNA [15]. Another interesting base modification is the 2-thio dT. When incorporated in the correct position in the DNA gap of an ASO, it was shown to provide allele specificity for an ON directed toward *Huntingtin* mRNA [16]. Substitutions have also been introduced on purine bases, for example the 2,6 diaminopurine which stabilizes the hybridization to thymine and uracil through its capacity to form an extra hydrogen bond [17].

3.2 Sugar and Phosphodiester Modifications

Among the sugar modifications the 2′-F and the 2′-*O*-Me substitutions in the ribose 2′ position were the first to be reported (*see* Fig. 1), and these have been frequently used in various classes of RNA-targeting ONs. Both modifications increase the binding affinity to a complementary RNA strand and also reduce sensitivity toward nucleases [14]. Chemical modifications at the 2′ position have also been reported to reduce the immunological response of administered ONs, at least in mice [18].

The 2′-*O*-MOE modification also provides an enhanced binding affinity and nuclease resistance, as compared to 2′-*O*-Me, and it has been used in two clinically approved ONs for the treatment of familial hypercholesterolaemia [19] and in spinal muscular atrophy (SMA) [20].

Similar to PNA, LNA-containing ONs have high affinity toward complementary sequences, and display a strong mismatch discrimination toward both DNA and RNA, and significantly increases stability toward nucleases. A number of LNA modifications have later been synthesized, adding further to the chemical spectra of locked RNA analogs which improve the affinity, specificity and biological effects when inserted into ONs [21]. Of specific interest are those where the 2′-oxygen has been substituted by an amine resulting in a 2′-amino-LNA, thus further influencing the sugar conformation and the net charge of the corresponding ON [22]. A closely related modification is the 2′-4′ constrained ethylene bridged nucleic acid, ENA, which has also been used in gapmers and in splice-switching ASOs [23]. LNA of different types are extensively being used in all types of clinically relevant ONs. The use of a few LNAs in the seed region of siRNA was lately shown to reduce off-target effects [24], and has also been introduced in the passenger strand of so called small internally segmented interfering (sisi) RNA [25]. The UNA modification, despite a slightly destabilizing property when incorporated inside an ON, has also been used in sisiRNA [25] as well as in aptamers [26] and as antimir [27].

All these RNA analogs are commonly combined with a phosphodiester linkage modification, most frequently the phosphorothioate (PS) linkage with a sulphur atom substituting one of the nonbridging oxygens in the phosphate group [3]. Other linker modifications used are the N3′-5′ phosphoramidate (NP) linkage which stabilizes the ONs but does not support activation of RNase H [28], and the N3′-P5′-thio-phosphoramidate linkage which has been used in the clinically tested telomerase antagonist GRN163L (Imetelstat) [29].

The PS linkage is stable against nucleases but has also the important property of binding to serum proteins, which prolongs the ON half-life in serum. The PS linkage also influences positively the cellular internalization of modified ONs [30]. These properties have resulted in the frequent use of the PS linkage in therapeutic ONs. A concern is that toxicity events, like complement activation, reported for PS containing ONs [31, 32], and platelet reduction have been described both in a nonhuman primate [33] and in a few patients [34] treated with PS containing ASOs.

3.3 Additional Backbone Modifications

In addition to the numerous RNA analogs tested and used in therapeutic ONs, several completely different chemistries have been used as backbone entities for the nucleobases. Among these we will only discuss the PMO [35], the PNA [7], and the tricyclo-DNA(tc-DNA) [12] chemical modifications.

Since PMOs are highly resistant to nucleases and have good base-pairing properties they have been used in ASOs to modify splicing of pre-mRNA [36, 37]. PMO oligomers have also been utilized to reduce specific gene expression by blocking the RNA interaction with proteins involved in, for example, viral translation and to block viral RNA replication [38, 39]. Due to the uncharged backbone, PMO oligomers require assistance to be efficiently taken up into cells, unless given in very high doses. The uncharged backbone, however, allows for the attachment of charged cell-penetrating peptides, which may increase the future clinical usage of this chemistry, for a recent review *see* [39]. The safety of the PMO chemistry has been shown in clinical trials (e.g., for the approved compound eteplirsen [40]), and peptide-conjugated PMOs have been shown to be active in two different disease mouse models, for X-linked agammaglobulinemia [41] and SMA [42].

PNAs, being composed of an uncharged peptide-like *N*2-aminoethyl-glycine backbone, are normally synthesized with one or several charged amino acids at the terminals, in order to improve their solubility. PNA oligomers display high binding affinity and specificity toward their corresponding RNA or DNA targets, but are not taken up spontaneously by cells unless attached to positively charged cell-penetrating peptides [43]. The PNA chemistry has had an impact on diagnostic applications as probes in quantitative PCR and in fluorescence in situ hybridization (PNA-FISH) [44]. Furthermore, promising reports are emerging on the possibility to develop PNA as specific antibacterial compounds, [45] and as anticancer drugs through, for example, blocking the activity of oncomiRs [46, 47], for a recent review *see* [48].

The tc-DNA is another interesting modification which has been tested as ASOs; for example, it was found to be as efficient as a 2′-*O*-MOE gapmer in silencing the *scavenger receptor B1 (SR-B1)* mRNA [49]. This modification has also been introduced in ONs acting as splice-modifying [50], and as translation-blocking [51]. Interestingly, tc-DNA ONs have a broad in vivo distribution, which distinguish them from most of the other ON analogs. Gapmers containing tc-DNA have been used, for example, to downregulate human huntingtin expression in mice carrying a human mutated *HTT* gene. The ability of splice-switching tc-DNA ONs to cross the blood–brain barrier (BBB) has also been confirmed by the increased wild type *SMN* mRNA levels in mouse brain after weekly subcutaneous injections [52]. For a review over tc-DNAs *see* [53].

4 Approved Therapeutic ONs and Therapeutics in Late-Stage Clinical Trials.

For obvious reasons, the first ON therapeutics that entered clinical trials had the early-on discovered modifications such as the PS backbone, 2′-*O*-Me and 2′-F sugar modifications. Accordingly, the first FDA approved ON drug fomivirsen (Vitravene) consisted of unmodified DNA nucleotides with a PS backbone [54]. However, studies on its mode of action indicated multiple pathways including RNase H mediated cleavage and/or steric blocking [55]. In the end, Fomivirsen only became a transient success due to the reduced need for treatment in the approved indication (CMV retinitis in HIV infection), as the underlying cause was better treated using other drugs. The next ON drug to be approved was Pegaptanib (Macugen) for treatment of Macular degeneration, a polyethylene glycol (PEG) conjugated aptamer with mostly 2′-*O*-Me and 2′-F RNA modifications and with phosphodiester backbone [56]. The first approved gapmer ON was Mipomersen (Kynamro) for treatment of Hypercholesterolemia. Like the later approved Inotersen (Tegsedi) for treatment of Transthyretin amyloidosis, Mipomersen contains 2′-*O*-MOE RNA in the flanking sequences surrounding the central DNA region, combined with PS linkages throughout the ON, and 5-Methyl cytosines [54, 57, 58].

The two approved splice-switch ONs Eteplirsen (Exondys 51) and Nusinersen (Spinraza) are also modified using the early-discovered modifications, PMO and 2′-*O*-MOE PS-backbone respectively [59, 60]. The first siRNA approved, Patisiran (Onpattro) for treatment of Transthyretin amyloidosis, consists of mixed RNA/2′-*O*-Me RNA strands with DNA overhangs (two nucleotides on each strand) with phosphodiester backbones. Since the cellular uptake of siRNA is limited, Patisiran requires an LNP (Lipid nanoparticle) formulation to reach the intracellular space [61]. All approved ONs with the indications and the corresponding approval dates are listed in Table 2 together with their ON-class.

Other ONs in late-stage clinical trials include RG6042 (IONIS-HTTRx) [62] and Volanosorsen (Waylivra) [34], two 2′-*O*-MOE RNA PS gapmers targeting huntingtin mRNA (*HTT*) in Huntington's disease (HD) and apolipoprotein (ApoC-III) in familial chylomicronemia syndrome (FCS), respectively. Two PMO splice-switch ONs named Golodirsen and Casimersen for the treatment

Table 2
List of approved ON therapeutics up to date

ON drug	ON Class	Approved	Indication
Fomivirsen (Vitravene)	ASO	1998 (FDA) 1999 (EMA)	CMV retinitis
Pegaptanib (Macugen)	Aptamer	2004 (FDA)	Macular degeneration
Mipomersen (Kynamro)	Gapmer ASO	2013 (FDA)	Hyper cholesterolemia
Eteplirsen (Exondys 51)	Splice-switch ASO	2016 (FDA)	Duchenne muscular dystrophy
Defibrotide (Defitelio)[a]	ssDNA/aptamer	2016 (FDA)	VOD in HSCT
Nusinersen (Spinraza)	Splice-switch ASO	2017 (FDA)	Spinal muscular atrophy
Patisiran (Onpattro)	siRNA	2018 (FDA/EMA)	Transthyretin amyloidosis
Inotersen (Tegsedi)	Gapmer ASO	2018 (FDA/EMA)	Transthyretin amyloidosis

CMV Cytomegalovirus, *VOD* Veno-occlusive disease, *HSCT* Human stem cell transplantation
[a]The mechanism of action is debated

of Duchenne muscular dystrophy (DMD) are currently in phase III clinical trials [63]. In general, many of the ON therapeutics that are upcoming clinical candidates in the pipelines use more elaborated combinations of modifications, and/or carry targeting ligands to reach the desired cell type or tissue for increased uptake. Such ONs include the late-stage clinical siRNAs Inclisiran [64], Givosiran and Revusiran [65], all using a mixture of 2′-*O*-MOE and 2′-F RNA and terminal PS backbones in either one or both strands, conjugated with the *N*-acetylgalactosamine (GalNAc) ligand for increased hepatocyte uptake through the asialoglycoprotein receptor (ASGPR). Imetelstat is another late-stage clinical ON for the treatment of certain cancers, especially myelodysplastic syndromes. This ON has a thio-phosphoramidate (NPS) backbone conjugated with a palmitoyl (C16) lipid group in the 5′ end [66].

5 Concluding Remarks

Oligonucleotides have become important tools in molecular biology, in diagnostic procedures and also as therapeutics. Crucial for this development has been the development of new chemistries. Many synthetic nucleic acid derivatives have been generated over the years and several modifications have been introduced in ONs and tested in biological systems. While oligonucleotides have been approved as medicines there are many remaining challenges, especially regarding tissue-specific delivery and pharmacological properties.

Acknowledgments

This work was supported by the Swedish Research Council, the Stockholm County Council, Hjärnfonden, and Vinnova/SweLife.

References

1. Reist EJ, Benitez A, Goodman L (1964) The synthesis of some 5-′-thiopentofuranosylpyrimidines. J Org Chem 29(3):554–558
2. Codington JF, Doerr IL, Fox JJ (1964) Nucleosides. XVIII. Synthesis of 2-′-fluorothymidine, 2′-fluorodeoxyuridine, and other 2′-halogeno-2′-deoxy nucleosides. J Org Chem 29(3):558–564
3. Eckstein F (1966) Nucleoside phosphorothioates. J Am Chem Soc 88:4292–4294
4. Bobst AM, Rottman F, Cerutti PA (1969) Effect of the methylation of the 2′-hydroxyl groups in polyadenylic acid on its structure in weakly acidic and neutral solutions and on its capability to form ordered complexes with polyuridylic acid. J Mol Biol 46(2):221–234
5. Martin P (1995) Ein neuer zugang zu 2′-O-alkylribonucleosiden und eigenschaften deren oligonucleotide. Helv Chim Acta 78 (2):486–504
6. Summerton J, Weller D (1997) Morpholino antisense oligomers: design, preparation, and properties. Antisense Nucleic Acid Drug Dev 7(3):187–195
7. Nielsen PE, Egholm M, Berg RH, Buchardt O (1991) Sequence-selective recognition of DNA by strand displacement with a thymine-substituted polyamide. Science 254 (5037):1497–1500
8. Nielsen P, Dreioe LH, Wengel J (1995) Synthesis and evaluation of oligodeoxynucleotides containing acyclic nucleosides: introduction of three novel analogues and a summary. Bioorg Med Chem 3(1):19–28
9. Obika S, Nanbu D, Hari Y, Morio K-I, In Y, Ishida T et al (1997) Synthesis of 2′-O, 4′-C-methyleneuridine and -cytidine. Novel bicyclic nucleosides having a fixed C3′-endo sugar puckering. Tetrahedron Lett 38:8735–8738
10. Koshkin AA, Singh SK, Nielsen P, Rajwanshi VK, Kumar R, Meldgaard M et al (1998) Synthesis of the adenine, cytosine, guanine, 5-methylcytosine, thymine and uracil bicyclonucleoside monomers, oligomerisation, and unprecedented nucleic acid recognition. Tetrahedron 54:3607–3630
11. Seth PP, Siwkowski A, Allerson CR, Vasquez G, Lee S, Prakash TP et al (2009) Short antisense oligonucleotides with novel 2′-4′ conformationaly restricted nucleoside analogues show improved potency without increased toxicity in animals. J Med Chem 52 (1):10–13
12. Renneberg D, Leumann CJ (2002) Watson-crick base-pairing properties of tricyclo-DNA. J Am Chem Soc 124(21):5993–6002
13. Lundin KE, Gissberg O, Smith CI (2015) Oligonucleotide therapies: the past and the present. Hum Gene Ther 26(8):475–485
14. Smith CIE, Zain R (2019) Therapeutic oligonucleotides: state of the art. Annu Rev Pharmacol Toxicol 59:605–630
15. Terrazas M, Kool ET (2009) RNA major groove modifications improve si RNA stability and biological activity. Nucleic Acids Res 37 (2):346–353
16. Ostergaard ME, Kumar P, Nichols J, Watt A, Sharma PK, Nielsen P et al (2015) Allele-selective inhibition of mutant huntingtin with 2-thio- and C5- triazolylphenyl-deoxythymidine-modified antisense oligonucleotides. Nucleic Acid Ther. 25(5):266–274
17. Wan WB, Seth PP (2016) The medicinal chemistry of therapeutic oligonucleotides. J Med Chem 59(21):9645–9667
18. Henry S, Stecker K, Brooks D, Monteith D, Conklin B, Bennett CF (2000) Chemically modified oligonucleotides exhibit decreased immune stimulation in mice. J Pharmacol Exp Ther 292(2):468–479
19. Raal FJ, Santos RD, Blom DJ, Marais AD, Charng MJ, Cromwell WC et al (2010) Mipomersen, an apolipoprotein B synthesis inhibitor, for lowering of LDL cholesterol concentrations in patients with homozygous familial hypercholesterolaemia: a randomised, double-blind, placebo-controlled trial. Lancet 375(9719):998–1006
20. Gidaro T, Servais L (2019) Nusinersen treatment of spinal muscular atrophy: current knowledge and existing gaps. Dev Med Child Neurol 61(1):19–24

21. Lundin KE, Hojland T, Hansen BR, Persson R, Bramsen JB, Kjems J et al (2013) Biological activity and biotechnological aspects of locked nucleic acids. Adv Genet 82:47–107
22. Lou C, Samuelsen SV, Christensen NJ, Vester B, Wengel J (2017) Oligonucleotides containing aminated 2′-amino-LNA nucleotides: synthesis and strong binding to complementary DNA and RNA. Bioconjug Chem 28 (4):1214–1220
23. Lee T, Awano H, Yagi M, Matsumoto M, Watanabe N, Goda R et al (2017) 2′-O-methyl RNA/ethylene-bridged nucleic acid chimera antisense oligonucleotides to induce dystrophin exon 45 skipping. Genes (Basel) 8(2)
24. Iribe H, Miyamoto K, Takahashi T, Kobayashi Y, Leo J, Aida M et al (2017) Chemical modification of the si RNA seed region suppresses off-target effects by steric hindrance to base-pairing with targets. ACS Omega 2 (5):2055–2064
25. Mook O, Vreijling J, Wengel SL, Wengel J, Zhou C, Chattopadhyaya J et al (2010) In vivo efficacy and off-target effects of locked nucleic acid (LNA) and unlocked nucleic acid (UNA) modified si RNA and small internally segmented interfering RNA (sisi RNA) in mice bearing human tumor xenografts. Artif DNA PNA XNA 1(1):36–44
26. Kotkowiak W, Lisowiec-Wachnicka J, Grynda J, Kierzek R, Wengel J, Pasternak A (2018) Thermodynamic, anticoagulant, and Antiproliferative properties of thrombin binding aptamer containing novel UNA derivative. Mol Ther Nucleic Acids. 10:304–316
27. Ferino A, Miglietta G, Picco R, Vogel S, Wengel J, Xodo LE (2018) Micro RNA therapeutics: design of single-stranded mi R-216b mimics to target KRAS in pancreatic cancer cells. RNA Biol 15(10):1273–1285
28. Heidenreich O, Gryaznov S, Nerenberg M (1997) RNase H-independent antisense activity of oligonucleotide N3′--> P 5′ phosphoramidates. Nucleic Acids Res 25(4):776–780
29. Schrank Z, Khan N, Osude C, Singh S, Miller RJ, Merrick C et al (2018) Oligonucleotides targeting telomeres and telomerase in cancer. Molecules 23(9)
30. Eckstein F (2014) Phosphorothioates, essential components of therapeutic oligonucleotides. Nucleic Acids Ther 24(6):374–387
31. Iannitti T, Morales-Medina JC, Palmieri B (2014) Phosphorothioate oligonucleotides: effectiveness and toxicity. Curr Drug Targets 15(7):663–673
32. Henry SP, Seguin R, Cavagnaro J, Berman C, Tepper J, Kornbrust D (2016) Considerations for the characterization and interpretation of results related to alternative complement activation in monkeys associated with oligonucleotide-based therapeutics. Nucleic Acids Ther 26(4):210–215
33. Narayanan P, Shen L, Curtis BR, Bourdon MA, Nolan JP, Gupta S et al (2018) Investigation into the mechanism (s) that leads to platelet decreases in cynomolgus monkeys during administration of ISIS 104838, a 2-′-MOE-modified antisense oligonucleotide. Toxicol Sci 164(2):613–626
34. Crooke ST, Baker BF, Witztum JL, Kwoh TJ, Pham NC, Salgado N et al (2017) The effects of 2′-O-methoxyethyl containing antisense oligonucleotides on platelets in human clinical trials. Nucleic Acids Ther 27(3):121–129
35. Stirchak EP, Summerton JE, Weller DD (1989) Uncharged stereoregular nucleic acid analogs: 2. Morpholino nucleoside oligomers with carbamate internucleoside linkages. Nucleic Acids Res 17(15):6129–6141
36. Yokota T, Duddy W, Partridge T (2007) Optimizing exon skipping therapies for DMD. Acta Myol 26(3):179–184
37. Du L, Gatti RA (2011) Potential therapeutic applications of antisense morpholino oligonucleotides in modulation of splicing in primary immunodeficiency diseases. J Immunol Methods 365(1–2):1–7
38. Deas TS, Binduga-Gajewska I, Tilgner M, Ren P, Stein DA, Moulton HM et al (2005) Inhibition of flavivirus infections by antisense oligomers specifically suppressing viral translation and RNA replication. J Virol 79 (8):4599–4609
39. Nan Y, Zhang YJ (2018) Antisense Phosphorodiamidate Morpholino oligomers as novel antiviral compounds. Front Microbiol 9:750
40. Lim KR, Maruyama R, Yokota T (2017) Eteplirsen in the treatment of Duchenne muscular dystrophy. Drug Des Devel Ther 11:533–545
41. Bestas B, Moreno PM, Blomberg KE, Mohammad DK, Saleh AF, Sutlu T et al (2014) Splice-correcting oligonucleotides restore BTK function in X-linked agammaglobulinemia model. J Clin Invest 124(9):4067–4081
42. Hammond SM, Hazell G, Shabanpoor F, Saleh AF, Bowerman M, Sleigh JN et al (2016) Systemic peptide-mediated oligonucleotide therapy improves long-term survival in spinal muscular atrophy. Proc Natl Acad Sci U S A 113(39):10962–10967
43. Lundin KE, Good L, Stromberg R, Graslund A, Smith CI (2006) Biological activity and biotechnological aspects of peptide nucleic acid. Adv Genet 56:1–51

44. Gupta A, Mishra A, Puri N (2017) Peptide nucleic acids: advanced tools for biomedical applications. J Biotechnol 259:148–159
45. Narenji H, Gholizadeh P, Aghazadeh M, Rezaee MA, Asgharzadeh M, Kafil HS (2017) Peptide nucleic acids (PNAs): currently potential bactericidal agents. Biomed Pharmacother 93:580–588
46. Babar IA, Cheng CJ, Booth CJ, Liang X, Weidhaas JB, Saltzman WM et al (2012) Nanoparticle-based therapy in an in vivo micro RNA-155 (mi R-155)-dependent mouse model of lymphoma. Proc Natl Acad Sci U S A 109(26):E1695–E1704
47. Brognara E, Fabbri E, Aimi F, Manicardi A, Bianchi N, Finotti A et al (2012) Peptide nucleic acids targeting mi R-221 modulate p27Kip1 expression in breast cancer MDA-MB-231 cells. Int J Oncol 41 (6):2119–2127
48. Montazersaheb S, Hejazi MS, Nozad CH (2018) Potential of peptide nucleic acids in future therapeutic applications. Adv Pharm Bull 8(4):551–563
49. Murray S, Ittig D, Koller E, Berdeja A, Chappell A, Prakash TP et al (2012) Tricyclo DNA-modified oligo-2′-deoxyribonucleotides reduce scavenger receptor B1 mRNA in hepatic and extra-hepatic tissues--a comparative study of oligonucleotide length, design and chemistry. Nucleic Acids Res 40(13):6135–6143
50. Relizani K, Goyenvalle A (2018) Use of Tricyclo-DNA antisense oligonucleotides for exon skipping. Methods Mol Biol 1828:381–394
51. Ivanova G, Reigadas S, Ittig D, Arzumanov A, Andreola ML, Leumann C et al (2007) Tricyclo-DNA containing oligonucleotides as steric block inhibitors of human immunodeficiency virus type 1 tat-dependent trans-activation and HIV-1 infectivity. Oligonucleotides 17(1):54–65
52. Robin V, Griffith G, Carter JL, Leumann CJ, Garcia L, Goyenvalle A (2017) Efficient SMN rescue following subcutaneous Tricyclo-DNA antisense oligonucleotide treatment. Mol Ther Nucleic Acids 7:81–89
53. Aupy P, Echevarria L, Relizani K, Goyenvalle A (2017) The use of Tricyclo-DNA oligomers for the treatment of genetic disorders. Biomedicine 6(1)
54. Geary RS, Henry SP, Grillone LR (2002) Fomivirsen: clinical pharmacology and potential drug interactions. Clin Pharmacokinet 41 (4):255–260
55. Anderson KP, Fox MC, Brown-Driver V, Martin MJ, Azad RF (1996) Inhibition of human cytomegalovirus immediate-early gene expression by an antisense oligonucleotide complementary to immediate-early RNA. Antimicrob Agents Chemother 40(9):2004–2011
56. Ng EW, Shima DT, Calias P, Cunningham ET Jr, Guyer DR, Adamis AP (2006) Pegaptanib, a targeted anti-VEGF aptamer for ocular vascular disease. Nat Rev Drug Discov 5 (2):123–132
57. Geary RS, Baker BF, Crooke ST (2015) Clinical and preclinical pharmacokinetics and pharmacodynamics of mipomersen (kynamro ((R))): a second-generation antisense oligonucleotide inhibitor of apolipoprotein B. Clin Pharmacokinet 54(2):133–146
58. Yu RZ, Grundy JS, Henry SP, Kim TW, Norris DA, Burkey J et al (2015) Predictive dose-based estimation of systemic exposure multiples in mouse and monkey relative to human for antisense oligonucleotides with 2′-o-(2-methoxyethyl) modifications. Mol Ther Nucleic Acids 4:e218
59. Sazani P, Ness KP, Weller DL, Poage DW, Palyada K, Shrewsbury SB (2011) Repeat-dose toxicology evaluation in cynomolgus monkeys of AVI-4658, a phosphorodiamidate morpholino oligomer (PMO) drug for the treatment of duchenne muscular dystrophy. Int J Toxicol 30(3):313–321
60. Hua Y, Sahashi K, Hung G, Rigo F, Passini MA, Bennett CF et al (2010) Antisense correction of SMN2 splicing in the CNS rescues necrosis in a type III SMA mouse model. Genes Dev 24(15):1634–1644
61. Yang J (2019) Patisiran for the treatment of hereditary transthyretin-mediated amyloidosis. Expert Rev Clin Pharmacol 12(2):95–99
62. Shen X, Corey DR (2018) Chemistry, mechanism and clinical status of antisense oligonucleotides and duplex RNAs. Nucleic Acids Res 46(4):1584–1600
63. Rodrigues M, Yokota T (2018) An overview of recent advances and clinical applications of exon skipping and splice modulation for muscular dystrophy and various genetic diseases. Methods Mol Biol 1828:31–55
64. Khvorova A (2017) Oligonucleotide therapeutics – a new class of cholesterol-lowering drugs. N Engl J Med 376(1):4–7
65. Zimmermann TS, Karsten V, Chan A, Chiesa J, Boyce M, Bettencourt BR et al (2017) Clinical proof of concept for a novel hepatocyte-targeting gal NAc-si RNA conjugate. Mol Ther 25(1):71–78
66. Jackson SR, Zhu CH, Paulson V, Watkins L, Dikmen ZG, Gryaznov SM et al (2007) Anti-adhesive effects of GRN163L – an

oligonucleotide N3′->P 5′ thio-phosphoramidate targeting telomerase. Cancer Res 67(3):1121–1129

67. Hamel Y, Lacoste J, Frayssinet C, Sarasin A, Garestier T, Francois JC et al (1999) Inhibition of gene expression by anti-sense C-5 propyne oligonucleotides detected by a reporter enzyme. Biochem J 339(Pt 3):547–553
68. Wagner RW, Matteucci MD, Grant D, Huang T, Froehler BC (1996) Potent and selective inhibition of gene expression by an antisense heptanucleotide. Nat Biotechnol 14 (7):840–844
69. Kamiya Y, Donoshita Y, Kamimoto H, Murayama K, Ariyoshi J, Asanuma H (2017) Introduction of 2,6-diaminopurines into Serinol nucleic acid improves anti-mi RNA performance. Chembiochem 18(19):1917–1922
70. Monia BP, Lesnik EA, Gonzalez C, Lima WF, McGee D, Guinosso CJ et al (1993) Evaluation of 2′-modified oligonucleotides containing 2′-deoxy gaps as antisense inhibitors of gene expression. J Biol Chem 268 (19):14514–14522
71. Goemans N, Mercuri E, Belousova E, Komaki H, Dubrovsky A, McDonald CM et al (2018) A randomized placebo-controlled phase 3 trial of an antisense oligonucleotide, drisapersen, in Duchenne muscular dystrophy. Neuromuscul Disord 28(1):4–15
72. Maruyama R, Touznik A, Yokota T (2018) Evaluation of exon inclusion induced by splice switching antisense oligonucleotides in SMA patient fibroblasts. J Vis Exp 135
73. Lima JF, Carvalho J, Pinto-Ribeiro I, Almeida C, Wengel J, Cerqueira L et al (2018) Targeting mi R-9 in gastric cancer cells using locked nucleic acid oligonucleotides. BMC Mol Biol 19(1):6
74. Krutzfeldt J, Rajewsky N, Braich R, Rajeev KG, Tuschl T, Manoharan M et al (2005) Silencing of micro RNAs in vivo with 'antagomirs'. Nature 438(7068):685–689
75. Nulf CJ, Corey D (2004) Intracellular inhibition of hepatitis C virus (HCV) internal ribosomal entry site (IRES)-dependent translation by peptide nucleic acids (PNAs) and locked nucleic acids (LNAs). Nucleic Acids Res 32(13):3792–3798
76. Edwards SL, Poongavanam V, Kanwar JR, Roy K, Hillman KM, Prasad N et al (2015) Targeting VEGF with LNA-stabilized G-rich oligonucleotide for efficient breast cancer inhibition. Chem Commun (Camb) 51 (46):9499–9502
77. Elle IC, Karlsen KK, Terp MG, Larsen N, Nielsen R, Derbyshire N et al (2015) Selection of LNA-containing DNA aptamers against recombinant human CD73. Mol BioSyst 11 (5):1260–1270
78. Volk DE, Lokesh GLR (2017) Development of phosphorothioate DNA and DNA thioaptamers. Biomedicine 5(3)
79. Faria M, Spiller DG, Dubertret C, Nelson JS, White MR, Scherman D et al (2001) Phosphoramidate oligonucleotides as potent antisense molecules in cells and in vivo. Nat Biotechnol 19(1):40–44
80. Gryaznov SM (2010) Oligonucleotide n3′--> p 5′ phosphoramidates and thiophoshoramidates as potential therapeutic agents. Chem Biodivers 7(3):477–493
81. Gao X, Shen X, Dong X, Ran N, Han G, Cao L et al (2015) Peptide nucleic acid promotes systemic dystrophin expression and functional rescue in dystrophin-deficient mdx mice. Mol Ther Nucleic Acids 4:e255
82. Siwkowski AM, Malik L, Esau CC, Maier MA, Wancewicz EV, Albertshofer K et al (2004) Identification and functional validation of PNAs that inhibit murine CD40 expression by redirection of splicing. Nucleic Acids Res 32(9):2695–2706
83. Doyle DF, Braasch DA, Simmons CG, Janowski BA, Corey DR (2001) Inhibition of gene expression inside cells by peptide nucleic acids: effect of mRNA target sequence, mismatched bases, and PNA length. Biochemistry 40(1):53–64

Chapter 2

Tissue-Specific Delivery of Oligonucleotides

Xin Xia, Nicolette Pollock, Jiehua Zhou, and John Rossi

Abstract

From the initial discovery of short-interfering RNA (siRNA) and antisense oligonucleotides for specific gene knockdown at the posttranscriptional level to the current CRISPR-Cas9 system offering gene editing at the genomic level, oligonucleotides, in addition to their biological functions in storing and conveying genetic information, provide the most prominent solutions to targeted gene therapies. Nonetheless, looking into the future of curing cancer and acute diseases, researchers are only cautiously optimistic as the cellular delivery of these polyanionic biomacromolecules is still the biggest hurdle for their therapeutic realization. To overcome the delivery obstacle, oligonucleotides have been encapsulated within or conjugated with delivery vehicles for enhanced membrane penetration, improved payload, and tissue-specific delivery. Such delivery systems include but not limited to virus-based vehicles, gold-nanoparticle vehicles, formulated liposomes, and synthetic polymers. In this chapter, delivery challenges imposed by biological barriers are briefly discussed; followed by recent advances in tissue-specific oligonucleotide delivery utilizing both viral and nonviral delivery vectors, discussing their advantages, and how judicious design and formulation could improve and expand their potential as delivery vehicles.

Key words Oligonucleotide therapeutics, Tissue-specific, Phagocytosis, EPR, Endosomal escape, Ligands, Antibodies, Aptamers

1 Introduction

For the past two decades, the ever-growing potential of gene therapy has drawn substantial efforts from all research fields [1–13]. Although the concept of introducing exogenous oligonucleotides into target cells and subsequently correcting for the incorrectness and/or strengthening the weakness is well known, its implementation is challenging, as multiple biological barriers need to be conquered prior to the effectuation of the therapeutic effects. The introduction of exogenous oligonucleotides can be achieved through sequence engineering into viral transfer vector and delivery via viral transduction so that the therapeutics are expressed endogenously. This methodology has been widely applied to post-transcriptional gene modulation with antisense RNAs. Alternatively, oligonucleotides can be delivered by synthetic vector via

Olof Gissberg et al. (eds.), *Oligonucleotide-Based Therapies: Methods and Protocols*, Methods in Molecular Biology, vol. 2036, https://doi.org/10.1007/978-1-4939-9670-4_2, © Springer Science+Business Media, LLC, part of Springer Nature 2019

electrostatic complexation and transported across the cell membrane through endocytosis. Regardless of the category of delivery vehicles to be employed, a successful delivery strategy should be able to protect oligonucleotide therapeutics from serum degradation and macrophage phagocytosis, transfer them across the cellular membrane, facilitate their endosomal escape, and possibly deliver them into the nucleus if transcriptional regulation is desired.

For viral-based delivery strategy, engineered biological systems such as bacteriophages [14–16] and recombinant viruses [17–22] have been widely utilized for transmembrane delivery of nucleic acids, based on their invasive nature. Further, retroviral-based delivery strategies enable nucleus penetration and stable expression of the therapeutics endogenously. Regardless of the effectiveness of gene transfer, the viral delivery itself has been considered nonspecific toward host cell types, as well as immunogenic which limits the possibility of repetitive or strengthening dosing. Moreover, nucleus delivery by the retroviral-based system is a double-edged sword, as the tendency of random gene integration by the retroviral system may lead to unforeseen gene disorder [13, 23–28].

On the other hand, synthetic vectors have also demonstrated with great potential to deliver oligonucleotides therapeutics such as siRNA, small antisense oligonucleotides, mRNA, and even plasmid DNA into intracellular spaces [29–33]. Categories of synthetic delivery vehicles include but not limited to lipid nanoparticles (LNP), polymeric nanoparticles, and polymersomes [8, 12, 34–37]. Additionally, synthetic delivery vehicles composed with biological building blocks have also shown great promises in engineered oligonucleotide delivery; examples of such systems include but not limited to protein cage, cell-penetrating peptides, and aptamers. Key advantages of synthetic vectors over viral vectors are their facile manufacturing process with limited batch-to-batch variation, and more importantly the flexibility in chemical modification for targeted gene delivery [8, 34–36, 38–40]. Further, the various synthetic vectors can be used in combination for synergistic enhancement of the delivery efficiency. However, for synthetic vectors to be widely accepted and utilized, improvements on delivery efficiency have to be made to be comparable to viral transduction, as nowadays the majority of the clinical trials on gene therapy still employ viral gene transfer [40].

In this chapter, following an introduction on challenges of transmembrane oligonucleotides deliveries, the most recent developments on both nonviral and viral delivery systems are discussed, with a special focus on vector engineering for tissue-specific delivery of therapeutic oligonucleotides.

2 Therapeutic Oligonucleotides

The discovery of posttranscriptional gene silencing via RNA interference (RNAi) has motivated the scientific development of an array of oligonucleotide therapeutics, with foundational milestones made by Baulcombe [41] and Tuschi [42]. siRNAs and miRNA mimetics have been frequently interrogated in laboratories and in clinical trials, aiming at treating abnormal gene functions [29, 43–52]. In recent years, oligonucleotide therapies have expanded beyond the traditional RNAi pathway. Expression knockdown via RNase H-mediated transcript degradation has been reported prior to RNAi and has regained focus during recent years [53–57]; additionally blunt translational inhibition via steric-blocking oligonucleotides has also been proved effective in gene expression inhibition [58–62]. Besides direct targeting on coding transcripts, targeting long noncoding RNAs (lncRNAs) has emerged as a novel approach for gene regulation. LncRNAs execute a substantial repertoire of biological functions, including transcriptional regulation, posttranscriptional regulation as well as epigenetic regulation. Hence, oligonucleotides targeting lncRNAs carry more of tuning expression profiles than straightforward expression knockdowns [46, 63–66].

Oligonucleotides exploiting the RNAi pathway are processed, and the antisense strand is loaded onto the RNA-induced silencing complex (RISC). Formed RISC complexes target mRNA transcripts in a sequence-specific manner, either fully complementary regarding siRNA or partially complementary regarding miRNA mimetics [29, 30, 67] (Fig. 1a). However, due to the complexity of human genome composition and the abundance of transcripts within the cellular compartment, foreseeable off-target effects can be speculated as the major side effect, along with the immunogenicity resulting from toll-like receptor activation [68–70]. Expression downregulation observed upon deliveries of siRNA or miRNA mimetics are the result of mRNA cleavage by Argonaute II and subsequent degradation, which hinders protein translation. Argonaute II protein only nicks mRNA strand at the predictable location along the double-stranded region; therefore, antisense strands remains complexed within RISC and are anticipated to fulfill multiple turnovers prior to degradation and clearance. Typically, expression downregulation upon siRNA or miRNA mimetic administration can be observed up to 7 days [71, 72].

RNase H-mediated gene knockdown is an alternative to the RNAi pathway. RNase H belongs to a family of non-sequence-specific endonucleases, which exists in both nucleus and cytoplasm and cleaves RNA at RNA/DNA hybrid duplex region. The original functions of RNase H are to remove RNA primers during lagging strand replication prior to Okazaki fragment ligation and maintain

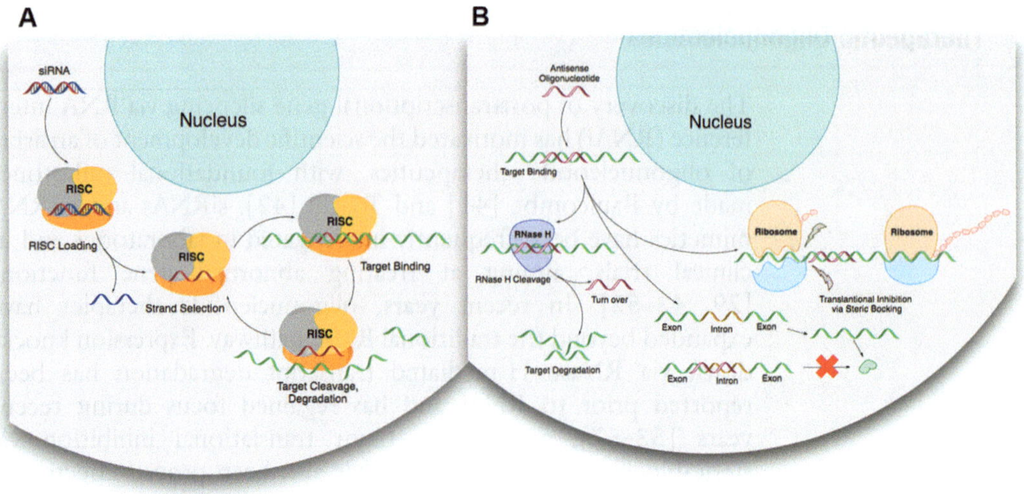

Fig. 1 Cellular mechanisms of oligonucleotide therapeutics. (**a**). RNAi pathway. Delivered siRNA complex is firstly recognized by RNA induced silencing complex (RISC). Upon loading onto the RISC complex, the antisense is selected, while the sense strand is unloaded and subjected to degradation. The antisense-loaded RISC hence can bind the targeted gene transcript, leads to transcript cleavage and cellular degradation. The antisense-loaded RISC can fulfill multiple rounds of gene silencing until the stability of loaded antisense is compromised. (**b**) Other pathways. Antisense oligonucleotides can also function through non-RNAi pathways. Typically employed gene regulation pathway is through RNase H mediated transcript degradation. The delivered antisense oligonucleotide can sequence specifically recognize the targeted gene transcript. The duplex hybrid is designed to adopt DNA–RNA topology and hence can be identified by endogenous RNase H. RNase H nicks the transcript while leaving the antisense intact for multiple turnovers. Additionally, fully modified antisense oligonucleotides that endure long-term serum exposure can be used to associate with transcript consistently until cellular recycling. The strong thermodynamic profile of the hybrid hampers ribosomal sliding along the mRNA chain, hence preventing or aborting the protein translation

genome stability [73–75]. Oligonucleotides utilizing RNase H-mediated mRNA degradation generally display backbones mimicking DNA, hence guiding the cleavage at the desired location on the transcripts [54, 56]. Similar to siRNA and others exploiting RNAi pathway, the antisense oligonucleotides for RNase H pathways are capable for multiple rounds of transcript cleavage (Fig. 1b). Having said that, the downsides of RNase H-recruiting oligonucleotide therapy that may be less fruitful compared to the RNAi pathway is the unclear mechanism of RNase H cleavage and whether there is a sequence preference [76], only until recently, a brief sequence preference landscape of RNase H has been published [77].

Apparently, cleavage-initiated mRNA degradation is not the sole method to achieve expression knockdown, as the biophysical approach has also been proved effective in regulating gene expression. Steric blocking oligonucleotides resemble roadblocks for protein translation, as they are chemically modified to acquire high stability upon mRNA hybridization [58, 60, 61, 78]. Protein synthesis by cellular translation machinery is impeded once it encounters the hybrid region; as a result, translation is stalled and the target gene expression is downregulated without transcript degradation. Not only translation impediment but steric-blocking oligonucleotides also succeed in altering pre-mRNA splicing patterns, giving the merit of its undegradable gene modulation strategy (Fig. 1b).

Only one-fifth of the cellular transcripts are gene encoding, and recent results indicate that the abundant noncoding transcripts are, in fact, critical in autogenous regulation of cellular function. The biological destinies of the 20% coding transcripts are modulated by the abundant 80% of noncoding transcripts, and with the emerging roles of noncoding transcripts in cancer and other diseases, targeting those noncoding transcripts is with equal if not more therapeutic value. Antisense oligonucleotides can be applied seamlessly to non-coding transcripts targeting, apart from gene knockdown that typically observed aiming at coding transcripts, targeting noncoding transcripts yields various biological outcomes, such as altered expression profiles via alternative splicing, transcriptional modulation, gene upregulation, and epigenetic modifications [49].

The merit of oligonucleotide therapies is more apparent when noncoding transcripts are the target [45, 64]. Coding transcripts typically yield protein entities that are also available for small-molecule drugs or antibody targeting. On the other hand, noncoding sequences remain invisible for those traditional medicines. With oligonucleotides, treatments can be extended to an upper regulatory level as the noncoding transcripts dominating the protein synthesis are tagged and manipulated. What should also be kept in mind is the adverse side of oligonucleotide therapy, where burdensome delivery can yield undesired alteration in gene expression profiles that can be hazardous toward healthy tissues [40, 79].

3 Barriers for Oligonucleotide Delivery

Successful outcomes of gene therapy heavily depend on the delivery strategy exploited. Different from small-molecule drug delivery, encapsulation or complexation of oligonucleotides with delivery vehicles is not typically considered as great challenges, as polyanionic oligonucleotides can be readily complexed through electrostatic interactions [6, 31, 80]. However, the unstable nature of oligonucleotides compared to chemical drugs urges novel formulation strategies or material engineering for enhanced protection, against the phagocytic system, nuclease degradation, and endosomal/lysosomal digestion. Conjointly, also applicable to the delivery of any therapeutics, directing therapeutics to specific sites with adequate potencies remains formidable, as nonspecific localization of therapeutics inevitably lowers efficacious dosage at disease loci and causes side effects.

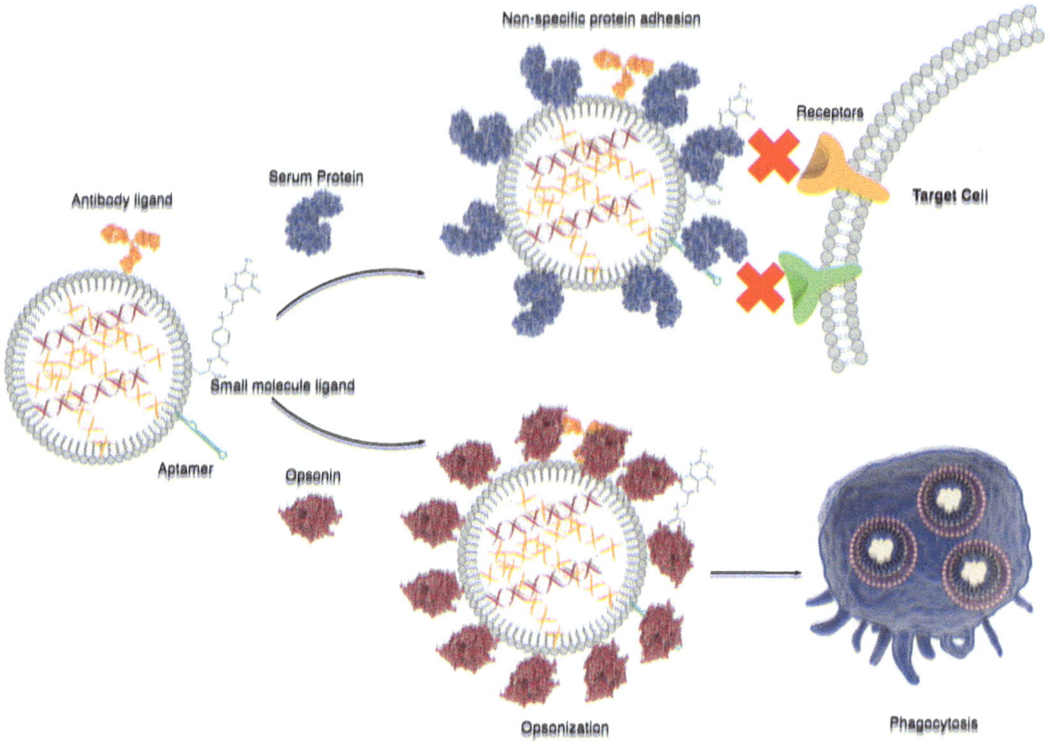

Fig. 2 Formation of protein corona in the systemic circulation and the adverse impact on therapeutic delivery. Protein corona can form tightly surrounding the administered therapeutics in the blood circulation. Abundant serum proteins mask the tissue-specific ligands, such as antibodies (shown in orange on delivery particle), aptamers (*green*) and small molecules, rendering them incapable of being recognized by the cell surface receptors (shown in yellow and green on the target cell). Additionally, foreign objects can turn on the radar of the immune system, leads to opsonization and the formation of opsonin cage around the delivery complex. Opsonin modifications attract phagocytic cells and result in the delivery complexes being engulfed and destroyed through phagocytosis

3.1 Mononuclear Phagocyte System

As one of the most critical defense barriers, mononuclear phagocyte system (MPS) is composed of cells from myeloid lineages, majorly monocytes in blood circulation and resident tissue macrophages in lymph nodes and liver [81–83]. Cells belonging to MPS are phagocytic and clear out foreign pathogens and cell debris via a cellular marking process named opsonization (Fig. 2). Labeling microbes, pathogens, and dead cells with opsonin generate a protein corona that neutralizes the innate negative charge on the biological membrane, hence permitting favorable interactions with surface receptors presented on the phagocytic immune cells [79, 84].

Specifically for synthetic vectors, clearance of delivered oligonucleotides through MPS explains the frequently observed discrepancies between in vitro and in vivo results. Depending on the chemical nature of the synthetic vector, the degree and kinetics of opsonization vary from seconds to days. Once devoured, both the delivery vehicle and the cargo are digested under oxidative conditions, and small digested pieces are cleared through renal filtration [71, 85], while the nondegradable portions are permanently stored in the MPS organs [40]. In the short term, MPS suppresses therapeutic efficacies; however, profound pathological damages to the MPS tissues resulting from digestive debris accumulation are more concerning.

Engineering the surface of synthetic vectors for oligonucleotides delivery has hence become a perpetual effort in minimizing the MPS suppression of therapeutic efficacies. Biomimetic surfaces resembling either red blood cells or lymphocytes are developed to enhance the stability and circulation time. Chemically, PEGylation is a classic strategy to install an additional hydration layer to the delivery complex and hence subdue the opsonin adhesion [86–90]. Yet, PEGylation fails to serve as the universal solution. As demonstrated by Dawson and coworkers, even with optimum PEGylation confirmed in in vitro conditions, the site-specific targeting by transferrin is still sequestered due to the formation of protein corona [91]. One could speculate that both the degree of PEGylation and the chemical nature of the delivery vector jointly determine the final therapeutic outcome.

3.2 Extravasation

Survival from blood circulation does not necessarily mean a successful delivery, as extravasation of the delivery complexes from the systemic circulation to the targeted tissue imposes another major challenge. The final biodistribution of the therapeutics is dominated by the size and the chemical properties of the delivery complexes.

When considering the size of the delivery complexes, naked oligonucleotides or small oligonucleotide-ligand conjugates are typically cleared through the glomerular filtration system due to their relatively small size (3–6 nm). Ironically, protein corona formation in the bloodstream yields sizes larger than the renal clearance threshold, which offers a diverted route for the delivery complex only if it survives from the scrutiny of MPS. Alternatively, to synthetically increase the size of the delivery complex, and hence avoid the loss of oligonucleotides from urine excretion has been investigated for decades. A seminal work by Maeda and coworkers on enhanced permeability and retention (EPR) has enlightened material scientists as to taking advantages of the leaky vasculatures found in tumor and inflammatory tissues [92–94]. Delivery complexes sized from 20 to 100 nm are considered to be most efficient in tumor targeting (Fig. 3). For a while, this EPR effect seems to be the panacea for curing cancer, as it offers effective extravasation right at the targeting tissue. Controversially, EPR has shown only modest enhancement for tumor-specific delivery, and comparatively lessened random tissue distribution, not to mention the slow accumulation of oligonucleotide therapeutics to the efficacious concentration at the target tissue [94–96].

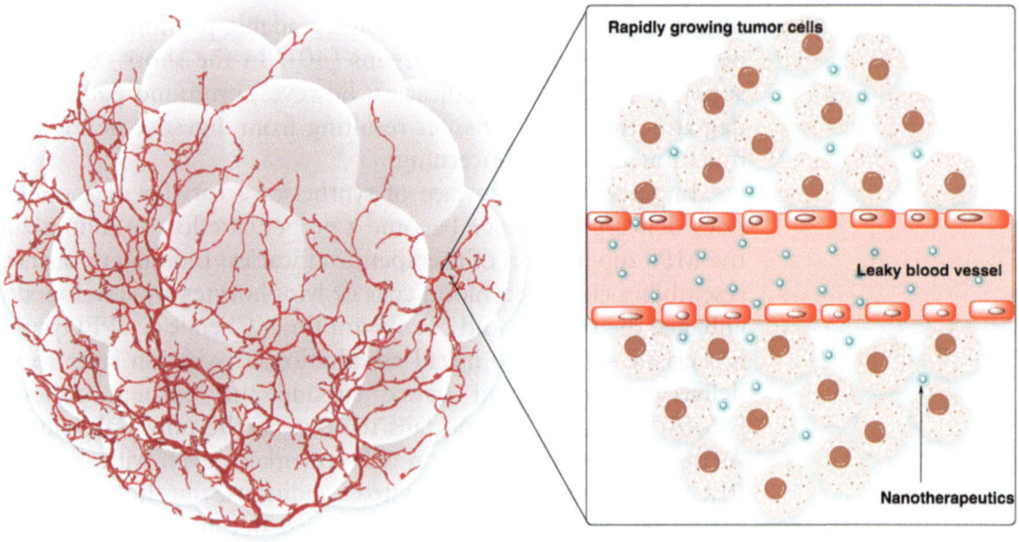

Fig. 3 Enhanced permeation and retention. To support massive tumor cell proliferation, angiogenesis is generally upregulated at the disease loci. Blood vessels in and surrounding the tumor regions are characterized by leaky vasculature, which offers an advantage for delivery of nanometer-sized therapeutics (shown as blue spheres). The nanotherapeutics can travel in the blood circulation, and preferentially enter tumor tissues due to the observed EPR effect

The suboptimal delivery outcomes for passive delivery of oligonucleotides through EPR effect can be explained with high intratumoral pressure during tumor expansion. Besides EPR reported by Meada, pathological features during tumorigenesis include poor lymphatic drainage and elevated mechanic forces [97–99]. With the nutrients supplied by hypervascular blood vessels, tumor cell proliferation appears to be unrestricted, leads to increased solid pressure due to tissue expansion, and high interstitial fluid pressure (IFP) resulting from poor lymphatic drainage [100]. Solid pressure provides a mechanical force that compresses flexible vessels and matrix, hence restraining the intratumoral circulation. Additionally, IFP generates a counteracting pressure gradient across the vessel epithelial, further preventing the passive delivery of the payload.

3.3 Endocytosis and Endosomal Escape

Upon extravasation, membrane transversal delivery of oligonucleotides into the intracellular space is a challenge, and the efficiency of the delivery is heavily dependent on the surface properties of the delivery vehicle.

The transmembrane motion can be passive without active transporters, such as diffusion if the hydrophobic material is utilized or absorbed when the cationic surface is presented by the delivery vehicle. As a result, less predictable delivery efficiency can be expected due to nonspecific adherence of the delivery complexes, which can occur at a higher frequency.

A superior alternative is through active endocytosis, which requires the extracellular interactions of the delivery vehicle with cell surface receptors. There are several reasons why endocytosis is a better choice for oligonucleotide therapeutic delivery. First, the delivery efficiency is more of a biological nature, depending on the strength of the chosen recognition pair. Second, tissue-specific delivery can be achieved if the tissue or disease-specific biomarker has been selected as the surface receptor. Third, the delivery efficiency can be constantly improved through ligand optimizations, such as antibody selection, aptamer evolution, and chemical modifications.

Despite the apparent merit of receptor-mediated endocytosis on oligonucleotide delivery, the intracellular destiny of delivered oligonucleotide remains formidable. Once being engulfed, the delivery complexes are entrapped within vesicles inversely coated with the cell membrane, termed the endosome [101]. For the typical endocytosis pathway, internalized molecules are transported through a series of distinct membrane compartments, associated with this process are increased acidity and oxidative stress within those membrane compartments. For oligonucleotides, the harsh conditions within the endosome result in expedited degradation (Fig. 4). Installations of functional moieties onto the synthetic vectors for proton buffering have been demonstrated to be effective. Such materials are protonated and subsequently expanded in size once acidity increases within the endosome, therefore destabilize the endosomal membrane and facilitate the endosomal escape [36, 102–105].

Exactly how much of the therapeutics survives the endosomal escape process is hard to evaluate, as it is a course that competes with time. Furthermore, depending on the functional moieties used, the oligonucleotides encapsulated or loaded, as well as the overall biophysical characters of the loaded delivery complexes, proton sponge mediated escape may yield unfruitful, and the majority of the payload ends up recycled via degradation process.

3.4 Others Barriers

As oligonucleotide therapies progress, targeting neuropathology has become more intriguing. However, as a critical self-protection strategy, blood–brain barrier composed with tight junctions that prevent passive diffusion of molecules into the brain [106]. The general tactic to achieve therapeutic delivery across blood–brain barrier (BBB) is to lipidize the therapeutics by encapsulating the drug within hydrophobic vehicles [107]; however, this is a more of a passive approach and generally exhibits nonspecific biodistribution. Delivery molecules that act as "Trojan horses" specifically targeting the BBB transporter to facilitate the molecule influx offer alternative approaches, however the reactions of brain

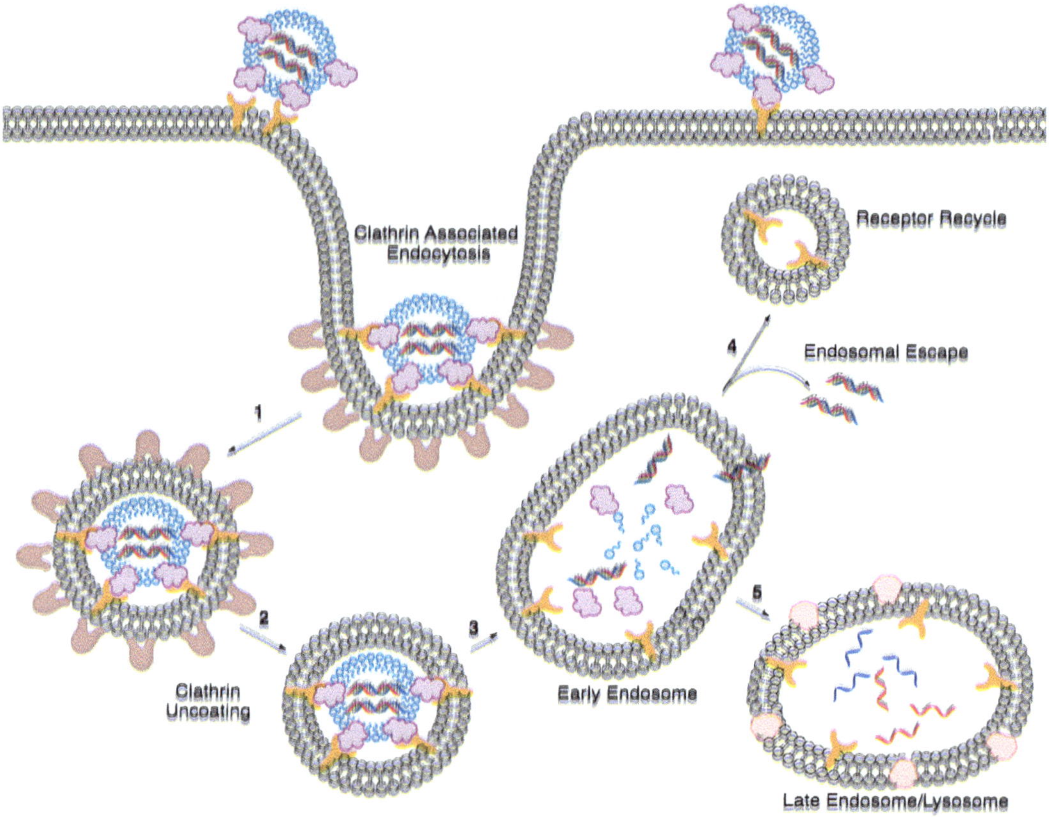

Fig. 4 Endocytosis and endosomal escape. Ligand–receptor interaction typically initiates endocytosis. The contact of ligand and surface receptor recruit intracellular clathrin protein. (1) The cell membrane starts to fold inward until a reversed bilayer particle containing the delivery complex is formed inside the cell. The endocytosed lipid vesicle is coated with clathrin. (2) Clathrin uncoats and recycles. (3) pH starts to decrease in the early endosome. At this stage, preferably delivery complexes disassemble and oligonucleotides escape from the endosome. (4) At this stage preferably delivery complexes disassemble and olionucleotides escape from the endosome. (5) As endosome matures into late endosome and lysosome, the high acidity environment within the vesicle degrades encapsulated complexes that fail to escape

epithelial cells as well as the routes of final transcytosis remain unpredictable [108, 109].

Another foreseeable difficulty of oligonucleotide delivery is specificity, especially for treating blood pathologies. Absence of the EPR effects that offers semispecific delivery of oligonucleotides to the tumor and inflammatory regions, treatments for blood pathologies without the presences of solid tumor have to rely on target-driven delivery to minimize the off-target effect. Additionally, the circulating delivery complexes in the bloodstream are extremely vulnerable for MPS clearance, hence highly competitive recognition pairs are in high demand.

4 Efforts in Tissue-Specific Oligonucleotides Delivery

As discussed in the details above, oligonucleotide therapeutics hold great promises in treating gene malfunctions at transcriptional and translational levels, apart from traditional medicines that tag only gene products. However, the delivery of oligonucleotides endures the same general challenges.

The majority of the delivery strategies employ positively charged synthetic vectors in order to condensate the polyanionic oligonucleotides, while novel approaches for sequence-specific oligonucleotide docking are under development. To escape MPS clearance, chemical moieties functioning as camouflage are installed, such as polysaccharides, mimetic lipids, and self-antigens. As for delivery specificity, which has been an everlasting endeavor, various tissue-specific ligands are discovered, optimized and displayed on the surface of the delivery vehicles. The exactitude of delivery locations greatly minimizes the possibility of the off-target effects, lowering cytotoxicity, if there is any; additionally, the narrow biodistribution conferred by specific delivery decreases the dosing amount and effectively prevents the onset of somatic resistance. The following section will be focused on advances made in the tissue-specific delivery of oligonucleotides.

4.1 Passive Delivery Strategy

Although generally not being considered as effectual tissue-specific delivery, passive delivery strategies [110], based on EPR effect as well as acid tumor microenvironment, have been somewhat proved to be attainable and semispecific [94, 95, 100] (Fig. 3).

With the leaky vasculature signatures in the EPR effect, nanosized delivery complexes are able to accumulate near the tumor tissue, resulting in improved tissue penetration. In order to effectively utilize EPR effect, the size of the delivery vehicles has to reside with 20–100 nm range to mitigate from renal clearance and liver accumulation [111]. Surface modifications are necessary to survive MPS clearance and have prolonged circulation time [96, 112]. The most widely employed modification is PEGylation, where the PEG layer provides enhanced solubility while the hydrate sheath shields opsonization or nonspecific adherence from circulatory serum proteins [79, 86, 113–116]. Besides decorating with PEG, nanoparticles presenting self-peptides [117] or biomimetic bilayers [118–123] are alternative tactics for immune system evasion.

Compared to delivery systems only exploring the EPR effect, a more active targeting method takes advantage of the increased acidity near the tumor and inflammatory tissues [124, 125]. The delivery system can still be coated with MPS evasive materials like PEG but through pH-sensitive chemistry [126]. The idea is to have the more voluminous delivery complexes disassemble at abnormally acidified loci so that the condensed core loaded with oligonucleotides can be launched for tissue penetration [127–130]. This method is still considered as passive delivery; however, it evaluates two parameters at the same time for a more specific delivery into tumor tissues.

4.2 Stimuli-Responsive Tissue Targeting

Another major class of tissue-specific delivery strategy relies on external forces, such as heat and magnetic field, to guide the localization of oligonucleotides [111].

Thermo-responsive delivery takes advantage of novel materials that change their physical states upon temperature changes [131, 132]. One example is that materials with upper critical solution temperature (UCST) close to physiological temperature can load therapeutics at room temperature, relying on either the hyperthermic character of tumor/inflammatory tissues or external heat application, and therapeutic unloading can be controlled at the defined region [133, 134].

Magnetofection utilizes delivery particles with paramagnetic property, through the application of a strong external magnetic field near the target tissue, and loaded paramagnetic particles are then able to accumulate in the targeted tissue [135, 136]. Magnetofection is distinctly different from MRI imaging with magnetic contrasting reagents in that the latter relies on EPR for preferred tumor accumulation [137–139].

Other examples of external stimuli are ultrasound agitation and light irradiation, [140–142] the latter requires the decoration of light-sensitive chemical moieties. Similar to heat and magnetic induction, these delivery methods are only semispecific. External forces are applied to an estimated region, not a defined tissue; the depth of targeted tissue regarding the body surface where the forces are applied dominates the delivery efficiency; further delivery via external stimulations are also unavailing in treating blood diseases where no defined disease loci is presented.

Similar to tactics using EPR effect, there are also delivery strategies designed according to altered redox profiles within tumor regions, in which redox-sensitive chemical linkages are installed within the delivery vehicle, and the increased intracellular glutathione concentration would facilitate the release of loaded therapeutics, such as oligonucleotides [111, 143–145]. Nevertheless, this redox-responsive delivery cannot be categorized as tissue-specific delivery, as the redox response only occurs following the translocation of the delivery complexes into the intracellular spaces.

4.3 Ligand-Driven Oligonucleotide Delivery

A more tailored method is demanded to differentiate not just normal regions and diseased regions, but into more details to tell apart from normal cells and diseased cells; further, it should be smart enough to seek its target and mitigate around nonspecific distribution. The innate biological system has presented us an ideal prototype—receptor-mediated endocytosis. The binding of extracellular ligands onto cell surface receptors initiates the internalization of ligands via endocytosis pathways. Chemical conjugation of cargos or delivery complexes with tissue-specific ligands has been proved inept in altering the endocytosis biology; on the contrary, the conjugated macromolecules are internalized with superb efficiency compared to passive delivery via EPR and other routes [146]. The following section will be focused on three categories of ligands frequently exploited in the delivery field: small-molecule ligands, protein ligands, and oligonucleotide ligands.

4.3.1 Small-Molecule Ligands

Naturally occurring small-molecule ligands such as folate [147–149], glucose [150], galactose [151–154], and *N*-acetylgalactosamine [155–158] have been frequently conjugated with oligonucleotides or delivery complexes, and interrogated for the delivery specificity and efficiency. They share a common feature of targeting ubiquitously expressed surface receptors; hence, tumor-specific deliveries via those ligands heavily depend on the differences of receptor expression profiles between healthy and diseased tissues.

The folate receptor is one of the most exploited exoplasmic receptors for therapeutic delivery (Fig. 5). The natural ligand for folate receptor is folate that belongs to the vitamin B family. Folate is considered essential for the human body, as its derivative tetrahydrofolate is the starting material for various biological molecules,

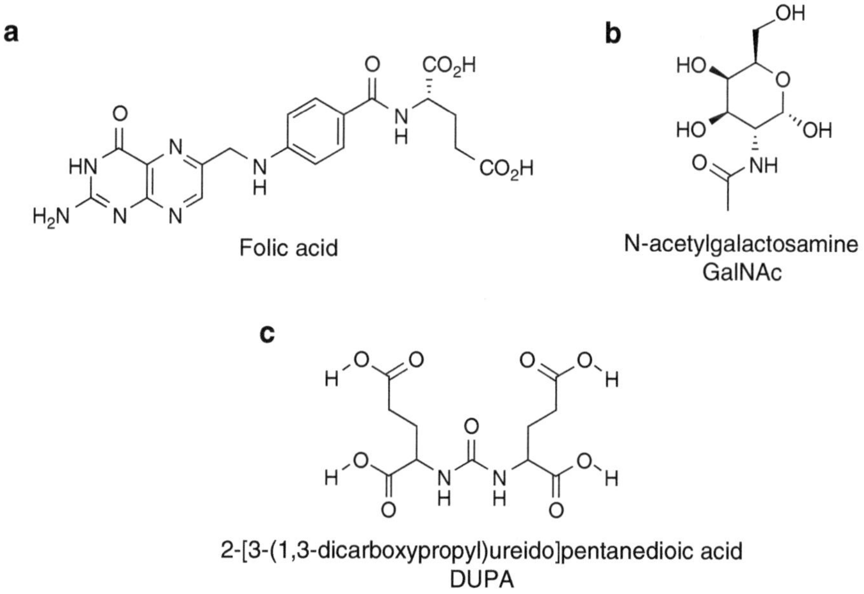

Fig. 5 Small-molecule ligands. Small-molecule ligands frequently exploited in tissue-specific oligonucleotide delivery. (**a**) Folic acid (folate) for folate receptor targeting; (**b**) GalNAc or ASGPR targeting of the liver; (**c**) DUPA for PSMA targeting

such as purines, pyrimidines, and amino acids. Folate is solely supplied from the dietary input and its biological concentration remains steady. Therefore, in order to support the much higher proliferation rate of malignant cells, folate receptors are overly expressed so that malignant cells can acquire more proportion of folate [159]. This makes targeting the folate receptor a straightforward tactic, even though the normal cells do express the folate receptor, the degree of overexpression statistically drives all folate-conjugated therapeutics into the disease loci. Both folate and its derivatives have been conjugated directly onto the oligonucleotide [160–162] or linked to the synthetic vectors [163–166] for oligonucleotide delivery, majorly focusing on siRNAs.

Another receptor that has drawn great attention is the asialoglycoprotein receptor (ASGPR). ASGPR is a type of exoplasmic glycoprotein-binding lectin mainly expressed in liver cells. Targeting ASGPRs for therapeutic delivery has become a trendy strategy in treating liver diseases and hematopoietic deficiencies [167]. However, efficacious delivery via ASPGR endocytosis pathway is nothing but challenging. First, ASGPR merely recognizes generalized glycosylation features of a ligand, although various carbohydrates have been reported to function as ligands for oligonucleotide delivery via ASGPR-mediated endocytosis [153, 154, 168, 169], a single ligand with superb binding affinity has not been identified (Fig. 5). Second, biological sugars in great abundance like glucose are competitive inhibitors of delivery ligand. Third, as the liver is the major metabolism site and oftentimes presents a high degree of nonspecific deposit of delivery complexes, targeting the liver has become somehow peculiar. To tackle these limitations, delivery ligands have been conjugated to present multivalency [153–155, 157, 168–172]. As anticipated, multivalent ligand displays have shown synergistic promotion of oligonucleotide delivery efficiencies both in vitro and in vivo [71].

Alternatively, disease-specific small-molecule ligands are more appealing since they are designed to recognize particular malignancy biomarkers, therefore off-target delivery to healthy tissues is minimized, which also means a lower dose may be used for better potency and decreased risk for resistance. One successful example is urea-based ligand 2-[3-(1,3-dicarboxypropyl)ureido]pentanedioic acid (DUPA), which specifically recognizes prostate specific membrane antigen (PSMA) (Fig. 5). DUPA and its derivatives have been conjugated to siRNA [161, 173], and siRNA-loading lipid nanoparticles [174]. Additionally, Levitzki et al. have tethered DUPA with polyethyleneimine (PEI) and demonstrated that PEI-DUPA condensated poly(I:C) is only able to specifically induce apoptosis in prostate cancer cells in vitro and in vivo, and no toxic immune stimulation has been observed [175, 176].

4.3.2 Protein and Polypeptide Ligands

Naturally occurring protein ligands can be explored for tissue-specific delivery. For some protein ligands, the targeted surface receptors are not cancer cell exclusive. However, the differences in expression profiles enable the cancer cells to absorb the majority of protein-conjugated delivery complexes. A frequent conjugation strategy is to link the targeting warhead with synthetic vectors, which condenses the oligonucleotide therapeutics. However, direct conjugations of protein ligands with oligonucleotides may mask the efficiency of the payloads, due to the significantly bigger sizes of proteins compared to oligonucleotides.

Epidermal growth factor (EGF) is one of the protein ligands commonly employed for therapeutic delivery purposes. Its natural receptor epidermal growth factor receptor (EGFR) is overexpressed in a wide variety of cancer cells. Additionally, the association of EGF to EGFR yield efficacious internalization of the ligand hence is in favor of engineering EGF-mediated delivery systems [177]. Yu et al. have demonstrated the successful delivery of TNFα encoding plasmid via a poly(amidoamine) (PAMAM) dendrimer with multivalent EGF display, which yields tenfold higher delivery efficiency compare to naked dendrimer control [178]. The in vivo efficacy of EGF conjugates was further proved by Levitzki and Wagner in glioblastoma and A431 xenograft animal models. In both cases, EGF is conjugated to PEI via polyethylene glycol (PEG) linkers for tumor-specific delivery of immunostimulatory dsRNA poly(I:C) [179, 180].

Oligonucleotide delivery through transferrin receptor-mediated endocytosis has also been highlighted in numerous studies. The interaction of transferrin with transferrin receptor is the major route of cellular iron uptake, which is through receptor-mediated endocytosis of Fe^{3+}-loaded transferrin [181] Like EGFR, transferrin receptor is highly expressed on the surfaces of various cancer cell as a mechanism to support cell growth [182, 183]. Transferrin-conjugates have been employed to deliver pDNA [184, 185], DNAzyme [186], siRNA [187, 188], and antisense oligonucleotides [189]. Further, transferrin-conjugated delivery systems exhibit great potential in targeted delivery of therapeutics to the brain. The BBB, paved with tight junctions, functions as the protective shield for the central nervous system (CNS). BBB only displays selective permeability for molecules critical for CNS function, typically through active receptor-mediated endocytosis [106]. The high-density expression profile of transferrin receptor has been supported by scientific evidence, therefore making the transferrin receptor a preferred target for therapeutic delivery into the brain [107, 190–192].

Antibodies selected for disease-specific or function-specific antigens offer enhanced targeting efficiency and less random tissue distribution. The specificity of antibodies is highly dependent on the production methods, and monoclonal antibodies with high affinity and specificity are preferred for therapeutic delivery [193]. Generally, antibody-conjugated systems display high specificity and improved therapeutic effects compared to naked delivery systems [194–200]. To further improve the targeting efficiency and reduce possible side effects from nonspecific interactions made with the antibody constant region, Fab fragments are used instead of the whole antibody [201–205]. Take anti-HIV oligonucleotide therapy as an example; in the study reported by Kumar et al., appending the delivery complexes with anti-CD7 antibody enabled antiviral siRNA delivery to $CD7^+$ mature T-cells, and prolonged viral suppression has been observed in HIV-infected humanized mice [206]. Alternatively, instead of tagging the cells susceptible for viral infection, tagging the infected cells with anti-HIV antibody offers an alternative route of treating infectious diseases. As demonstrated by Lieberman and coworkers, siRNA delivery via conjugated delivery system decorated with anti-HIV *Env* can exert a similar therapeutic effect [201].

Short polypeptides either derived from biological systems or systematically designed, can also execute specific binding toward cell surface proteins, and they hold several advantages over protein-based macromolecular ligands. Truncation from biological proteins to yield high-affinity small peptide ligands is a routinely applied strategy. Bhatia and coworkers conjugated the F3 peptide, derived from high-mobility-group proteins, onto a quantum dot and demonstrated the successful delivery of siRNA to cancer cells [207]. Brain-targeting RVG29 derived from rabies virus can drive transcytosis of conjugated DNA [208]. Similarly, the hypothalamic-specific 30-amino acid peptide leptin 30 is truncated from full-length hypothalamic hormone leptin and has been employed to deliver therapeutics across BBB [80]. On the other hand, small natural polypeptides can be directly employed as the delivery ligand. Angiopep-2, which targets low-density lipoprotein receptor-related protein (LRP) presented on the BBB, has been conjugated with various synthetic vectors to deliver oligonucleotides to the brain [209–212]. Chlorotoxin, a 36-amino acid peptide toxin from scorpion venom, has preferential localization to glioma cells and specific blockage of chloride ion channels [213], and both siRNA [214, 215] and pDNA [216, 217] have been successfully delivered via systems utilizing chlorotoxin as delivery ligands. The small size of polypeptide ligands allows chemical modifications to enhance their serum stability, typically through retro-inverso isomerization [218, 219]. Alternatively, polypeptide ligands can be identified through phage display method, examples are hepatocellular carcinoma targeting SP94 [220] and EGFR targeting GE11 [221].

4.3.3 Oligonucleotide Ligands and Aptamer Ligands

Oligonucleotides not only carry therapeutic properties, but they can also be employed as ligands for tissue-specific delivery. One frequently applied ligand is CpG oligonucleotide. Immunostimulatory CpG oligonucleotides activate Toll-like receptor 9 (TLR9), which is exclusively expressed on the surface of B cells and plasmacytoid dendritic cells (pDCs). Using CpG as delivery ligands, Kortylewski et al. report potent antitumor immune response upon CpG-guided delivery of STAT 3 specific siRNA into $TLR9^+$ immune cells [222, 223].

A great portion of oligonucleotide ligands are aptamers, which were discovered in the early 1990s and have since shown promising clinical applications for human diseases such as cancer, AIDS, and other diseases such as macular degeneration [224, 225]. Aptamers are characterized as short, single-stranded ribonucleic acid (RNA) and deoxyribonucleic acid (ssDNA) oligonucleotides that can fold into distinct secondary and tertiary structures. As a result of their three-dimensional structures, aptamers are able to bind to molecular targets with high affinity and specificity [226, 227]. Targeted delivery through aptamer–oligonucleotide conjugates may be used for gene therapy, immunotherapy, chemotherapy, photodynamic therapy, as well as phototherapy [228].

Aptamers are obtained through an in vitro screening process called systematic evolution of ligands by exponential enrichment (SELEX) (Fig. 6). Briefly, a random ssDNA or ssRNA library is generated, and the library is then incubated with a target molecule. Nonbinding sequences are then separated through methods such as electrophoresis gel, nitrocellulose filter binding, or a bead-based capture system. The eluted aptamers are then amplified through polymerase chain reaction (PCR) when working with DNA aptamer selection, or reverse transcription PCR (RT-PCR) and RNA transcription when working with RNA aptamer selection. The SELEX cycle process is repeated 8–16 times to obtain high-affinity binding nucleic acid enrichment through the repeated cycles. The final aptamers are then selected through cloning and high-throughput sequencing techniques, such as Sanger sequencing. During the library generation, the quality and design should be taken into careful consideration to obtain equal motif amounts of the four nucleotides to widen the investigation of the sequence [229]. During the selection process, short randomized regions (N20), as well as larger randomized regions (N40) are used for sequence coverage and greater intricacy for three-dimensional structure and folds [230]. The average amount of randomized regions used during experimentation is generally 20–60 nucleotides; however, isolated aptamers through the SELEX process have ranged from eight nucleotides [231] to 228 nucleotides in length [232].

Targeted oligonucleotide delivery using aptamers has shown to be a promising method, majorly due to ability of aptamers to have

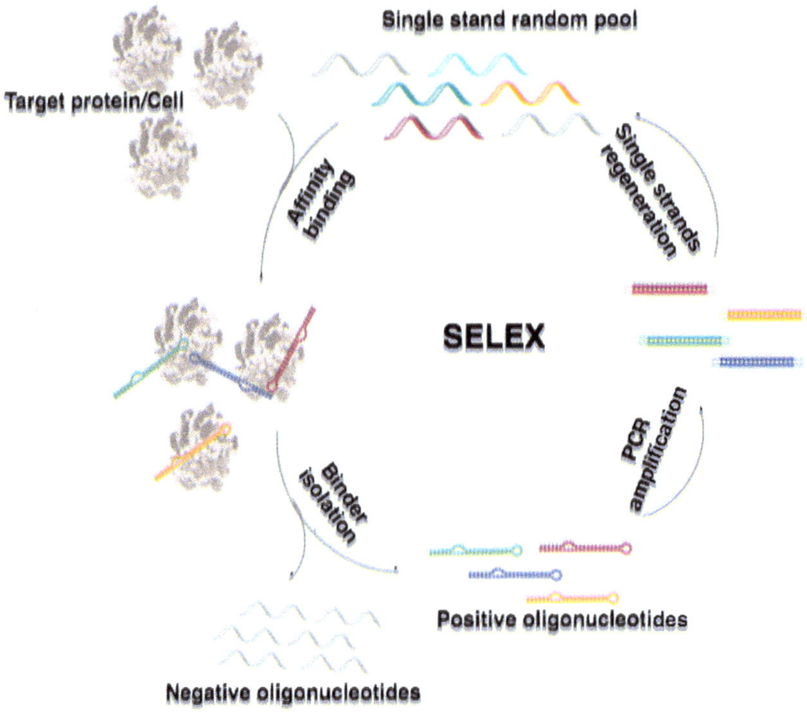

Fig. 6 Systematic evolution of ligands by exponential enrichment (SELEX). SELEX starts with a pool of single-stranded oligonucleotides with random sequences. The initial pool is subjected to either protein target or a typical type of cells, and the incubation yields the separation of binding sequences from nonbinding sequences. The isolated binding sequences are then subjected to error-prone PCR amplification, to maintain the main folding structure while generating mutations mimicking natural evolution. Subsequently, the double-stranded PCR pool is transformed into single-stranded oligonucleotide pool, via either exonuclease digestion for DNA or transcription for RNA. The pool is then subjected to another round of binding selection with a tuned selecting condition in order to enhance the binding affinity. During rounds of SELEX, only the strong binding sequences, either from the original pool or generated from error-prone PCR amplification, can be enriched

low toxicity, low immunogenicity, high specificity and affinity, as well as their ability to be easily modified through their chemical structures [233] Additional advantages of using aptamers for targeted drug delivery include their ability to be synthesized in high volumes and their ability to have a low, if at all any batch variation [226, 234].

The majority of aptamer-conjugated delivery systems for oligonucleotides are through direct conjugation by placing an inert spacer sequence in between the aptamer sequence and the oligonucleotide [40, 235, 236]. Additional guide strand annealing, however, is required if siRNA is the payload [3, 4, 237, 238]. As the result of a target-driven selection process, aptamer-mediated delivery is tissue-specific [4] or even cell-type specific [3, 237, 239, 240]. For example, Rossi and coworkers reported a series of delivery endeavors since their initial discovery of anti-gp120 aptamer [237, 241–243]. This anti-gp120 aptamer specifically recognizes

HIV-1 *Env* glycoprotein and has potential in targeting infected $CD4^+$ T-cells. It has been proved that the aptamer alone has antiviral potency to some degree; hence, one can speculate that oligonucleotide delivery using anti-gp120 aptamer as ligand can exert synergistic inhibitory effects [237]. Tan and coworkers reported their revolutionary whole cell-based SELEX [244], which has offered a new strategy in selecting aptamers befitting innate biological environments. The identified sgc8 aptamer is able to differentiate the cell surface characters among various leukemia cells. Using the indirect conjugation method, sgc8 was docked onto purified AAV viral vector, furthermore overcoming the major obstacle of unspecificity from AAV-mediated gene delivery [245].

Despite the advantages of using aptamers for targeted drug delivery, some solvable limitations and challenges when using aptamers for targeted drug delivery are their potential for cross-reactivity in respect to the therapeutic application, for example, aptamers have the potential to interact with other proteins. However, this biological challenge may be avoided through the SELEX process by introducing a structurally similar negative selection step [246]. Another challenge when using aptamers for targeted drug delivery is their potential for degradation; however, there have been many methods that allow for protection against aptamer degradation, such as through the use of chemically modified nucleobases during SELEX [247]. Other limitations and challenges that are present when using aptamers for therapeutic drug delivery are therapeutic cost and formulation, biostability, and pharmacokinetics [4]. However, one of the main challenges with using aptamers for targeted drug delivery is the therapeutic outcome when using aptamers selected on nonnative conditions, rather than native conditions. For example, if the SELEX process is done under nonnative or nonphysiological conditions, challenges may persist as the recombinant proteins may not be able to fold into the correct structural configuration. As a result, targets that are in the native configuration may not be recognized through the selected aptamers [248].

5 Challenges in Tissue-Specific Oligonucleotide Delivery

Tissue-specific delivery of oligonucleotide has great potential in solving issues such as poor bioavailability, suboptimal membrane penetration, random tissue distribution, and so on. However, the future is shadowed by several challenges in this tissue-specific delivery strategy, and one can only be cautiously optimistic that all the challenges can be conquered.

5.1 Finding the Right Target

The prerequisite for almost all tissue-specific delivery strategy is good ligand–receptor pair. Exploring ubiquitously expressed surface receptors offers ease in finding the pairing ligand; furthermore, improvements on ligand association affinity can be easily achieved using the natural ligand as a design prototype. However, using those ligand–receptor pairs can be tricky. To avoid broad tissue distribution, the expression profile of targeted receptor has to be magnitude higher in disease tissues comparing to healthy tissues. Hence, by assuming the ligand conjugates exert the same affinity to their receptors from all expressing tissues, from a statistical point of view, a higher proportion of the ligand conjugates will be absorbed to the disease loci. Another big concern is that the delivery efficiency can be compromised due to competitive inhibitions from the receptors natural ligand. ASGPR, for example, is a lectin that binds glycosylated ligands. Although trivalent GalNAc conjugation exhibits improved hepatocyte uptake, biological sugars can also bind the receptor and be competitive inhibitory if in greater concentration [167, 249].

There are cases that targeting ubiquitously expressed surface receptors can be beneficial. Take folate receptor as an example, which has α and β two isoforms. Among two isoforms, the β-isoform of the folate receptor has recently become a novel target. Besides being overexpressed on the surface of various cancer cells, β-isoform is the only type of folate receptor expressed on the exoplasmic surface of activated macrophages that have been recruited to cancer and inflammatory sites [250–252]. This expression profile of β-isoform offers great potential to deliver therapeutics to both the tumor cells and the tumor-associated macrophages. Since not all malignant cells express folate receptors [253], targeting tumor regions indirectly through activated macrophage is able to facilitate the diagnosis. Recent research evidence indicates the cancer-promoting functions of tumor-associated macrophage; hence, targeting activated macrophages around the tumor region is an additional merit of targeting the folate receptor β-isoform. Yet there are no natural ligands exclusively for the β-isoform, hence this imposes another challenge regarding proper ligand selection.

Alternatively, to mitigate the issues of off-target delivery, utilizing disease-specific receptors offers the best option. However, this also can be most challenging, as disease biomarker discovery is a formidable process and oftentimes yield less fruitful than anticipated [254]. Even with a successful identification, it takes tremendous effort to further determine the intracellular pathway and to find a delivery-compatible ligand.

Sometimes, even with a disease-specific target, the delivery efficiency can be disappointing. The absolute expression level of a target also plays an essential role in determining the final outcome of targeted delivery strategies [146]. Especially for disease biomarkers, the absolute number of exoplasmic receptors can be oftentimes extremely low, even with a strong ligand–receptor pair, during a given period of time the total concentration of internalized therapeutics is far below the effective concentration [255]. If taken an additional measure on receptor recycling profiles, disease-specific receptors that take longer time to resurface to the membrane yields unproductive for delivery purposes [256, 257].

5.2 Finding the Right Ligands

With the right target, identifying a high-affinity ligand holds the key to an efficient delivery. Generally, for ubiquitously expressed receptors, there is already a selection of ligands available. However, to achieve ideal delivery outcomes, selected ligands have to exert superb binding affinity over all the counterparts. One tactic is to construct multivalent ligand clusters to achieve cooperative binding [14, 156, 163, 169]. One unique method worth mentioning is the chimeric display of two different ligands to narrow down the tissue distribution [161]. Thomas et al. employed dual labeling with both folate and DUPA; folate drives the delivery vehicles to inflammatory sites, while DUPA further directs the delivery to only the PSMA-positive cells. Thermodynamically speaking, ligand–receptor interaction is diffusion controlled, and the degree of Brownian motion is inversely correlated to the size of the molecule, therefore larger ligands present a slower association rate comparing to smaller ligands. Based on the thermodynamic model of ligand–receptor binding, truncation of the larger ligands to its minimum active fragments can yield improved binding kinetics. This ligand optimization approach has been implemented in multiple delivery systems with protein, peptide, or aptamer ligands. An additional merit of functional truncation is that it offers opportunities for multivalent ligand construction if the yielded fragment is small in size. For example, RGD tripeptide is the minimum recognition sequence of fibronectin that binds integrins and promoting cell adhesion to the extracellular matrix [258], and it has been demonstrated as a potent ligand for site-specific delivery of oligonucleotides [113, 138, 259, 260].

Oftentimes neither the natural ligands nor the further improved ones fail to execute decent delivery efficiencies, or with a novel, disease-specific target, selecting a new ligand for the receptor is hence demanded. The first challenge in selecting a suitable ligand is to determine the chemical property of the ligand. Small-molecule ligands, protein/peptide ligands, and aptamer ligands do not behave equivalently, and the choice of which heavily depends on the surface character of the target. If the targeting site on the receptor is small and concave, one chooses an antibody-based ligand could render it incapable of binding; on the other hand, a large flat surface is more suitable for macromolecular ligands. Second, the selection conditions for suitable ligands have to closely mimic native biological conditions. Despite antibody selection, routinely, targeted receptors are isolated or overexpressed on the surface of immortalized cells. Although convenient, this type of selection methods ignores the critical role of posttranslational modifications of proteins on their recognition capability. With HIV-1 Env gp120 as an example, the native gp120 is coated with mannose glycans, however, the glycosylation patterns are significantly altered when expressed in various cell lines [261–263]. Third, natural binders of receptors have to be taken into consideration during ligand selection otherwise they might turn out to be competitive inhibitors of selected ligands. Competitive inhibition can be troublesome if the natural binder of the receptor is biologically abundant or has higher affinity, as the inhibitory effect can be easily overridden [264, 265].

Pressure applied during the ligand selection process is typically related to binding kinetics, in other words, it is the binding affinity that has been selected. The dilemma is that a strong binder does not equal to efficient endocytic activity. Selected ligands can be antagonists for the receptor, therefore, reduce the degree of intracellular activities upon receptor association. Hence, antagonizing ligands themselves can be therapeutic but are not qualified for delivery purposes. Additionally, the endosomal escape of ligand-conjugated therapeutics should be more kinetically advanced compared to receptor recycling; this allows both efficient intracellular delivery of the therapeutics and full regeneration of receptors. For this reason, ligands with superb binding affinity might be less effective in the intracellular release, therefore hampering the delivery efficiency [146].

5.3 Finding the Right Conjugation Chemistry

Another major challenge in tissue-specific delivery is to construct effective delivery complexes, generally via chemical conjugation. Ligand conjugation onto delivery vectors has fewer restrictions, as the oligonucleotide payloads are typically encapsulated within the core hence lack of contacts with the surroundings. The chemical conjugation simply requires suitable linker to make distance between the ligand and particle surface so that the ligands are free to rotate and adapt to optimum binding orientation and conformation.

On the other hand, direct chemical conjugation of ligands onto the payload imposes more challenges. The central principle for direct conjugation is that both the receptor targeting property of the ligand and the therapeutic activity of the payload needs to be preserved. Linker length in between these two components heavily depends on their sizes and chemical natures. Strategy-wise, longer linkers are preferred to connect larger protein ligands and oligonucleotides so that the protein ligand can adopt the optimal conformation without masking the therapeutic domain; further, nonspecific adherence of oligonucleotides to the protein ligand should be avoided. The more challenging situation is when both ligands and the therapeutics are oligonucleotides, as frequently observed that the folding topology of oligonucleotide ligands, especially aptamer, determines their recognition activity; henceforth, proper strategy has to be taken so that each component folds independently and correctly. Tactics utilize oligonucleotide "sticky bridge" linker have been reported to link receptor-targeting aptamers with siRNA. "Sticky bridge" is a segment of duplex RNA hybridized through an annealing process; each strand of the duplex is covalently linked with either the ligand or the therapeutics [241, 266]. The exact sequence of "sticky bridge" requires thermodynamic simulations to ensure the avoidance of nonspecific hybridization with the functional component, hence alters when different functional components are employed. However, it is advantageous as each component can adopt their optimum folding prior to the duplex formation [240].

For both conjugation schemes, chemical linkers may be more facile to use, and typically no thermodynamic simulation is required. Chemically inert linkers such as PEG linker present adequate flexibility and hydrophilicity. Bioconjugation methodologies such as copper-free "Click" chemistry [267], disulfide exchange [207, 268], and ester–amide exchange [269–271] have been frequently employed but not as carefree as one would assume. Protein ligands may be rich in primary amine or thiol-presenting amino acids on the surface; hence, bioconjugation through disulfide linkage or ester–amide exchange can yield random and multiple conjugations onto one ligand molecule. Copper-free click chemistry, on the other hand, leaves a bulky cyclooctyne chemical moiety, which can potentially influence the flexibility of the linker or even possibly disturb the functional folding of the oligonucleotide.

The last challenge in the conjugation process is to choose the conjugation sites on both the ligand and the oligonucleotide. The conjugation sites on siRNA, dsRNA, or microRNA should not interfere with the oligonucleotide biological processing so as the conjugation sites on ligands do not disturb the recognition interface between the ligand and the receptor.

6 Conclusion

On top of the potent gene modulations exerted by oligonucleotide therapeutics, tissue-specific delivery of these potent drugs makes them more appealing. The specific delivery strategy can effectively lower the administered doses of therapeutics and decrease the risk of resistance formation and off-target side effects. However, to achieve tissue-specific delivery, challenges are imposed. For example, identification of unique surface receptors according to disease type is critically essential, and it is slightly different from the trendy biomarker discovery. The identified receptor is not only indicative of the disease type but also should be adequately expressed for delivery purposes. Ligands selected against identified receptors should be effectively internalized through endocytosis without any off-target bindings. Further, even with the ideal ligand–receptor pair, suboptimal choices on conjugation chemistry can have an adverse impact on the overall delivery efficiency. Hence, tissue-specific delivery of oligonucleotides still has a long way to go, and multidisciplinary and collaborative efforts should be emphasized.

References

1. Montecalvo A, Larregina AT, Shufesky WJ et al (2012) Mechanism of transfer of functional microRNAs between mouse dendritic cells via exosomes. Blood 119:756–766
2. Furusawa M, Nishimura T, Yamaizumi M et al (1974) Injection of foreign substances into single cells by cell fusion. Nature 249:449–450
3. McNamara JO, Andrechek ER, Wang Y et al (2006) Cell type–specific delivery of siRNAs with aptamer-siRNA chimeras. Nat Biotechnol 24:1005–1015
4. Dassie JP, Liu X-Y, Thomas GS et al (2009) Systemic administration of optimized aptamer-siRNA chimeras promotes regression of PSMA-expressing tumors. Nat Biotechnol 27:839–849
5. Rice RR, Muirhead AN, Harrison BT et al (2005) Simple, robust strategies for generating DNA-directed RNA interference constructs, RNA interference. Elsevier, Amsterdam, pp 405–419
6. Jiang H-L, Choi Y-J, Cho M-H et al (2010) Chitosan and chitosan derivatives as DNA and siRNA carriers, Chitin, chitosan, oligosaccharides and their derivatives. CRC Press, London, pp 377–390
7. Aied A, Greiser U, Pandit A et al (2013) Polymer gene delivery: overcoming the obstacles. Drug Discov Today 18:1090–1098
8. Mitragotri S, Burke PA, Langer R (2014) Overcoming the challenges in administering biopharmaceuticals: formulation and delivery strategies. Nat Rev Drug Discov 13:655–672
9. Naldini L (2015) Gene therapy returns to centre stage. Nature 526:351–360
10. Naldini L (2011) Ex vivo gene transfer and correction for cell-based therapies. Nat Rev Genet 12:301–315
11. Wittrup A, Lieberman J (2015) Knocking down disease: a progress report on siRNA therapeutics. Nat Rev Genet 16:543–552
12. Stewart MP, Sharei A, Ding X et al (2016) In vitro and ex vivo strategies for intracellular delivery. Nature 538:183–192
13. Yin H, Kanasty RL, Eltoukhy AA et al (2014) Non-viral vectors for gene-based therapy. Nat Rev Genet 15:541–555
14. Larocca D, Burg MA, Jensen-Pergakes K et al (2002) Evolving phage vectors for cell targeted gene delivery. Curr Pharm Biotechnol 3:45–57
15. Smith GP (1985) Filamentous fusion phage: novel expression vectors that display cloned antigens on the virion surface. Science 228:1315–1317
16. Poul MA, Marks JD (1999) Targeted gene delivery to mammalian cells by filamentous bacteriophage. J Mol Biol 288:203–211
17. Davidson BL, Harper SQ (2005) Viral delivery of recombinant short hairpin RNAs. Methods Enzymol 392:145–173
18. Kay MA, Glorioso JC, Naldini L (2001) Viral vectors for gene therapy: the art of turning infectious agents into vehicles of therapeutics. Nat Med 7:33–40
19. Di Giusto DL, Krishnan A, Li L, et al (2010) RNA-based gene therapy for HIV with lentiviral vector modified CD34 cells in patients undergoing transplantation for AIDS-related lymphoma. Issues Sci Transl Med 2(36): 36ra43
20. Thomas CE, Ehrhardt A, Kay MA (2003) Progress and problems with the use of viral vectors for gene therapy. Nat Rev Genet 4:346–358
21. Gao G-P, Alvira MR, Wang L et al (2002) Novel adeno-associated viruses from rhesus monkeys as vectors for human gene therapy. Proc Natl Acad Sci U S A 99:11854–11859
22. Daya S, Berns KI (2008) Gene therapy using adeno-associated virus vectors. Clin Microbiol Rev 21:583–593
23. Pack DW, Hoffman AS, Pun S et al (2005) Design and development of polymers for gene delivery. Nat Rev Drug Discov 4:581–593
24. Mintzer MA, Simanek EE (2009) Nonviral vectors for gene delivery. Chem Rev 109:259–302

25. Rosenberg SA, Restifo NP (2015) Adoptive cell transfer as personalized immunotherapy for human cancer. Science 348:62–68
26. June CH, Riddell SR, Schumacher TN (2015) Adoptive cellular therapy: a race to the finish line. Sci Transl Med 7:280ps7
27. Seow Y, Wood MJ (2009) Biological gene delivery vehicles: beyond viral vectors. Mol Ther 17:767–777
28. Li S-D, Huang L (2006) Gene therapy progress and prospects: non-viral gene therapy by systemic delivery. Gene Ther 13:1313–1319
29. Zimmermann TS, Lee ACH, Akinc A et al (2006) RNAi-mediated gene silencing in non-human primates. Nature 441:111–114
30. Scherer LJ, Rossi JJ (2003) Approaches for the sequence-specific knockdown of mRNA. Nat Biotechnol 21:1457–1465
31. Gonzalez H, Hwang SJ, Davis ME (1999) New class of polymers for the delivery of macromolecular therapeutics. Bioconjug Chem 10:1068–1074
32. Liu Y, Wenning L, Lynch M (2004) New poly (D-glucaramidoamine) s induce DNA nanoparticle formation and efficient gene delivery into mammalian cells. J Am Chem Soc 126 (24):7422–7423
33. Park JS, Yi SW, Kim HJ et al (2016) Receptor-mediated gene delivery into human mesenchymal stem cells using hyaluronic acid-shielded polyethylenimine/pDNA nanogels. Carbohydr Polym 136:791–802
34. Akinc A, Lynn DM, Anderson DG et al (2003) Parallel synthesis and biophysical characterization of a degradable polymer library for gene delivery. J Am Chem Soc 125:5316–5323
35. Green JJ, Langer R, Anderson DG (2008) A combinatorial polymer library approach yields insight into nonviral gene delivery. Acc Chem Res 41:749–759
36. Putnam D, Gentry CA, Pack DW et al (2001) Polymer-based gene delivery with low cytotoxicity by a unique balance of side-chain termini. Proc Natl Acad Sci U S A 98:1200–1205
37. Oberli MA, Reichmuth AM, Dorkin JR et al (2017) Lipid Nanoparticle Assisted mRNA Delivery for Potent Cancer Immunotherapy. Nano Lett 17:1326–1335
38. Yu AC, Chen H, Chan D et al (2016) Scalable manufacturing of biomimetic moldable hydrogels for industrial applications. Proc Natl Acad Sci U S A 113:14255–14260
39. Dahlman JE, Kauffman KJ, Xing Y et al (2017) Barcoded nanoparticles for high throughput in vivo discovery of targeted therapeutics. Proc Natl Acad Sci U S A 114:2060–2065
40. Whitehead KA, Langer R, Anderson DG (2009) Knocking down barriers: advances in siRNA delivery. Nat Rev Drug Discov 8:129–138
41. Hamilton AJ, Baulcombe DC (1999) A species of small antisense RNA in posttranscriptional gene silencing in plants. Science 286:950–952
42. Zamore PD, Tuschl T, Sharp PA et al (2000) RNAi: double-stranded RNA directs the ATP-dependent cleavage of mRNA at 21 to 23 nucleotide intervals. Cell 101:25–33
43. Han M-H, Goud S, Song L et al (2004) The Arabidopsis double-stranded RNA-binding protein HYL1 plays a role in microRNA-mediated gene regulation. Proc Natl Acad Sci U S A 101:1093–1098
44. Iorio MV, Ferracin M, Liu C-G et al (2005) MicroRNA gene expression deregulation in human breast cancer. Cancer Res 65:7065–7070
45. Ling H, Fabbri M, Calin GA (2013) MicroRNAs and other non-coding RNAs as targets for anticancer drug development. Nat Rev Drug Discov 12:847–865
46. Roberts TC, Wood MJA (2013) Therapeutic targeting of non-coding RNAs. Essays Biochem 54:127–145
47. Hobert O (2008) Gene regulation by transcription factors and microRNAs. Science 319:1785–1786
48. Xia H, Mao Q, Paulson HL et al (2002) siRNA-mediated gene silencing in vitro and in vivo. Nat Biotechnol 20:1006–1010
49. Morris KV, Chan SW-L, Jacobsen SE et al (2004) Small interfering RNA-induced transcriptional gene silencing in human cells. Science 305:1289–1292
50. Meister G, Tuschl T (2004) Mechanisms of gene silencing by double-stranded RNA. Nature 431:343–349
51. Chendrimada TP, Gregory RI, Kumaraswamy E et al (2005) TRBP recruits the dicer complex to Ago2 for microRNA processing and gene silencing. Nature 436:740–744
52. McManus MT, Sharp PA (2002) Gene silencing in mammals by small interfering RNAs. Nat Rev Genet 3:737–747
53. Liang X-H, Sun H, Nichols JG et al (2017) RNase H1-dependent antisense oligonucleotides are robustly active in directing RNA cleavage in both the cytoplasm and the nucleus. Mol Ther 25:2075–2092
54. Nowotny M, Gaidamakov SA, Crouch RJ et al (2005) Crystal structures of RNase H bound

to an RNA/DNA hybrid: substrate specificity and metal-dependent catalysis. Cell 121:1005–1016
55. Inoue H, Hayase Y, Iwai S et al (1987) Sequence-dependent hydrolysis of RNA using modified oligonucleotide splints and RNase H. FEBS Lett 215:327–330
56. Walder RY, Walder JA (1988) Role of RNase H in hybrid-arrested translation by antisense oligonucleotides. Proc Natl Acad Sci U S A 85:5011–5015
57. Vickers TA, Koo S, Bennett CF et al (2003) Efficient reduction of target RNAs by small interfering RNA and RNase H-dependent antisense agents. A comparative analysis. J Biol Chem 278:7108–7118
58. Bonham MA, Brown S, Boyd AL et al (1995) An assessment of the antisense properties of RNase H-competent and steric-blocking oligomers. Nucleic Acids Res 23:1197–1203
59. Kole R, Krainer AR, Altman S (2012) RNA therapeutics: beyond RNA interference and antisense oligonucleotides. Nat Rev Drug Discov 11:125–140
60. Morcos PA (2007) Achieving targeted and quantifiable alteration of mRNA splicing with Morpholino oligos. Biochem Biophys Res Commun 358:521–527
61. Woolf TM (1995) To Cleave or Not To Cleave: Ribozymes and Antisense. Antisense Res Dev 5:227–232
62. Dias N, Dheur S, Nielsen PE et al (1999) Antisense PNA tridecamers targeted to the coding region of ha-ras mRNA arrest polypeptide chain elongation1. J Mol Biol 294:403–416
63. Lennox KA, Behlke MA (2016) Cellular localization of long non-coding RNAs affects silencing by RNAi more than by antisense oligonucleotides. Nucleic Acids Res 44:863–877
64. Lee JT (2012) Epigenetic regulation by long noncoding RNAs. Science 338:1435–1439
65. Mercer TR, Mattick JS (2013) Structure and function of long noncoding RNAs in epigenetic regulation. Nat Struct Mol Biol 20:300–307
66. Huarte M (2015) The emerging role of lncRNAs in cancer. Nat Med 21:1253–1261
67. Kher G, Trehan S, Misra A (2011) 7- Antisense Oligonucleotides and RNA Interference. In: Misra A (ed) Challenges in delivery of therapeutic genomics and proteomics. Elsevier, London, pp 325–386
68. Karikó K, Bhuyan P, Capodici J et al (2004) Exogenous siRNA mediates sequence-independent gene suppression by signaling through toll-like receptor 3. Cells Tissues Organs 177:132–138
69. Takeda K, Kaisho T, Akira S (2003) Toll-like receptors. Annu Rev Immunol 21:335–376
70. Kawai T, Akira S (2010) The role of pattern-recognition receptors in innate immunity: update on Toll-like receptors. Nat Immunol 11:373–384
71. Nair JK, Attarwala H, Sehgal A et al (2017) Impact of enhanced metabolic stability on pharmacokinetics and pharmacodynamics of GalNAc-siRNA conjugates. Nucleic Acids Res 45:10969–10977
72. Sashital DG, Doudna JA (2010) Structural insights into RNA interference. Curr Opin Struct Biol 20:90–97
73. Murante RS, Henricksen LA, Bambara RA (1998) Junction ribonuclease: an activity in Okazaki fragment processing. Proc Natl Acad Sci U S A 95:2244–2249
74. Liu B, Hu J, Wang J et al (2017) Direct visualization of RNA-DNA primer removal from Okazaki fragments provides support for flap cleavage and exonucleolytic pathways in eukaryotic cells. J Biol Chem 292 (12):4777–4788
75. Qiu J, Qian Y, Frank P et al (1999) Saccharomyces cerevisiae RNase H(35) functions in RNA primer removal during lagging-strand DNA synthesis, most efficiently in cooperation with Rad27 nuclease. Mol Cell Biol 19:8361–8371
76. Cerritelli SM, Crouch RJ (2009) Ribonuclease H: the enzymes in eukaryotes. FEBS J 276:1494–1505
77. Kielpinski LJ, Hagedorn PH, Lindow M et al (2017) RNase H sequence preferences influence antisense oligonucleotide efficiency. Nucleic Acids Res 45:12932–12944
78. Resina S, Kole R, Travo A et al (2007) Switching on transgene expression by correcting aberrant splicing using multi-targeting steric-blocking oligonucleotides. J Gene Med 9:498–510
79. Owens DE 3rd, Peppas NA (2006) Opsonization, biodistribution, and pharmacokinetics of polymeric nanoparticles. Int J Pharm 307:93–102
80. Liu Y, Li J, Shao K et al (2010) A leptin derived 30-amino-acid peptide modified pegylated poly-L-lysine dendrigraft for brain targeted gene delivery. Biomaterials 31:5246–5257
81. Rosales C, Uribe-Querol E (2017) Phagocytosis: a fundamental process in immunity. Biomed Res Int 2017:9042851

82. Sansonetti PJ (2000) Phagocytosis, a cell biology view. J Cell Sci 113:3355–3356
83. Aderem A (2003) Phagocytosis and the Inflammatory Response. J Infect Dis 187: S340–S345
84. Czuprynski CJ (2016) Opsonization and Phagocytosis. In: Vohr H-W (ed) Encyclopedia of immunotoxicology. Springer, Berlin, Heidelberg, pp 674–676
85. Choi HS, Liu W, Misra P et al (2007) Renal clearance of quantum dots. Nat Biotechnol 25:1165–1170
86. Harris JM, Chess RB (2003) Effect of pegylation on pharmaceuticals. Nat Rev Drug Discov 2:214–221
87. Hatakeyama H, Akita H, Harashima H (2011) A multifunctional envelope type nano device (MEND) for gene delivery to tumours based on the EPR effect: a strategy for overcoming the PEG dilemma. Adv Drug Deliv Rev 63:152–160
88. Mishra S, Webster P, Davis ME (2004) PEGylation significantly affects cellular uptake and intracellular trafficking of non-viral gene delivery particles. Eur J Cell Biol 83:97–111
89. Suk JS, Xu Q, Kim N et al (2016) PEGylation as a strategy for improving nanoparticle-based drug and gene delivery. Adv Drug Deliv Rev 99:28–51
90. Webber MJ, Appel EA, Vinciguerra B et al (2016) Supramolecular PEGylation of biopharmaceuticals. Proc Natl Acad Sci U S A 113:14189–14194
91. Salvati A, Pitek AS, Monopoli MP et al (2013) Transferrin-functionalized nanoparticles lose their targeting capabilities when a biomolecule corona adsorbs on the surface. Nat Nanotechnol 8:137–143
92. Matsumura Y, Maeda H (1986) A new concept for macromolecular therapeutics in cancer chemotherapy: mechanism of tumoritropic accumulation of proteins and the antitumor agent smancs. Cancer Res 46:6387–6392
93. Maeda H, Wu J, Sawa T et al (2000) Tumor vascular permeability and the EPR effect in macromolecular therapeutics: a review. J Control Release 65:271–284
94. Fang J, Nakamura H, Maeda H (2011) The EPR effect: Unique features of tumor blood vessels for drug delivery, factors involved, and limitations and augmentation of the effect. Adv Drug Deliv Rev 63:136–151
95. Prabhakar U, Maeda H, Jain RK et al (2013) Challenges and key considerations of the enhanced permeability and retention effect for nanomedicine drug delivery in oncology. Cancer Res 73:2412–2417
96. Nakamura Y, Mochida A, Choyke PL et al (2016) Nanodrug delivery: is the enhanced permeability and retention effect sufficient for curing cancer? Bioconjug Chem 27:2225–2238
97. Jain RK (2001) Normalizing tumor vasculature with anti-angiogenic therapy: a new paradigm for combination therapy. Nat Med 7:987–989
98. Ferretti S, Allegrini PR, Becquet MM et al (2009) Tumor interstitial fluid pressure as an early-response marker for anticancer therapeutics. Neoplasia 11:874–881
99. Northey JJ, Przybyla L, Weaver VM (2017) tissue force programs cell fate and tumor aggression. Cancer Discov 7:1224–1237
100. Greish K (2010) Enhanced permeability and retention (EPR) effect for anticancer nanomedicine drug targeting. Methods Mol Biol 624:25–37
101. Doherty GJ, McMahon HT (2009) Mechanisms of endocytosis. Annu Rev Biochem 78:857–902
102. Mishra S, Heidel JD, Webster P et al (2006) Imidazole groups on a linear, cyclodextrin-containing polycation produce enhanced gene delivery via multiple processes. J Control Release 116:179–191
103. Varkouhi AK, Scholte M, Storm G et al (2011) Endosomal escape pathways for delivery of biologicals. J Control Release 151:220–228
104. Stewart MP, Lorenz A, Dahlman J et al (2016) Challenges in carrier-mediated intracellular delivery: moving beyond endosomal barriers. Wiley Interdiscip Rev Nanomed Nanobiotechnol 8:465–478
105. Akinc A, Thomas M, Klibanov AM et al (2005) Exploring polyethylenimine-mediated DNA transfection and the proton sponge hypothesis. J Gene Med 7:657–663
106. Obermeier B, Daneman R, Ransohoff RM (2013) Development, maintenance and disruption of the blood-brain barrier. Nat Med 19:1584–1596
107. Pardridge WM (2007) shRNA and siRNA delivery to the brain. Adv Drug Deliv Rev 59:141–152
108. Pardridge WM (2002) Drug and gene targeting to the brain with molecular Trojan horses. Nat Rev Drug Discov 1:131–139
109. Georgieva JV, Hoekstra D, Zuhorn IS (2014) Smuggling drugs into the brain: an overview of ligands targeting transcytosis for drug

delivery across the blood-brain barrier. Pharmaceutics 6:557–583
110. Bertrand N, Wu J, Xu X et al (2014) Cancer nanotechnology: the impact of passive and active targeting in the era of modern cancer biology. Adv Drug Deliv Rev 66:2–25
111. Karimi M, Ghasemi A, Sahandi Zangabad P et al (2016) Smart micro/nanoparticles in stimulus-responsive drug/gene delivery systems. Chem Soc Rev 45:1457–1501
112. Blanco E, Shen H, Ferrari M (2015) Principles of nanoparticle design for overcoming biological barriers to drug delivery. Nat Biotechnol 33:941–951
113. Schiffelers RM, Ansari A, Xu J et al (2004) Cancer siRNA therapy by tumor selective delivery with ligand-targeted sterically stabilized nanoparticle. Nucleic Acids Res 32:e149
114. Veiman K-L, Künnapuu K, Lehto T et al (2015) PEG shielded MMP sensitive CPPs for efficient and tumor specific gene delivery in vivo. J Control Release 209:238–247
115. Kaul G, Amiji M (2005) Tumor-targeted gene delivery using poly(ethylene glycol)-modified gelatin nanoparticles: in vitro and in vivo studies. Pharm Res 22:951–961
116. Hu Y, Haynes MT, Wang Y et al (2013) A Highly efficient synthetic vector: nonhydrodynamic delivery of DNA to hepatocyte nuclei in vivo. ACS Nano 7:5376–5384
117. Rodriguez PL, Harada T, Christian DA et al (2013) Minimal "Self" peptides that inhibit phagocytic clearance and enhance delivery of nanoparticles. Science 339:971–975
118. Usman WM, Pham TC, Kwok YY et al (2018) Efficient RNA drug delivery using red blood cell extracellular vesicles. Nat Commun 9:2359
119. Villa CH, Anselmo AC, Mitragotri S et al (2016) Red blood cells: supercarriers for drugs, biologicals, and nanoparticles and inspiration for advanced delivery systems. Adv Drug Deliv Rev 106:88–103
120. Muzykantov VR (2010) Drug delivery by red blood cells: vascular carriers designed by mother nature. Expert Opin Drug Deliv 7:403–427
121. Parodi A, Quattrocchi N, van de Ven AL et al (2013) Synthetic nanoparticles functionalized with biomimetic leukocyte membranes possess cell-like functions. Nat Nanotechnol 8:61–68
122. Hu Q, Sun W, Qian C et al (2015) Anticancer platelet-mimicking nanovehicles. Adv Mater 27:7043–7050
123. Anselmo AC, Modery-Pawlowski CL, Menegatti S et al (2014) Platelet-like nanoparticles: mimicking shape, flexibility, and surface biology of platelets to target vascular injuries. ACS Nano 8:11243–11253
124. Kraus M, Wolf B (1996) Implications of acidic tumor microenvironment for neoplastic growth and cancer treatment: a computer analysis. Tumour Biol 17:133–154
125. Estrella V, Chen T, Lloyd M et al (2013) Acidity generated by the tumor microenvironment drives local invasion. Cancer Res 73:1524–1535
126. Danhier F, Feron O, Préat V (2010) To exploit the tumor microenvironment: passive and active tumor targeting of nanocarriers for anti-cancer drug delivery. J Control Release 148:135–146
127. Xia J, Tian H, Chen J et al (2016) pH-triggered sheddable shielding system for polycationic gene carriers. Polymers 8:141
128. Dimde M, Neumann F, Reisbeck F et al (2017) Defined pH-sensitive nanogels as gene delivery platform for siRNA mediated in vitro gene silencing. Biomater Sci 5:2328–2336
129. Sethuraman VA, Na K, Bae YH (2006) pH-responsive sulfonamide/PEI system for tumor specific gene delivery: an in vitro study. Biomacromolecules 7:64–70
130. Li H-J, Du J-Z, Liu J et al (2016) Smart superstructures with ultrahigh pH-sensitivity for targeting acidic tumor microenvironment: instantaneous size switching and improved tumor penetration. ACS Nano 10:6753–6761
131. Teotia AK, Sami H, Kumar A (2015) 1-Thermo-responsive polymers: structure and design of smart materials. In: zhang z (ed) switchable and responsive surfaces and materials for biomedical applications. Woodhead Publishing, Oxford, pp 3–43
132. Hoogenboom R (2014) Temperature-responsive polymers: properties, synthesis and applications. In: Aguilar MR, San Román J (eds) Smart polymers and their applications. Woodhead Publishing, Oxford, pp 15–44
133. Schmaljohann D (2006) Thermo- and pH-responsive polymers in drug delivery. Adv Drug Deliv Rev 58:1655–1670
134. Twaites BR, de las HAC, Cunliffe D et al (2004) Thermo and pH responsive polymers as gene delivery vectors: effect of polymer architecture on DNA complexation in vitro. J Control Release 97:551–566
135. Mykhaylyk O, Zelphati O, Rosenecker J et al (2008) siRNA delivery by magnetofection. Curr Opin Mol Ther 10:493–505

136. Scherer F, Anton M, Schillinger U et al (2002) Magnetofection: enhancing and targeting gene delivery by magnetic force in vitro and in vivo. Gene Ther 9:102–109
137. Bae KH, Lee K, Lee J et al (2011) Surface functionalized hollow manganese oxide nanoparticles for cancer targeted siRNA delivery and magnetic resonance imaging. J Control Release 152(Suppl 1):e133–e134
138. Lee JH, Lee K, Moon SH et al (2009) All-in-one target-cell-specific magnetic nanoparticles for simultaneous molecular imaging and siRNA delivery. Angew Chem Int Ed Engl 48 (23):4174–4179
139. Medarova Z, Pham W, Farrar C et al (2007) In vivo imaging of siRNA delivery and silencing in tumors. Nat Med 13:372–377
140. Torchilin VP (2014) Multifunctional, stimuli-sensitive nanoparticulate systems for drug delivery. Nat Rev Drug Discov 13:813–827
141. Kelley EG, Albert JNL, Sullivan MO et al (2013) Stimuli-responsive copolymer solution and surface assemblies for biomedical applications. Chem Soc Rev 42:7057–7071
142. Shen Y, Fu X, Fu W et al (2015) Biodegradable stimuli-responsive polypeptide materials prepared by ring opening polymerization. Chem Soc Rev 44:612–622
143. Becker AL, Orlotti NI, Folini M et al (2011) Redox-active polymer microcapsules for the delivery of a survivin-specific siRNA in prostate cancer cells. ACS Nano 5:1335–1344
144. Han L, Tang C, Yin C (2015) Dual-targeting and pH/redox-responsive multi-layered nanocomplexes for smart co-delivery of doxorubicin and siRNA. Biomaterials 60:42–52
145. Zhuang Y, Deng H, Su Y et al (2016) Aptamer-functionalized and backbone redox-responsive hyperbranched polymer for targeted drug delivery in cancer therapy. Biomacromolecules 17:2050–2062
146. Srinivasarao M, Low PS (2017) Ligand-targeted drug delivery. Chem Rev 117:12133–12164
147. Yang T, Li B, Qi S et al (2014) Co-delivery of doxorubicin and Bmi1 siRNA by folate receptor targeted liposomes exhibits enhanced anti-tumor effects in vitro and in vivo. Theranostics 4:1096–1111
148. Yang C, Gao S, Kjems J (2014) Folic acid conjugated chitosan for targeted delivery of siRNA to activated macrophages in vitro and in vivo. J Mater Chem B Mater Biol Med 2:8608–8615
149. Lee H, Lytton-Jean AKR, Chen Y et al (2012) Molecularly self-assembled nucleic acid nanoparticles for targeted in vivo siRNA delivery. Nat Nanotechnol 7:389–393
150. Venturelli L, Nappini S, Bulfoni M et al (2016) Glucose is a key driver for GLUT1-mediated nanoparticles internalization in breast cancer cells. Sci Rep 6:21629
151. Murata J-I, Ohya Y, Ouchi T (1997) Design of quaternary chitosan conjugate having antennary galactose residues as a gene delivery tool. Carbohydr Polym 32:105–109
152. Kim TH, Kim SI, Akaike T et al (2005) Synergistic effect of poly(ethylenimine) on the transfection efficiency of galactosylated chitosan/DNA complexes. J Control Release 105:354–366
153. Thapa B, Kumar P, Zeng H et al (2015) Asialoglycoprotein receptor-mediated gene delivery to hepatocytes using galactosylated polymers. Biomacromolecules 16:3008–3020
154. Zacco E, Hütter J, Heier JL et al (2015) Tailored presentation of carbohydrates on a coiled coil-based scaffold for asialoglycoprotein receptor targeting. ACS Chem Biol 10:2065–2072
155. Matsuda S, Keiser K, Nair JK et al (2015) siRNA conjugates carrying sequentially assembled trivalent N-acetylgalactosamine linked through nucleosides elicit robust gene silencing in vivo in hepatocytes. ACS Chem Biol 10:1181–1187
156. Nair JK, Willoughby JLS, Chan A et al (2014) Multivalent N-acetylgalactosamine-conjugated siRNA localizes in hepatocytes and elicits robust RNAi-mediated gene silencing. J Am Chem Soc 136:16958–16961
157. Rajeev KG, Nair JK, Jayaraman M et al (2015) Hepatocyte-specific delivery of siRNAs conjugated to novel non-nucleosidic trivalent N-acetylgalactosamine elicits robust gene silencing in vivo. Chembiochem 16:903–908
158. Zhao L, Liu M, Wang J et al (2015) Chondroitin sulfate-based nanocarriers for drug/gene delivery. Carbohydr Polym 133:391–399
159. Xia W, Low PS (2010) Folate-targeted therapies for cancer. J Med Chem 53:6811–6824
160. Guo S, Huang F, Guo P (2006) Construction of folate-conjugated pRNA of bacteriophage phi29 DNA packaging motor for delivery of chimeric siRNA to nasopharyngeal carcinoma cells. Gene Ther 13:814–820
161. Thomas M, Kularatne SA, Qi L et al (2009) Ligand-targeted delivery of small interfering RNAs to malignant cells and tissues. Ann N Y Acad Sci 1175:32–39

162. Shim MS, Kwon YJ (2010) Efficient and targeted delivery of siRNA in vivo: In vivo siRNA delivery. FEBS J 277:4814–4827
163. York AW, Zhang Y, Holley AC et al (2009) Facile synthesis of multivalent folate-block copolymer conjugates via aqueous RAFT polymerization: targeted delivery of siRNA and subsequent gene suppression. Biomacromolecules 10:936–943
164. Arima H, Yoshimatsu A, Ikeda H et al (2012) Folate-PEG-appended dendrimer conjugate with α-cyclodextrin as a novel cancer cell-selective siRNA delivery carrier. Mol Pharm 9:2591–2604
165. Fernandes JC, Qiu X, Winnik FM et al (2012) Low molecular weight chitosan conjugated with folate for siRNA delivery in vitro: optimization studies. Int J Nanomedicine 7:5833–5845
166. York AW, Huang F, McCormick CL (2010) Rational design of targeted cancer therapeutics through the multiconjugation of folate and cleavable siRNA to RAFT-synthesized (HPMA-s-APMA) copolymers. Biomacromolecules 11:505–514
167. Roggenbuck D, Mytilinaiou MG, Lapin SV et al (2012) Asialoglycoprotein receptor (ASGPR): a peculiar target of liver-specific autoimmunity. Auto Immun Highlights 3:119–125
168. Nishikawa M, Takemura S, Takakura Y et al (1998) Targeted delivery of plasmid DNA to hepatocytes in vivo: optimization of the pharmacokinetics of plasmid DNA/galactosylated poly(L-lysine) complexes by controlling their physicochemical properties. J Pharmacol Exp Ther 287:408–415
169. Lepenies B, Lee J, Sonkaria S (2013) Targeting C-type lectin receptors with multivalent carbohydrate ligands. Adv Drug Deliv Rev 65:1271–1281
170. Medina SH, Tekumalla V, Chevliakov MV et al (2011) N-acetylgalactosamine-functionalized dendrimers as hepatic cancer cell-targeted carriers. Biomaterials 32:4118–4129
171. Rouet R, Thuma BA, Roy MD et al (2018) Receptor-mediated delivery of CRISPR-Cas9 endonuclease for cell-type-specific gene editing. J Am Chem Soc 140:6596–6603
172. Nakagawa O, Ming X, Huang L et al (2010) Targeted intracellular delivery of antisense oligonucleotides via conjugation with small-molecule ligands. J Am Chem Soc 132:8848–8849
173. Tai W, Li J, Corey E et al (2018) A ribonucleoprotein octamer for targeted siRNA delivery. Nat Biomed Eng 2:326–337
174. Lee JB, Zhang K, Tam YYC et al (2016) A Glu-urea-Lys ligand-conjugated lipid nanoparticle/siRNA system inhibits androgen receptor expression in vivo. Mol Ther Nucleic Acids 5:e348
175. Langut Y, Talhami A, Mamidi S et al (2017) PSMA-targeted polyinosine/polycytosine vector induces prostate tumor regression and invokes an antitumor immune response in mice. Proc Natl Acad Sci U S A 114:13655–13660
176. Li Y, Xu X-L, Zhao D et al (2015) TLR3 ligand poly IC attenuates reactive astrogliosis and improves recovery of rats after focal cerebral ischemia. CNS Neurosci Ther 21:905–913
177. Chen J, Gamou S, Takayanagi A et al (1994) A novel gene delivery system using EGF receptor-mediated endocytosis. FEBS Lett 338:167–169
178. Yu H, Nie Y, Dohmen C et al (2011) Epidermal growth factor–PEG functionalized PAMAM-Pentaethylenehexamine dendron for targeted gene delivery produced by click chemistry. Biomacromolecules 12:2039–2047
179. Shir A, Ogris M, Wagner E et al (2006) EGF receptor-targeted synthetic double-stranded RNA eliminates glioblastoma, breast cancer, and adenocarcinoma tumors in mice. PLoS Med 3:e6
180. Schaffert D, Kiss M, Rödl W et al (2011) Poly (I:C)-mediated tumor growth suppression in EGF-receptor overexpressing tumors using EGF-polyethylene glycol-linear polyethylenimine as carrier. Pharm Res 28:731–741
181. Jandl JH, Inman JK, Simmons RL et al (1959) Transfer of iron from serum iron-binding protein to human reticulocytes. J Clin Invest 38:161–185
182. Ponka P (2004) Iron and cell proliferation: another piece of the puzzle. Blood 104:2620–2621
183. Le NTV, Richardson DR (2002) The role of iron in cell cycle progression and the proliferation of neoplastic cells. Biochim Biophys Acta 1603:31–46
184. Koppu S, Oh YJ, Edrada-Ebel R et al (2010) Tumor regression after systemic administration of a novel tumor-targeted gene delivery system carrying a therapeutic plasmid DNA. J Control Release 143:215–221
185. Li H, Qian ZM (2002) Transferrin/transferrin receptor-mediated drug delivery. Med Res Rev 22:225–250
186. Pun SH, Tack F, Bellocq NC et al (2004) Targeted delivery of RNA-cleaving DNA

enzyme (DNAzyme) to tumor tissue by transferrin-modified, cyclodextrin-based particles. Cancer Biol Ther 3:641–650

187. Cardoso ALC, Simões S, de Almeida LP et al (2007) siRNA delivery by a transferrin-associated lipid-based vector: a non-viral strategy to mediate gene silencing. J Gene Med 9:170–183

188. Tietze N, Pelisek J, Philipp A et al (2008) Induction of apoptosis in murine neuroblastoma by systemic delivery of transferrin-shielded siRNA polyplexes for downregulation of Ran. Oligonucleotides 18:161–174

189. Yang X, Koh CG, Liu S et al (2009) Transferrin receptor-targeted lipid nanoparticles for delivery of an antisense oligodeoxyribonucleotide against Bcl-2. Mol Pharm 6:221–230

190. Wiley DT, Webster P, Gale A et al (2013) Transcytosis and brain uptake of transferrin-containing nanoparticles by tuning avidity to transferrin receptor. Proc Natl Acad Sci U S A 110:8662–8667

191. Huang R-Q, Qu Y-H, Ke W-L et al (2007) Efficient gene delivery targeted to the brain using a transferrin-conjugated polyethyleneglycol-modified polyamidoamine dendrimer. FASEB J 21:1117–1125

192. Wei L, Guo X-Y, Yang T et al (2016) Brain tumor-targeted therapy by systemic delivery of siRNA with Transferrin receptor-mediated core-shell nanoparticles. Int J Pharm 510:394–405

193. Firer MA, Gellerman G (2012) Targeted drug delivery for cancer therapy: the other side of antibodies. J Hematol Oncol 5:70

194. Ngamcherdtrakul W, Morry J, Gu S et al (2015) Cationic polymer modified mesoporous silica nanoparticles for targeted SiRNA delivery to HER2+ breast cancer. Adv Funct Mater 25:2646–2659

195. Wang CY, Huang L (1987) pH-sensitive immunoliposomes mediate target-cell-specific delivery and controlled expression of a foreign gene in mouse. Proc Natl Acad Sci U S A 84:7851–7855

196. Guo J, Russell EG, Darcy R et al (2017) Antibody-targeted cyclodextrin-based nanoparticles for siRNA delivery in the treatment of acute myeloid leukemia: physicochemical characteristics, in vitro mechanistic studies, and ex vivo patient derived therapeutic efficacy. Mol Pharm 14:940–952

197. Lee J, Yun K-S, Choi CS et al (2012) T cell-specific siRNA delivery using antibody-conjugated chitosan nanoparticles. Bioconjug Chem 23:1174–1180

198. Chen Y, Zhu X, Zhang X et al (2010) Nanoparticles modified with tumor-targeting scFv deliver siRNA and miRNA for cancer therapy. Mol Ther 18:1650–1656

199. Bäumer S, Bäumer N, Appel N et al (2015) Antibody-mediated delivery of anti-KRAS-siRNA in vivo overcomes therapy resistance in colon cancer. Clin Cancer Res 21:1383–1394

200. Di Paolo D, Brignole C, Pastorino F et al (2011) Neuroblastoma-targeted nanoparticles entrapping siRNA specifically knockdown ALK. Mol Ther 19:1131–1140

201. Song E, Zhu P, Lee S-K et al (2005) Antibody mediated in vivo delivery of small interfering RNAs via cell-surface receptors. Nat Biotechnol 23:709–717

202. Sugo T, Terada M, Oikawa T et al (2016) Development of antibody-siRNA conjugate targeted to cardiac and skeletal muscles. J Control Release 237:1–13

203. Laroui H, Viennois E, Xiao B et al (2014) Fab'-bearing siRNA TNFα-loaded nanoparticles targeted to colonic macrophages offer an effective therapy for experimental colitis. J Control Release 186:41–53

204. Gao J, Liu W, Xia Y et al (2011) The promotion of siRNA delivery to breast cancer overexpressing epidermal growth factor receptor through anti-EGFR antibody conjugation by immunoliposomes. Biomaterials 32:3459–3470

205. Lu H, Wang D, Kazane S et al (2013) Site-specific antibody-polymer conjugates for siRNA delivery. J Am Chem Soc 135:13885–13891

206. Kumar P, Ban H-S, Kim S-S et al (2008) T cell-specific siRNA delivery suppresses HIV-1 infection in humanized mice. Cell 134:577–586

207. Derfus AM, Chen AA, Min D-H et al (2007) Targeted quantum dot conjugates for siRNA delivery. Bioconjug Chem 18:1391–1396

208. Liu Y, Huang R, Han L et al (2009) Brain-targeting gene delivery and cellular internalization mechanisms for modified rabies virus glycoprotein RVG29 nanoparticles. Biomaterials 30:4195–4202

209. Ren J, Shen S, Wang D et al (2012) The targeted delivery of anticancer drugs to brain glioma by PEGylated oxidized multi-walled carbon nanotubes modified with angiopep-2. Biomaterials 33:3324–3333

210. Shao K, Huang R, Li J et al (2010) Angiopep-2 modified PE-PEG based polymeric micelles for amphotericin B delivery targeted to the brain. J Control Release 147:118–126

211. Gao H, Zhang S, Cao S et al (2014) Angiopep-2 and activatable cell-penetrating peptide dual-functionalized nanoparticles for

systemic glioma-targeting delivery. Mol Pharm 11:2755–2763
212. Huile G, Shuaiqi P, Zhi Y et al (2011) A cascade targeting strategy for brain neuroglial cells employing nanoparticles modified with angiopep-2 peptide and EGFP-EGF1 protein. Biomaterials 32:8669–8675
213. Deshane J, Garner CC, Sontheimer H (2003) Chlorotoxin inhibits glioma cell invasion via matrix metalloproteinase-2. J Biol Chem 278:4135–4144
214. Veiseh O, Kievit FM, Fang C et al (2010) Chlorotoxin bound magnetic nanovector tailored for cancer cell targeting, imaging, and siRNA delivery. Biomaterials 31:8032–8042
215. Costa PM, Cardoso AL, Mendonça LS et al (2013) Tumor-targeted Chlorotoxin-coupled nanoparticles for nucleic acid delivery to glioblastoma cells: a promising system for glioblastoma treatment. Mol Ther Nucleic Acids 2:e100
216. Kievit FM, Veiseh O, Fang C et al (2010) Chlorotoxin labeled magnetic nanovectors for targeted gene delivery to glioma. ACS Nano 4:4587–4594
217. Huang R, Ke W, Han L et al (2011) Targeted delivery of chlorotoxin-modified DNA--loaded nanoparticles to glioma via intravenous administration. Biomaterials 32:2399–2406
218. Wei X, Zhan C, Chen X et al (2014) Retro-inverso isomer of Angiopep-2: a stable d-peptide ligand inspires brain-targeted drug delivery. Mol Pharm 11:3261–3268
219. Wei X, Zhan C, Shen Q et al (2015) A D-peptide ligand of nicotine acetylcholine receptors for brain-targeted drug delivery. Angew Chem Int Ed Engl 127:3066–3070
220. Li Z, Zhao R, Wu X et al (2005) Identification and characterization of a novel peptide ligand of epidermal growth factor receptor for targeted delivery of therapeutics. FASEB J 19:1978–1985
221. Lo A, Lin C-T, Wu H-C (2008) Hepatocellular carcinoma cell-specific peptide ligand for targeted drug delivery. Mol Cancer Ther 7:579–589
222. Kortylewski M, Swiderski P, Herrmann A et al (2009) In vivo delivery of siRNA to immune cells by conjugation to a TLR9 agonist enhances antitumor immune responses. Nat Biotechnol 27:925–932
223. Zhang Q, Hossain DMS, Nechaev S et al (2013) TLR9-mediated siRNA delivery for targeting of normal and malignant human hematopoietic cells in vivo. Blood 121:1304–1315
224. Ni X, Castanares M, Mukherjee A et al (2011) Nucleic acid aptamers: clinical applications and promising new horizons. Curr Med Chem 18:4206–4214
225. Keefe AD, Pai S, Ellington A (2010) Aptamers as therapeutics. Nat Rev Drug Discov 9:537–550
226. Röthlisberger P, Hollenstein M (2018) Aptamer chemistry. Adv Drug Deliv Rev 134:3–21
227. Liao J, Liu B, Liu J et al (2015) Cell-specific aptamers and their conjugation with nanomaterials for targeted drug delivery. Expert Opin Drug Deliv 12:493–506
228. Zhu G, Niu G, Chen X (2015) Aptamer-drug conjugates. Bioconjug Chem 26:2186–2197
229. Blind M, Blank M (2015) Aptamer selection technology and recent advances. Mol Ther Nucleic Acids 4:e223
230. Velez TE, Singh J, Xiao Y et al (2012) Systematic evaluation of the dependence of deoxyribozyme catalysis on random region length. ACS Comb Sci 14:680–687
231. Kwon YS, Ahmad Raston NH, Gu MB (2014) An ultra-sensitive colorimetric detection of tetracyclines using the shortest aptamer with highly enhanced affinity. Chem Commun 50:40–42
232. Li Y, Geyer CR, Sen D (1996) Recognition of anionic porphyrins by DNA aptamers. Biochemistry 35:6911–6922
233. Jiang F, Liu B, Lu J et al (2015) Progress and challenges in developing aptamer-functionalized targeted drug delivery systems. Int J Mol Sci 16:23784–23822
234. Hirao I, Kimoto M, Lee KH (2018) DNA aptamer generation by ExSELEX using genetic alphabet expansion with a mini-hairpin DNA stabilization method. Biochimie 145:15–21
235. Esposito CL, Cerchia L, Catuogno S et al (2014) Multifunctional aptamer-miRNA conjugates for targeted cancer therapy. Mol Ther 22:1151–1163
236. Kim JK, Choi K-J, Lee M et al (2012) Molecular imaging of a cancer-targeting theragnostics probe using a nucleolin aptamer- and microRNA-221 molecular beacon-conjugated nanoparticle. Biomaterials 33:207–217
237. Zhou J, Li H, Li S et al (2008) Novel dual inhibitory function aptamer–siRNA delivery system for HIV-1 therapy. Mol Ther 16:1481–1489
238. Chu TC, Twu KY, Ellington AD et al (2006) Aptamer mediated siRNA delivery. Nucleic Acids Res 34:e73

239. Yoon S, Huang K-W, Reebye V et al (2016) Targeted delivery of C/EBPα -saRNA by pancreatic ductal adenocarcinoma (PDAC)-specific RNA aptamers Inhibits tumor growth in vivo. Mol Ther 24(6):1106–1116
240. Yoon S, Huang K-W, Reebye V et al (2017) Aptamer-drug conjugates of active metabolites of nucleoside analogs and cytotoxic agents inhibit pancreatic tumor cell growth. Mol Ther Nucleic Acids 6:80–88
241. Zhou J, Preston Neff C, Swiderski P et al (2013) Functional in vivo delivery of multiplexed anti-HIV-1 siRNAs via a chemically synthesized aptamer with a sticky bridge. Mol Ther 21:192–200
242. Zhou J, Li H, Zhang J et al (2011) Development of cell-type specific anti-HIV gp120 aptamers for siRNA delivery. In: J Vis Exp
243. Zhou J, Lazar D, Li H et al (2018) Receptor-targeted aptamer-siRNA conjugate-directed transcriptional regulation of HIV-1. Theranostics 8:1575–1590
244. Shangguan D, Li Y, Tang Z et al (2006) Aptamers evolved from live cells as effective molecular probes for cancer study. Proc Natl Acad Sci U S A 103:11838–11843
245. Wu Y, Zhang L, Cui C et al (2018) Enhanced targeted gene transduction: AAV2 vectors conjugated to multiple aptamers via reducible disulfide linkages. J Am Chem Soc 140:2–5
246. Lakhin AV, Kazakov AA, Makarova AV et al (2012) Isolation and characterization of high affinity aptamers against DNA polymerase iota. Nucleic Acid Ther 22:49–57
247. Lakhin AV, Tarantul VZ, Gening LV (2013) Aptamers: problems, solutions and prospects. Acta Naturae 5:34–43
248. Catuogno S, Esposito CL (2017) Aptamer cell-based selection: overview and advances. Biomedicines 5(3). pii: E49
249. Pranatharthiharan S, Patel MD, Malshe VC et al (2017) Asialoglycoprotein receptor targeted delivery of doxorubicin nanoparticles for hepatocellular carcinoma. Drug Deliv 24:20–29
250. Van Der Heijden JW, Oerlemans R, Dijkmans BAC et al (2009) Folate receptor β as a potential delivery route for novel folate antagonists to macrophages in the synovial tissue of rheumatoid arthritis patients. Arthritis Rheum 60:12–21
251. Tsuneyoshi Y, Tanaka M, Nagai T et al (2012) Functional folate receptor beta-expressing macrophages in osteoarthritis synovium and their M1/M2 expression profiles. Scand J Rheumatol 41:132–140
252. Nakashima-Matsushita N, Homma T, Yu S et al (1999) Selective expression of folate receptor β and its possible role in methotrexate transport in synovial macrophages from patients with rheumatoid arthritis. Arthritis Rheum 42:1609–1616
253. Parker N, Turk MJ, Westrick E et al (2005) Folate receptor expression in carcinomas and normal tissues determined by a quantitative radioligand binding assay. Anal Biochem 338:284–293
254. Rifai N, Gillette MA, Carr SA (2006) Protein biomarker discovery and validation: the long and uncertain path to clinical utility. Nat Biotechnol 24:971–983
255. Srinivasarao M, Galliford CV, Low PS (2015) Principles in the design of ligand-targeted cancer therapeutics and imaging agents. Nat Rev Drug Discov 14:203–219
256. Maxfield FR, McGraw TE (2004) Endocytic recycling. Nat Rev Mol Cell Biol 5:121–132
257. Bareford LM, Swaan PW (2007) Endocytic mechanisms for targeted drug delivery. Adv Drug Deliv Rev 59:748–758
258. Pierschbacher MD, Ruoslahti E (1984) Cell attachment activity of fibronectin can be duplicated by small synthetic fragments of the molecule. Nature 309:30–33
259. Alam MR, Ming X, Fisher M et al (2011) Multivalent cyclic RGD conjugates for targeted delivery of small interfering RNA. Bioconjug Chem 22:1673–1681
260. Kong L, Alves CS, Hou W et al (2015) RGD peptide-modified dendrimer-entrapped gold nanoparticles enable highly efficient and specific gene delivery to stem cells. ACS Appl Mater Interfaces 7:4833–4843
261. Pritchard LK, Spencer DIR, Royle L et al (2015) Glycan clustering stabilizes the mannose patch of HIV-1 and preserves vulnerability to broadly neutralizing antibodies. Nat Commun 6:7479
262. Sanders RW, Venturi M, Schiffner L et al (2002) The mannose-dependent epitope for neutralizing antibody 2G12 on human immunodeficiency virus type 1 glycoprotein gp120. J Virol 76:7293–7305
263. Raska M, Takahashi K, Czernekova L et al (2010) Glycosylation patterns of HIV-1 gp120 depend on the type of expressing cells and affect antibody recognition. J Biol Chem 285:20860–20869
264. Donkor DA, Bhakta V, Eltringham-Smith LJ et al (2017) Selection and characterization of a DNA aptamer inhibiting coagulation factor XIa. Sci Rep 7:2102

265. Seiwert SD, Stines Nahreini T, Aigner S et al (2000) RNA aptamers as pathway-specific MAP kinase inhibitors. Chem Biol 7:833–843
266. Zhou J, Rossi JJ, Shum KT (2015) Methods for assembling B-cell lymphoma specific and internalizing aptamer-siRNA nanoparticles via the sticky bridge. Methods Mol Biol 1297:169–185
267. Chan DPY, Deleavey GF, Owen SC et al (2013) Click conjugated polymeric immuno-nanoparticles for targeted siRNA and antisense oligonucleotide delivery. Biomaterials 34:8408–8415
268. Taratula O, Garbuzenko OB, Kirkpatrick P et al (2009) Surface-engineered targeted PPI dendrimer for efficient intracellular and intratumoral siRNA delivery. J Control Release 140:284–293
269. Kim E, Jung Y, Choi H et al (2010) Prostate cancer cell death produced by the co-delivery of Bcl-xL shRNA and doxorubicin using an aptamer-conjugated polyplex. Biomaterials 31:4592–4599
270. Kim HA, Nam K, Kim SW (2014) Tumor targeting RGD conjugated bio-reducible polymer for VEGF siRNA expressing plasmid delivery. Biomaterials 35:7543–7552
271. Wu X, Ding B, Gao J et al (2011) Second-generation aptamer-conjugated PSMA-targeted delivery system for prostate cancer therapy. Int J Nanomed 6:1747–1756

Part II

Protocols and Strategies

Chapter 3

Designing siRNA and Evaluating Its Effect on RNA Targets Using qPCR and Western Blot

Linda Vidarsdottir, Oksana Goroshchuk, Iryna Kolosenko, and Caroline Palm-Apergi

Abstract

The discovery of the RNA interference (RNAi) pathway followed by the usage of synthetic short-interfering RNAs (siRNA) has contributed greatly to the understanding of gene function. Carefully designed siRNAs can considerably improve siRNA specificity leading to more accurate and efficient gene silencing. Evaluation of gene knockdown is vital for optimization of siRNA efficacy. Here we describe the fundamental principles of siRNA design and strategies for evaluating gene knockdown.

Key words Gene silencing, RNA interference, Short-interfering RNA, qPCR, Western blot

1 Introduction

Short-interfering RNAs (siRNA) are double-stranded RNA (dsRNA) molecules that can suppress gene expression by interfering with messenger RNAs (mRNAs), resulting in inhibition of translation or by inhibiting functional noncoding RNA molecules [1–3]. In 1998 it was reported that short dsRNAs in *C. elegans* induced enhanced gene suppression over single stranded RNAs (ssRNA). This was explained by the processing of dsRNAs through the evolutionary conserved RNA interference (RNAi) pathway [2]. RNAi is a highly regulated posttranscriptional gene silencing mechanism, activated by dsRNA (i.e., microRNA and siRNAs) after processing into 21–25 nucleotide RNA molecules by a Ribonuclease III enzyme named Dicer. Once the siRNA has been processed, the transactivation responsive RNA-binding protein (TRBP) recognizes the 2′-OH of the siRNA molecule and loads it into the RNA-induced silencing complex (RISC), a multiprotein complex. Inside RISC, the siRNA molecule is unwound into two ssRNAs assigned as the passenger strand and the guide strand (or the antisense strand). Argonaute 2 (Ago2), the catalytic protein

Olof Gissberg et al. (eds.), *Oligonucleotide-Based Therapies: Methods and Protocols*, Methods in Molecular Biology, vol. 2036, https://doi.org/10.1007/978-1-4939-9670-4_3, © Springer Science+Business Media, LLC, part of Springer Nature 2019

component of RISC, binds to the guide strand and cleaves the passenger strand [4]. Complementary mRNA is recognized by the guide strand through its seed sequence, corresponding to nucleotides 2–8 counted from the 5′ end [5]. When the guide strand is bound to a sequence-specific mRNA target, the catalytic endonuclease Ago2 cleaves the mRNA [6]. This pathway is highly efficient, as one guide RNA can induce cleavage of numerous target mRNAs.

The naturally occurring RNAi pathway can be utilized by synthetic, exogenous siRNAs and is successfully used in biomedical research for studying gene function. However, optimizing specificity and potency of siRNAs can be challenging. Numerous publications have addressed this by reporting on various algorithms that can predict functional siRNAs and their off-target effects. A variety of parameters have been shown to improve gene silencing and one should try to incorporate as many of them as possible into the siRNA design. Location and density of certain bases are some of the most important factors contributing to improved siRNA function [7–9].

Evaluating efficient knockdown by siRNAs can be performed using quantitative polymerase chain reaction (qPCR) and/or Western blot depending on the target gene. Off-target evaluation of siRNA can be predicted by algorithms or Blast as siRNAs can affect mRNA targets with limited sequence similarities [10]. In addition, folding of the target mRNA molecule should be considered as it can play a part in siRNA accessibility to the mRNA strand [11, 12]. Therefore, using multiple siRNAs for the same target is useful to verify that the correct phenotype caused by the knockdown is observed. Here we will describe the process of designing siRNAs and how to evaluate gene silencing after mRNA knockdown.

2 Materials

2.1 siRNA Design

1. Computer with an internet access.
2. Algorithm based on various parameters to predict siRNA design (*see* Subheading 3.1).
3. siRNAs can be ordered from commercial sources (e.g., Dharmacon, Ambion, IDT) (*see* **Note 1**).

2.2 Evaluation of siRNA Efficiency by qPCR

1. RNeasy mini kit from Qiagen. Prepare the RPE buffer according to the instruction manual by adding four volumes of ethanol (96–100%). Make sure to put a mark on the bottle "Ethanol added." Keep all kit components at room temperature or as directed by the manufacturer (*see* **Note 2**).

2. 70% ethanol: mix 35 mL of 100% ethanol with 15 mL of RNase-free water (*see* **Note 3**).
3. Prepare a set of RNase-free, DNase-free eppendorf tubes corresponding to the number of samples (*see* **Note 4**).
4. High-speed microcentrifuge with a cooling function.
5. NanoDrop™ (Thermo Fisher Scientific) or other spectrophotometer capable of determining RNA concentration in small volumes.
6. RNase-free water (*see* **Note 5**).
7. cDNA synthesis kit: M-MLV Reverse Transcriptase (RT) (200 U/mL), 5× or 10× RT buffer, 10 mM dNTP mix (mixture of 2.5 mM of dATP, dTTP, dGTP, and dCTP) and 0.1 M DTT.
8. PCR tubes or plates.
9. Tabletop centrifuge for tubes and PCR strips.
10. Thermal cycler.
11. Optical plate (96- or 384-well depending on the available real-time PCR machine and the number of samples).
12. Repeater pipette and appropriate filter tips (capable to dispense 7.5 μL).
13. 8- or 12-channel pipette and appropriate filter tips (capable of dispensing 2.5 μL).
14. Adhesive film.
15. Adhesive film applicator.
16. PCR Master Mix (e.g., TaqMan Fast Universal or SYBR Green) (*see* **Notes 6** and **7**).
17. TaqMan target gene assays (can be ordered predesigned or custom made) or SYBR Green qPCR primers (commercial or custom-designed).
18. Plate centrifuge.
19. qPCR machine.

2.3 Evaluation of siRNA Efficiency by Western Blot

Prepare all solutions using ultrapure water (purified deionized water 18 MΩ-cm at 25 °C). Store prepared solutions at room temperature (if not directed otherwise) or at the temperature recommended by the manufacturer. Follow the waste disposal regulations while discarding waste materials.

1. Radioimmunoprecipitation Assay (RIPA) buffer: 50 mM Tris–HCl, pH 7.4, 150 mM NaCl, 1 mM EDTA, pH 8.0, 1% NP-40, 1% Glycerol. Mix and adjust pH with HCl and store at 4 °C.

2. 1 mM dithiothreitol (DTT) in ultrapure water. Store at −20 °C.
3. Phosphatase inhibitor (*see* **Note 8**).
4. Protease inhibitor (*see* **Note 9**).
5. Lysis buffer: 1× RIPA buffer, 1 mM DTT, 1× phosphatase inhibitor, 1× protease inhibitor.
6. Protein Assay Bradford Dye reagent concentrate. Store at 4 °C.
7. Bovine serum albumin (BSA).
8. 96-well plate with clear flat bottom.
9. Spectrophotometer.
10. Precast polyacrylamide Bis–Tris gel. The percentage of the gel is determined by the size of the target protein.
11. Lithium dodecyl sulfate (LDS) sample buffer (4×) (Invitrogen) (*see* **Note 10**).
12. 2-(*N*-morpholino)ethanesulfonic acid (MES) buffer. Prepare 1× from 50 mL of stock buffer (Life Technologies) by adding 950 mL ultrapure water
13. Prestained protein standards. Keep according to manufacturer's recommendations (*see* **Note 11**).
14. NuPage Antioxidant (Invitrogen). Store at 4 °C.
15. Transfer buffer with ethanol: 50 mL Transfer buffer 20× (Life Technologies) + 100 mL ethanol +850 mL ultrapure water. Store at 4 °C.
16. 10× Tris-buffer saline (10× TBS): 1.5 M NaCl, 0.1 M Tris–HCl, pH 7.4. Store at 4 °C.
17. TBST: 1× TBS, 0.1% Tween (*see* **Note 12**).
18. Blocking buffer (*see* **Note 13**).
19. 10% sodium dodecyl sulfate (SDS) in ultrapure water (*see* **Note 14**).
20. Polyvinylidene difluoride (PVDF) or nitrocellulose membrane.
21. 3 mm filter paper (*see* **Note 15**).
22. Primary antibodies (*see* **Note 16**).
23. Secondary antibodies (*see* **Note 17**).
24. Gel knife.
25. High-speed microcentrifuge with a cooling function.
26. Dry bath or heating block for tubes.
27. Spectrophotometer.
28. Protein gel electrophoresis and transfer chamber system.
29. Imaging system.

3 Methods

3.1 Designing siRNAs for Gene Silencing

Time should be considered when designing siRNA. siRNA designed with your own in-house algorithm (using parameters described in this section) may take about 1–2 days while it will take less than an hour using an online siRNA design center (*see* **Note 18**).

1. Open the UCSC genome browser (https://genome.ucsc.edu) to access your target gene (*see* **Note 19**).
2. The genome browser should be set to default settings (*see* **Note 20**).
3. Select Genomes -> Human GRCh38/hg38 and enter gene name or position in the search term box and press "Go." If designing siRNA for a mouse gene, change the genome from the dropdown menu. For other organisms, *see* **Note 21**. Select a transcript variant and choose the FASTA format and save the sequence to a new document (*see* **Note 22**).
4. A list with transcript names will appear; select a transcript and the genome browser opens up to the location of that transcript (*see* **Note 23**).
5. One gene can give rise to various transcript variants and it is important for efficient gene silencing to target as many of them as possible (*see* **Note 24**). From the tracks available under "mRNA and EST," select "dense" under "Human mRNA" to display various mRNA transcripts. View and compare the transcripts displayed in the browser under Human mRNA from GenBank.
6. Select a target site that includes as many transcripts as possible within the open reading frame (ORF). Avoid intronic parts, the 5′ UTR and the 3′ UTR of protein coding genes as a target site [7].
7. Avoid single-nucleotide polymorphisms (SNPs) as targeting efficiency could differ between cell lines that have different SNPs [13]. The default setting on the UCSC genome browser will display common SNPs.
8. If possible, avoid targeting sites that are overlapping with antisense transcripts (*see* **Note 25**). Generally, siRNAs exhibit strand bias and only the guide strand should be processed and responsible for targeting of mRNAs. However, there is always a possibility that the guide strand is cleaved and the passenger strand is loaded into RISC.
9. When the optimal location is found select an appropriate number of nucleotides (i.e., 100–1000, enough for a siRNA online design center to come up with few different designs of high

quality, if not satisfactory select a different area). Zoom in or left click and drag the mouse (the mouse cursor needs to be on the grid). Select "Zoom in." Retrieve the DNA sequence by Select view - > DNA - > get DNA (*see* **Notes 26** and **27**).

10. Convert your DNA to RNA using online converter (available from multiple sources (i.e., http://www.attotron.com/cybertory/analysis/trans.htm).
11. Copy the RNA sequence and go to **step 12** for using commercially available web-tools or alternatively go to **step 13** for following your own in-house algorithm.
12. Use an online software to predict siRNA sequences. The online tools for designing siRNA are based on various published algorithms. Many of these are commercial websites that can also provide you with synthesized siRNAs. Following websites/companies are an example of sites that can be used for siRNA predictions: (siDESIGN Center (Dharmacon); siDirect [14]; siRNA Target Finder (GeneScript). A majority of the online siRNA design tools allows you to some extent to manually enter desired parameters (many of those mentioned in **step 13**).
13. Use your own in house algorithm based on the following parameters for optimal siRNA design.
    (a) *siRNA length*: The length of siRNA is typically a 19 nucleotide duplex with 2-nucleotide 3′ overhangs on each strand. Start by searching your target RNA for AA nucleotides as siRNA with 3′ overhanging UU dinucleotides have shown to be more effective [15] and select a 21 nucleotide sequence (*see* **Note 28**).
    (b) *G/C content*: Find a sequence for the siRNA that has a low G/C content between 30% and 52% [7, 16]. Also, avoid GC stretch of more than 9 nucleotides in length (*see* **Note 29**).
    (c) *Internal repeats*: Internal repeats and palindromes sequences within the siRNA can result in hairpin-like structures and should therefore be avoided. These structures can be predicted by melting temperature (T_m). High (>60 °C) internal T_m of siRNA correlates with hairpin structure and therefore decreases knockdown efficiency [16]. Copy either the guide strand or the passenger strand sequence and paste into the search box of an online oligonucleotide sequence calculator (i.e., OligoEvaluator (http://www.oligoevaluator.com) to get the T_m for your siRNA.

(d) *Base preference*: Base preferences of nucleotides at specific positions can improve gene silencing of siRNAs. Preference for an A/U at the 5′ end of the antisense strand will facilitate efficient and selective strand entry into RISC and therefore a preference for G/C at the 5′ sense strand is recommended. Sense strands with U at position 10 have shown enhanced gene silencing presumably due to activation of RISC that favors cleavage of 3′ U rather than A, G or C [16].

(e) *Avoid immune stimulatory and cytotoxic motifs*: The motifs "GUCCUUCAA" and "UGUGU" can cause an immune response and the motif "UGGC" has shown to cause cytotoxic effects [17–19].

(f) *Avoid termination signals*: Avoid stretches of more than four consecutive Ts as it may induce a termination signal.

14. Systematically arrange several siRNA designs in an excel file and select sequences that meets the criteria given in **step 13**. Select several target sequences [2–5] from different sites of your gene to maximize the chance of finding efficient siRNA.

15. Estimate the off-target effect of your sequences by using a web-based software (i.e., http://dharmacon.horizondiscovery.com/resources/tools-and-calculators/sirna-seed-locator/) to identify matches within the seed sequence. Blast searches will only give you a crude estimate of off-targets and should be used with seed sequence detection. Most siRNA prediction software packages will estimate possible off-targets continuously when designing siRNAs, as off target effects are difficult to predict with certainty.

16. Order (*see* **Note 30**) 3–5 different siRNAs (preferably targeting different sites of the target mRNA transcript) in order to find an optimal siRNA that efficiently silences your gene of interest. Currently, many high-impact journals request that the phenotype of one siRNA is verified by another siRNA, targeting the same gene.

17. Design a scrambled version of your sequence to be used as a negative control or buy a commercially available negative control.

18. Design or order an efficient siRNA as a positive control to optimize the transfection efficiency (*see* **Note 31**).

19. Upon siRNA transfection the siRNA concentration, transfection reagent and cell density need to be adjusted for optimal effect. Cell culture and delivery methods are not described in this chapter (*see* **Note 32**).

3.2 Evaluation of siRNA Efficiency by qPCR

Clean a working bench with a solution that destroys RNase or with ethanol. Use a set of pipettes designated for RNA work. Always use filter tips. Minimize the possibilities for contamination by closing the reagents immediately after use.

3.2.1 RNA Extraction (See Notes 33 and 34)

Extract RNA using, an established extraction method. For kits containing minispin columns, the protocol usually consists of the following steps:

1. Lyse the cells by adding 350 μL of the lysis buffer to the cell pellet and resuspend by pipetting until there are no visible cell debris left (*see* **Note 35**).
2. Precipitate RNA by adding equal amount (350 μL) of 70% ethanol to the lysis buffer and mix well for liquids to mix properly.
3. Load 700 μL of the lysate mixture to the spin column and spin down at 10,000 × *g*.
4. Discard the flow-through and wash the column with wash buffers, usually 2–3× (*see* **Note 36**).
5. Add 30 μL of RNase-free water to the center of the column and let it stand for 1 min at room temperature. Spin down at 10,000 × *g* to elute the RNA (*see* **Notes 37** and **38**).

3.2.2 Measure RNA Concentration

From this step on work on ice at all times.

1. Blank the machine (for example, NanoDrop™) by using the same water source as used to elute RNA from the spin columns (*see* **Note 5**).
2. Measure RNA concentration (use 1 μL RNA), record the data for each sample including the 260/280 and the 260/230 ratios (*see* **Note 39**).

3.2.3 cDNA Preparation

1. Dilute RNA in RNase-free H_2O to a final concentration of 50 ng/μL (*see* **Note 40**).
2. Prepare the Reverse Transcription Master Mix. Thaw the kit components on ice. Keep the reverse transcriptase on ice.
3. To calculate the volumes of the different mix components, use the template in Table 1 (*see* **Note 41**). Include one extra sample that will serve as a negative control and that does not contain the reverse transcriptase (*see* **Note 42**).
4. Use a repeater pipette to transfer 10 μL of the Master mix to the premarked PCR tubes.
5. Add 10 μL of the prediluted RNA.
6. Close the caps of the PCR tubes tightly. Mix gently and spin down briefly.

Table 1
Reagent volumes for cDNA preparation

Component	Volume (μL) for one reaction	Volume (μL) for X reactions
5× reverse transcription buffer	4	4X
10 mM dNTPs	1	1X
10 μM random primers	1	1X
Reverse transcriptase (e.g., M-MLV)	1	1X
0.1 M DTT	1	1X
RNase-free water	Up to 20 μL	
Total	20 μL	20X

7. Use a thermal cycler to run the following program for the M-MLV reverse transcriptase (otherwise, follow the instruction manual for your reverse transcription kit): 25 °C for 10 min, 37 °C for 30 min, 95 °C for 5 min and hold at 4 °C.
8. After the run is completed, spin the tubes and store the cDNA at −20 °C.
9. (Optional) DNA may be diluted 1:1 with RNase free water to decrease pipetting error in next step.

3.2.4 Quantitative PCR (TaqMan-Based Assay)

To normalize the expression of your gene of interest, one or several housekeeping genes (HG) may be used. A HG should have a stable expression in the investigated system and not vary in response to the siRNA. Beta-actin and GAPDH are commonly used, however, they are not always optimal. Check the literature and expression databases to choose an appropriate HG [20].

1. Decide the format for the qPCR run (96- or 384-well plate) and prepare a plate layout (*see* **Notes 43**).
2. While working on ice, prepare the Master Mix for the qPCR reaction for your target gene and the appropriate HG. The number of reactions needed for an assay in duplicates equals to 2× the number of samples +2 for noRT controls +2 no template controls +2 extra (overhead). The volumes of the individual reaction components can easily be calculated using the template presented in Table 2.
3. Mix the Master Mix gently and spin down.
4. Use a repeater pipette and transfer 7.5 μL of the Master Mix to a corresponding well in a 96-well clear bottom PCR plate.

Table 2
Reagents and volumes for TaqMan qPCR reactions

Reagent	Volume (μL) for one sample	Volume (μL) for X samples
2× TaqMan fast universal PCR master mix	5	5X
20× target gene assay	0.5	0.5X
Nuclease-free water	2	2X
Total volume	7.5	7.5X

5. Use a multichannel pipette (0.5–10 μL) to transfer 2.5 μL of the prediluted cDNA to the PCR plate containing the Master Mix.
6. Carefully seal the plate with an optical adhesive film. Avoid wrinkling!
7. Spin the plate down in a plate centrifuge, 2 min at 1000 × *g*, 4 °C.
8. Run the following program on a qPCR machine:
   (a) 95 °C for 20 s, 40 cycles of 95 °C for 1 s and 60 °C for 20 s.
9. Examine the melting curves and amplification plots visually after the run is complete (*see* **Note 44**).
10. Analyze the data using the Comparative C_T method ($2^{-\Delta\Delta CT}$) [21]. Briefly, the analysis consists of the following steps:
    (a) Export the C_T values to, for example, MS Excel.
    (b) Calculate the mean values for technical duplicates or triplicates.
    (c) Calculate ΔC_T by subtracting the mean C_T for the reference gene from the mean C_T of the target gene.
    (d) To calculate $\Delta\Delta C_T$, decide which sample will serve as a control. For RNAi experiments it is usually samples transfected with a scrambled or a negative siRNA control. Subtract the ΔC_T of the control from the ΔC_T for all samples. ΔC_T of the control should be 0 after this operation.
    (e) Calculate mRNA relative expression by $2^{-\Delta\Delta CT}$ (*see* **Notes 45** and **46**).

3.3 Evaluating siRNA Efficiency by Western Blot

3.3.1 Prepare Samples

1. Put frozen cell pellets in an icebox and add 25 μL lysis buffer per 4×10^6 cells. Adjust the volume according to the number of cells (*see* **Note 47**).
2. Mix the samples until no debris is visible. Incubate on ice for 10–30 min.
3. Cool the microcentrifuge to 4 °C while incubating.
4. Centrifuge the microcentrifuge tubes at 7500 × *g*, for 10 min at 4 °C.
5. Gently remove the tubes from the centrifuge and place them immediately on ice.
6. Transfer the supernatants into new tubes prechilled on ice and discard the pellets (see **Note 48**).
7. Perform Bradford assay in a 96 well microtiter plate to measure the protein concentration (*see* **Note 49**).
8. Prepare a BSA protein standard (1 mg/mL). Make a standard curve by diluting BSA in 40 μL Bradford reagent and PBS into at least five different concentrations over a range of 0–20 μg in a total volume of 200 μL for each concentration. For blank (0) point use 160 μL PBS and 40 μL Bradford reagent. For sample preparation, take 159 μL PBS + 40 μL Bradford reagent +1 μL of lysate for each sample (*see* **Note 50**).
9. Measure the absorbance at 595 nm in a plate spectrophotometer and calculate the protein concentration using Excel (*see* **Note 51**).
10. Turn on a heating block set at 85 °C. Prepare the samples by adding 30 μg protein to each tube and adjust according to the well-volume of the gel (*see* **Notes 52** and **53**).
11. Heat the samples in the heating block or dry bath at 85 °C for 5 min (*see* **Note 54**).
12. Remove the samples from the heating block and centrifuge 500 × *g* 1 min at room temperature.

3.3.2 Polyacrylamide Gel Electrophoresis

1. Choose and prepare a precast polyacrylamide Bis–Tris gel (*see* **Note 55**).
2. Prepare and assemble the electrophoresis equipment. Fill the inner chamber with 200 mL of running buffer suitable for your protein size (e.g., 1× MES running buffer). Before adding 600 mL of buffer to the outer chamber check that there is no buffer leakage from the inner chamber.
3. Load the sample (*see* **Notes 56** and **57**).
4. Load the appropriate prestained protein standard.
5. Add 500 μL antioxidant to the running buffer in the inner chamber (*see* **Note 58**).

6. Perform gel electrophoresis at constant 200 V for 45–90 min depending on protein size and percentage of the gel (*see* **Note 59**).

3.3.3 Blotting and Staining

1. After gel electrophoresis, cut the PVDF membrane and two sheets of 3 mm filter paper according to the size of the gel (*see* **Notes 60** and **61**).
2. Fill a tray with ice-cold transfer buffer and put sponges and two pieces of 3 mm filter papers to soak for 4–5 min. Always prewet PVDF marked membrane in ethanol for 2 min first and then in the ice-cold transfer buffer for 5 min.
3. Open the gel-cassette using a gel knife and ensure that the gel is kept on the back of the plastic plate. Carefully cut off the stacking gel and the thick part at the bottom using the gel knife. Cover the gel with one piece of already wet filter paper, flip over and put on the frontal cassette.
4. Put the PVDF membrane on the gel and cover the membrane with a second filter paper.
5. After sandwiching the gel and the membrane between the filter papers, air bubbles between the gel and membrane can be rolled out gently with a falcon tube (see **Note 62**).
6. Put three wet sponges in a deep back cassette and transfer the sandwiched gel on top of sponges.
7. Cover the sandwich with two wet sponges and the frontal cassette. Put the two cassettes together and place them in the blot chamber. Fixate in the blot chamber.
8. Add transfer buffer with ethanol to the transfer chamber. Add cold deionized water in the external chambers (*see* **Note 63**).
9. Run the transfer on ice at 40 V (expect a starting current of about 180 mA) for 60–90 min (*see* **Note 64**).
10. After the transfer is complete, turn off the system, discard all liquids in the transfer chamber and open the cassette. Use tweezers to carefully lift the membrane from the gel, place it in EtOH for 5–10 s and air-dry it for 15 min (*see* **Note 65**).
11. Reactivate the membrane after drying by washing once in 99% EtOH for 30 s.
12. Wash once in ultrapure water for 2 min.
13. Wash once in TBS for 3 min.
14. Block the membrane in Blocking Buffer and agitate at room temperature for 60 min (*see* **Note 66**).
15. Prepare the primary antibody by diluting it 1:1000 in TBST or as suggested in the manufacturer datasheet (*see* **Note 67**) and incubate the membrane with the antibody accordingly.

16. After incubation, wash the membrane three times for 15 min in a generous volume of TBST while agitating.
17. Dilute the secondary antibody in TBST +0.01% SDS according to the datasheet (see **Note 68**).
18. Incubate the membrane with the secondary antibody for 60–120 min with agitation at room temperature (*see* **Note 69**).
19. Wash the membrane two times for 10 min in TBST and one time for 5 min in TBS with agitation at room temperature (*see* **Note 70**).
20. Image the membrane using available imaging system (*see* **Notes 71** and **72**).

4 Notes

1. An in-house chemical synthesizer can also be used for generating siRNAs.
2. Alternatively, use other total mRNA extraction mini spin columns kits for RNA extraction from cells. Prelabel collection tubes and spin columns. Use an ethanol-resistant marker pen.
3. Prepare this solution in advance and keep at room temperature. In order to keep the solution clean, discard and prepare fresh solution on regular basis or aliquot to smaller volumes to avoid contamination that may occur when the tube is opened.
4. Prelabel the tubes with the date and a sample identifier. It is practical to mark both the lid and the tube itself.
5. RNase-free water used for RNA elution should be used as a blank measurement. Take out an aliquot of the RNase-free water that will be used for measurements to prevent contamination of the stock.
6. SYBR Green is an intercalating dye that binds dsDNA regardless of its origin (both specific and unspecific products); thus, it is important to analyze the final PCR products to detect possibly false positive results. The TaqMan technology is based on a sequence-specific fluorogenic probe that is quenched in the absence of specific product amplification. The advantage of TaqMan-based qPCR over SYBR Green qPCR is its high specificity. However, the cost of a Taqman-qPCR reaction is significantly higher than that of a SYBR Green qPCR reaction. Taqman qPCR is often more practical for genes that have paralogs (i.e., share a lot of structure with other genes) or for valuable primary patient cells. SYBR Green qPCR is also useful but only if the reaction is optimized.
7. TaqMan probes can be coupled to different dyes that allow detection of several products in the same tube (multiplexing).

8. Phosphatase inhibitors are necessary if the protein of interest contains a phosphorylation that should not be cleaved off.
9. Protease inhibitors are used to prevent degradation of proteins.
10. Prepare master mix with LDS and DTT taking 3–4 extra volumes and apply to empty wells to avoid formation of "a smile." Prepare 1–2 extra volumes to account for pipetting error.
11. It is recommended to have at least two prestained protein standards that can be detected on PVDF membrane and indicate different molecular weights.
12. Tween is very sticky and we recommend to cut off the end of a pipette tip for easier aspiration.
13. The choice of blocking buffer is defined by the available imaging system. For horseradish peroxidase system, blocking buffer should include 5% nonfat dry milk or BSA, diluted in TBST. Milk is not recommended for the studies on phosphoproteins (milk contains casein which is a phosphoprotein and can therefore cause high background when the phospho-specific antibody detects the casein). There are commercially available TBS- or PBS-based buffer solutions for infrared or near-infrared camera detection systems.
14. SDS precipitates at 4 °C. Keep at room temperature.
15. The PVDF membrane and filter papers should be prepared and cut in advance according to the size of the gel in use.
16. Preferably, use monoclonal antibodies (mouse, rabbit) to ensure specific binding to the target protein.
17. The choice should be defined by the available imaging system (e.g., horseradish peroxidase detecting system, infrared or near-infrared camera).
18. Predesigned siRNAs for the majority of protein coding genes are commercially available and could also be considered as an option.
19. It is also possible to retrieve the target gene sequence from gene databases.
20. The default settings are automatic when the UCSC genome browser is opened for the first time. To apply default settings, select "Genome Browser" -> "Reset all user settings."
21. Use the Entrez gene database (https://www.ncbi.nlm.nih.gov/gene/) to find your sequence. Search for your gene of interest by its name or Gene ID. Select the gene and organism. Under "Related information" select RefSeq RNAs.
22. The NCBI Reference Sequence project (RefSeq) provides prediction of annotated RNA sequences. Multiple RNA

transcripts can be generated from the same gene (i.e., caused by alternative splicing).

23. In most cases your sequence is highlighted in dark blue.

24. There is always a possibility that there are additional transcripts being produced by a gene that are not annotated in the genome browser.

25. Antisense transcripts are transcripts that overlap with other transcripts but have different directionality. Small arrows on the transcripts in the UCSC genome browser indicate the directionality of the transcripts.

26. The DNA that you will retrieve matches exactly what is displayed in the window of the UCSC browser.

27. Make sure that the DNA sequence you retrieve is from the correct strand. Select a transcript. The browser will open up an information site stating whether the RNA transcript originates from the − or + strand of the DNA.

28. Although 21 nucleotides are the default selection of the siRNA length, there are also reports on functional siRNA of different lengths [22–24].

29. The most efficient siRNAs (over 95% gene silencing) have low G/C content or between 30% and 52%.

30. Before ordering, visually compare the guide RNA sequence to your mRNA sequence. The guide RNA sequence should be complementary to your mRNA sequence.

31. Sequences for siRNA against housekeeping genes can be found in the literature or ordered on commercial website. Alternatively design a siRNA that targets a known gene (i.e., housekeeping gene) and has few or none off targets. After transfection of a positive siRNA control carefully monitor delivery cytotoxicity by counting the viable cell number.

32. Lipid based transfection reagents are most commonly used when transfecting siRNA to mammalian cells. Lentiviral vectors can be used for stable knockdowns. Cell confluency before transfection is typically around 60% and the optimal time from transfection to harvesting is about 24–72 h.

33. Extraction of good quality RNA is essential for the success of qPCR. Therefore, RNA extractions should be done carefully and RNA quality should be verified prior to setting up a qRT reaction. 24–72 h after transfection, collect the cells by trypsinization, scraping, or applying an RNA lysis buffer directly to the PBS-rinsed cells.

34. Avoid considerable changes in the temperature of the samples when spinning down the cells prior to lysis. For example, if

warm PBS is used, centrifuge at room temperature to avoid damaging the cell membranes.

35. The solution will become viscous due to the release of genomic DNA into the solution. Continue to mix by gently pipetting until the viscosity is reduced (and DNA is sheared).
36. To ensure good quality of RNA, spin empty columns once more after discarding the flow-through from the last washing step.
37. To increase the efficiency of the elution, heat the RNase-free water that is added to the column to 65 °C. It is also possible to make a second elution from the column if necessary by repeating the elution procedure and collecting the volume into a new tube. Mark the elution as 1 and 2 corresponding to the first and the second elution, respectively.
38. If SYBR Green is used for qPCR, RNA should be treated with DNase (e.g., TURBO DNA-free kit, Invitrogen) to avoid amplification of DNA since SYBR binds to dsDNA.
39. Relatively pure RNA will generate a typical bell-shaped peak. A 260/280 ratio of about 2.0 is an indicator of good RNA quality. Lower values may indicate contaminations with DNA or proteins. 260/230 ratio should be roughly the same as 260/280 or slightly higher. Considerably lower values may indicate contaminations with EDTA, phenol, etc. When RNA is extracted from low amount of starting material, it is sometimes hard to reach the desired 260/280 values. However, one should aim at getting at least 1.8. To trouble-shoot, RNA may be run on an agarose gel to identify if there is any DNA contamination.
40. A range of 50–500 ng of total RNA is optimal for the reverse transcription reaction. However, a note should always be made about the exact amount of RNA to perform a cross-experiment comparison.
41. When calculating the volumes of the kit components for the Master Mix, add two more samples as an overhead to account for pipetting dead volumes. When using a commercially available kit, follow the instructions in the manual for the volumes of reagents. Otherwise, use Table 1 as a reference.
42. Make a noRT negative control which includes all the components of the Master Mix except the reverse transcriptase. Transfer the reaction volume for the noRT sample into a PCR tube (9 μL) and substitute the reverse transcriptase with 1 μL of RNase-free H_2O. Add reverse transcriptase to the Master Mix. Mix gently and spin down using a tabletop centrifuge.

43. Each sample should be run in a technical duplicate or triplicate.
44. Melting curves should only have one peak corresponding to the amplification of the reaction product. The amplification plots for technical duplicates should be as close together as possible (C_T values should not differ more than 0.5 cycles. If the difference is larger, the data cannot be used and the experiment should be rerun).
45. After this operation, the expression of the target gene in the control will equal to 1. The expression of mRNA in other samples will now be presented as an increase or decrease compared to the chosen control. Knockdown efficiency of 80% is considered good.
46. Consider using additional negative controls. For example, including a "no template" control in addition to a "noRT" control. It will help trouble-shooting if any problem should occur.
47. Protein extraction should be performed on ice. Make sure that the cell pellet is completely resuspended in the lysis buffer by mixing with a pipette tip several times.
48. Samples can be frozen at −20 °C or −80 °C for later use or loaded onto a gel after the protein concentrations have been measured.
49. Here we use Bradford assay for protein concentration measurements, other assays are also available.
50. In case of very low protein concentration, prepare standard curve tenfold lower than recommended (starting with 0.1 μg/μL BSA instead of 1 μg/μL BSA). To increase the estimate of the R^2 value, increase the number of BSA dilutions for the standard curve.
51. For calculations: create a scatter plot based on the standard curve concentrations; set intercept at 0; display the equation and the R^2 value on the chart; calculate the sample protein concentrations using the obtained formula.
52. For 20 μL wells add 5 μL LDS, 2 μL DTT, 30 μg protein and fill up with ultrapure water to 20 μL total volume.
53. Turn on the heating block in advance and set the temperature to 85 °C and timer on 5 min.
54. Put a needle through the cap of the tube before putting it into the heating block to decrease pressure. Take the samples from the heating block on time to avoid evaporation.
55. Choose a gel percentage that is suitable for your protein size.
56. Before loading, make sure that the wells are empty and rinse them with running buffer twice. If possible, leave a space

between the ladder and samples to avoid mixing with the prestained protein standards.

57. If a Hamilton syringe is used, wash the syringe twice after each loading and three times after loading the ladder. The loading volume of the prestained protein ladder is 3–5 μL. Prestained protein ladders should be loaded last.
58. Antioxidants are important reagents that maintain proteins in a reduced state during electrophoresis.
59. Bubbles indicate that the gel is running. Make sure that the system does not get warm during electrophoresis. Run on ice or in a cold room, if possible, to ensure sharp and high-resolution bands.
60. PVDF membranes require careful pretreatment. During the transfer, always wear gloves: oils and proteins on the fingers will block efficient transfer and create dirty blots. Avoid touching the membrane with your fingers, use tweezers instead.
61. Mark the side of the first sample so it is easy to recognize after the transfer.
62. Ensure that there are no air bubbles by rolling the falcon round-bottom tube over the sponges while they are still in the tray with transfer buffer.
63. The remaining transfer buffer from the tray can be reused.
64. In case of transferring two gels simultaneously in two chambers, double the current of the system to 360 mA. Run transfer on ice to avoid overheating the system.
65. Membranes can be stored in dry condition or blocked after the reactivation.
66. Use Odyssey® Blocking buffer (TBS) when using near-infrared camera. Blocking prevents nonspecific background binding. If incubating in blocking buffer overnight, it is imperative to incubate at 4 °C to prevent contamination and destruction of the protein (important for phosphorylated proteins).
67. If the datasheet does not have a recommended dilution, try a range of dilutions (1:100–1:3000) and optimize it according to the results. Too much antibody will result in nonspecific bands. It is recommended to incubate the primary antibody overnight (no more than 18 h) at 4 °C. A higher antibody dilution and a prolonged incubation ensure specific binding. If it is necessary to check both phosphorylated and total protein expression, apply phospho-antibody first. Agitation of the antibody is recommended to enable adequate homogenous covering of the membrane and prevent uneven binding. Protect the membrane from light if using light sensitive antibody, by wrapping the box in foil or using a dark box.

68. Prepare secondary antibody in a tube. If the datasheet does not have a recommended dilution, try a range of dilutions (1:1000–1:20,000) and optimize the dilution according to the results. Too much antibody will result in nonspecific bands.
69. Agitation of the antibody solution is recommended to enable adequate homogenous covering of the membrane and prevent uneven binding.
70. Washing in TBS as a final step helps to remove residual antibodies and decrease possible background.
71. Adjust the protocol accordingly to the manufacturer's recommendations or requirements.
72. For example, horseradish peroxidase detecting system, infrared or near-infrared camera.

Acknowledgments

This study was supported by the Swedish Foundation for Strategic Research (C.P.A.) and the Swedish Childhood Cancer Foundation (C.P.A.).

References

1. Tuschl T (2001) RNA interference and small interfering RNAs. Chembiochem. 20(3):408-414doi: https://doi.org/10.1002/1439-7633(20010401)2:4<239::AID-CBIC239>3.0.CO;2-R (pii)
2. Fire A, Xu S, Montgomery MK et al (1998) Potent and specific genetic interference by double-stranded RNA in *Caenorhabditis elegans*. Nature 391(6669):806–811. https://doi.org/10.1038/35888
3. Johnsson P, Ackley A, Vidarsdottir L et al (2013) A pseudogene long-noncoding-RNA network regulates PTEN transcription and translation in human cells. Nat Struct Mol Biol 20(4):440–446. https://doi.org/10.1038/nsmb.2516
4. Martinez J, Patkaniowska A, Urlaub H et al (2002) Single-stranded antisense siRNAs guide target RNA cleavage in RNAi. Cell 110 (5):563–574. https://doi.org/10.1016/S0092-8674(02)00908-X
5. Ui-Tei K, Naito Y, Nishi K et al (2008) Thermodynamic stability and Watson-Crick base pairing in the seed duplex are major determinants of the efficiency of the siRNA-based off-target effect. Nucleic Acids Res 36 (22):7100–7109. https://doi.org/10.1093/nar/gkn902
6. Liu J, Carmell MA, Rivas FV et al (2004) Argonaute2 is the catalytic engine of mammalian RNAi. Science 305(5689):1437–1441. https://doi.org/10.1126/science.1102513
7. Elbashir SM, Harborth J, Weber K, Tuschl T (2002) Analysis of gene function in somatic mammalian cells using small interfering RNAs. Methods 26(2):199–213. https://doi.org/10.1016/S1046-2023(02)00023-3
8. Holen T, Amarzguioui M, Wiiger MT et al (2002) Positional effects of short interfering RNAs targeting the human coagulation trigger tissue factor. Nucleic Acids Res 30 (8):1757–1766. https://doi.org/10.1093/nar/30.8.1757
9. Khvorova A, Reynolds A, Jayasena SD (2003) Functional siRNAs and miRNAs exhibit strand bias. Cell 115(2):209–216. https://doi.org/10.1016/S0092-8674(03)00801-8
10. Jackson AL, Bartz SR, Schelter J et al (2003) Expression profiling reveals off-target gene regulation by RNAi. Nat Biotechnol 21 (6):635–637. https://doi.org/10.1038/nbt831
11. Tafer H, Ameres SL, Obernosterer G et al (2008) The impact of target site accessibility on the design of effective siRNAs. Nat

Biotechnol 26(83):578. https://doi.org/10.1038/nbt1404

12. Ameres SL, Martinez J, Schroeder R (2007) Molecular basis for target RNA recognition and cleavage by human RISC. Cell 130 (1):101–112. https://doi.org/10.1016/j.cell.2007.04.037
13. Fakhr E, Zare F, Teimoori-Toolabi L (2016) Precise and efficient siRNA design: a key point in competent gene silencing. Cancer Gene Ther 23(4):73–82
14. Naito Y, Yoshimura J, Morishita S, Ui-Tei K (2009) SiDirect 2.0: updated software for designing functional siRNA with reduced seed-dependent off-target effect. BMC Bioinformatics 10:392. https://doi.org/10.1186/1471-2105-10-392
15. Elbashir SM, Martinez J, Patkaniowska A et al (2001) Functional anatomy of siRNAs for mediating efficient RNAi in *Drosophila melanogaster* embryo lysate. EMBO J 20 (23):6877–6888. https://doi.org/10.1093/emboj/20.23.6877
16. Reynolds A, Leake D, Boese Q et al (2004) Rational siRNA design for RNA interference. Nat Biotechnol 22(3):326–330. https://doi.org/10.1038/nbt936
17. Fedorov Y, Anderson EM, Birmingham A et al (2006) Off-target effects by siRNA can induce toxic phenotype. RNA 12(7):1188–1196. https://doi.org/10.1261/rna.28106
18. Hornung V, Guenthner-Biller M, Bourquin C et al (2005) Sequence-specific potent induction of IFN-alpha by short interfering RNA in plasmacytoid dendritic cells through TLR7. Nat Med 11(3):263–270. https://doi.org/10.1038/nm1191
19. Judge AD, Sood V, Shaw JR et al (2005) Sequence-dependent stimulation of the mammalian innate immune response by synthetic siRNA. Nat Biotechnol 23(4):457–462. https://doi.org/10.1038/nbt1081
20. Sharan RN, Vaiphei ST, Nongrum S et al (2015) Consensus reference gene(s) for gene expression studies in human cancers: end of the tunnel visible? Cell Oncol 38(6):419–431
21. Schmittgen TD, Livak KJ (2008) Analyzing real-time PCR data by the comparative CT method. Nat Protoc 3(6):1101–1108. https://doi.org/10.1038/nprot.2008.73
22. Meade BR, Gogoi K, Hamil AS et al (2014) Efficient delivery of RNAi prodrugs containing reversible charge-neutralizing phosphotriester backbone modifications. Nat Biotechnol 32 (12):1256–1261. https://doi.org/10.1038/nbt.3078
23. Hagopian JC, Hamil AS, van den Berg A et al (2017) Induction of RNAi responses by short left-handed hairpin RNAi triggers. Nucleic Acid Ther 27(5):260–271. https://doi.org/10.1089/nat.2017.0686
24. Kim DH, Behlke MA, Rose SD et al (2005) Synthetic dsRNA dicer substrates enhance RNAi potency and efficacy. Nat Biotechnol 23 (2):222–226. https://doi.org/10.1038/nbt1051

Chapter 4

Antisense Oligonucleotides for Splice Modulation: Assessing Splice Switching Efficacy

Cristina S. J. Rocha

Abstract

Today, there are emerging numbers of oligonucleotide therapies being approved by the governmental authorities. These types of therapies present a different mode of action when compared to the traditional small molecules, acting at the RNA level instead of the protein level. In drug development, drug potency is defined by the drug affinity to the target biomolecule (target engagement), together with the ability to initiate a response at the molecular, cellular, tissue, or system level (efficacy). In oligonucleotide therapies, affinity and efficacy can be both easily evaluated by gene expression analysis. Although more advanced techniques can be used, this chapter presents a protocol to evaluate splice switching oligonucleotide efficacy that can be easily applied in a molecular biology laboratory without the need of advanced equipment. It describes all steps from sample preparation to data analysis.

Key words Splice modulation efficacy, Antisense oligonucleotides, RT-PCR, RNA isolation, Agarose electrophoresis, Splice switching oligonucleotides

1 Introduction

Human diseases are commonly associated with mutations that cause abnormal splicing, complete or partial exon loss or the retention of intronic sequences [1]. These mutations originate nonfunctional or deleterious protein isoforms, abnormal protein expression, or changes in the open reading frame [2]. Splice switching oligonucleotides (SSOs) can redirect toward the normal pre-mRNA splicing process and counteract the mutation biologic effects [3].

SSOs differ from their antisense counterparts by their mechanism of action and consequent chemistry modification requirements. SSOs are short, fully modified synthetic nucleic acids that bind complementary to the pre-mRNA sequence, blocking the RNA–RNA base-pairing or protein–RNA binding interactions that occur between components of the splicing machinery and the pre-mRNA [3]. This interference with the pre-mRNA splicing

Olof Gissberg et al. (eds.), *Oligonucleotide-Based Therapies: Methods and Protocols*, Methods in Molecular Biology, vol. 2036,
https://doi.org/10.1007/978-1-4939-9670-4_4,

mechanism makes it possible to select which exonic or intronic regions that will be incorporated in the final mRNA molecule, thus manipulating the protein production from a specific gene.

Nowadays, two SSOs based therapies are approved by FDA. Eteplirsen, designed to skip the exon 51 of the dystrophin protein, with application in Duchenne muscular dystrophy (DMD) [4] and nusinersen, that induces the inclusion of exon 7 in the *SMN2* mRNA, as therapeutic application for types 1, 2, and 3 spinal muscular atrophy (SMA) [5]. Although, several other studies are being developed for diseases like β-thalassemia, X-linked agammaglobulinemia [6], hypercholesterolemia [7], cancer, and neurodegenerative, inflammatory, and immunodeficiency diseases, among others [3].

To evaluate the SSO potency, the formation of the new mRNA splice isoforms needs to be determined. Splice isoforms do not always translate to proteins that can be identified by antibodies, so an analysis at the mRNA level by reverse transcription polymerase chain reaction (RT-PCR) is required. RT-PCR is composed of two distinct steps, the first strand cDNA synthesis and the PCR amplification [8]. First, the RNA is converted to a DNA template by a reverse transcriptase (RT) enzyme reaction through extension from one or more oligonucleotide primers. These primers can be a sequence specific primer; a series of random primers that hybridize along the length of the mRNA; or a primer directed toward the poly-A tail located at the 3′ end of most messenger RNA sequence [9]. In the case of SSOs-related studies, the use of the random primers for this step is preferential. After elongation, a double-stranded hybrid of RNA and DNA, called first-strand cDNA, is produced. This cDNA is then a suitable template for the PCR step and relative quantities of specific RNA templates can be determined by semiquantitative PCR.

Nowadays, advances in technology allowed the development of other more advanced and quantitative methods, like the reverse transcription quantitative real-time PCR (RT-qPCR) [10–16] and the digital droplet PCR (ddPCR) [17–20]. Unfortunately, these methods require specific and expensive equipment and are both based on TaqMan™ probes, which for certain specific sequences the design can be a challenge or even impossible. For these reasons, they will not be discussed in this chapter, but detailed information can be found in the references provided.

There are two steps at the RT-PCR workflow that I consider extremely important for successful results: the RNA samples preparation and the PCR primer design. Independently of the starting biological material (tissue or cell lines) after extraction, the RNA should be of high quality and integrity [21]. For the primer design the use of a primer design software is highly recommended [22]. Not only because attention to all normal parameters like CG content, primer dimer formation, secondary structures and no secondary products is required, but also because SSOs efficacy is focused on a specific region of the RNA sequence of interest, which restricts the primer design [8, 22, 23].

In this chapter, the protocol presented will be an adaptation of the protocol used for the assessment of an SSO specific for the *PCSK9* gene in cell lines [7], although directions for tissue analysis will also be provided in the respective notes.

2 Materials

2.1 RNA Isolation (See Note 1)

1. TRIzol™ Plus RNA Purification Kit and Phasemaker™ Tubes Complete System.
2. Chloroform.
3. 70% ethanol (in DEPC-treated water).
4. 100% ethanol.
5. PureLink™ DNase Set (*see* **Note 2**).
6. RNase decontamination solution.
7. Centrifuge and rotor capable of reaching of 12,000 × *g* and 4 °C.
8. RNase-free pipette tips.
9. 2 mL RNase-free microcentrifuge polypropylene tubes (*see* **Note 3**).
10. Agarose.
11. 1× TAE Buffer DEPC: 40 mM Tris, 20 mM acetic acid, 1 mM EDTA in DEPC-treated water.
12. RNA ladder (200–6000 bp size range) in 47.5% formamide, 0.0125% SDS, 0.0125% bromophenol blue, 0.0125% xylene cyanol FF, 0.0125% ethidium bromide, 0.75 mM EDTA.
13. 6× DNA Loading Dye: 10 mM Tris–HCl (pH 7.6), 0.03% bromophenol blue, 0.03% xylene cyanol FF, 0.15% orange G, 60% glycerol, 60 mM EDTA.
14. SYBR® Safe DNA Gel Stain 10,000× in DMSO.
15. NanoDrop Microvolume Spectrophotometer.
16. Electrophoresis equipment.
17. Power supply.
18. Gel documentation, or gel imaging system.

2.2 cDNA Synthesis

1. High-Capacity cDNA Reverse Transcription Kit including:
   (a) MultiScribe™ Reverse Transcriptase, 50 U/μL.
   (b) 10× RT Buffer.
   (c) 25× dNTP mix.

(d) 10× RT Random Primers.

2. RNase Inhibitor: 20 U/μL RNase Inhibitor, 20 mM HEPES--KOH, pH 7.6, 50 mM KCl, 8 mM DTT, 50% (v/v) glycerol.
3. Nuclease free water, molecular grade.
4. PCR tubes.
5. RNase-free filter pipette tips.
6. RNase-free microcentrifuge tubes.
7. PCR thermal cycler with heated lid.

2.3 RT-PCR

1. HotStarTaq Plus DNA Polymerase kit including the following:
   (a) HotStarTaq Plus DNA Polymerase 5 units/μL diluted in storage buffer: 20 mM Tris–HCl, 100 mM KCl, 1 mM DTT, 0.1 mM EDTA, 0.5% (v/v) Nonidet® P-40, 0.5% (v/v) Tween® 20, 50% glycerol (v/v), stabilizer, pH 9.0 at 20 °C.
   (b) HotStarTaq Plus DNA Polymerase 10× PCR Buffer with Tris–HCl, KCl, $(NH_4)_2SO_4$, 15 mM $MgCl_2$, pH 8.7 at 20 °C.
   (c) 25 mM $MgCl_2$ solution.
2. 10 mM of dNTP mix: (from 100 mM stock of dTTP, dATP, dGTP, dCTP, add 10 μL of each to 60 μL of nuclease-free water to make a 100 μL mix of dNTPs).
3. Primers for gene of interest at 5 μM (*see* **Note 4**).
   (a) *PCSK9* forward primer: 5′-TGGGGACCAACTTT GGCCGC.
   (b) *PCSK9* reverse primer: 5′-TGGCCTCAGCTGGTGG AGCT.
4. Primers for housekeeping gene at 5 μM (*see* **Note 5**).
   (a) *HPRT* forward primer: 5′-GACTTTGCTTTCCTTGGT CAG.
   (b) *HPRT* reverse primer: 5′-GGCTTATATCCAACACTT CGTGGG.
5. Nuclease-free water, molecular grade.
6. PCR tubes.
7. DNase-free filter pipette tips.
8. DNase-free microcentrifuge tubes.
9. PCR thermal cycler with heated lid.

2.4 Agarose Gel Electrophoresis

1. Agarose.
2. 1× TBE Buffer: 89 mM Tris, 89 mM boric acid, 2 mM EDTA.
3. SYBR® Safe DNA Gel Stain 10,000× in DMSO.

4. DNA Ladder (100–15,000 bp size range) 0.5 μg/μL in 10 mM Tris–HCl (pH 7.6), 1 mM EDTA.
5. 6× DNA Loading Dye, *see* Subheading 2.1, **item 13**.
6. DNase-free filter pipette tips.
7. DNase-free microcentrifuge tubes.
8. NanoDrop Microvolume Spectrophotometer.
9. Electrophoresis equipment.
10. Power supply.
11. Gel documentation, or gel imaging, system.
12. ImageJ Software.

3 Methods

3.1 RNA Isolation

Before you start, please be attentive to the following guidelines. Wear disposable gloves while handling reagents, RNA samples and tubes/columns to prevent RNase contamination from the surface of the skin. Change gloves frequently, particularly as the protocol progresses from crude extracts to more purified materials. Perform all steps at room temperature (20–25 °C), unless indicated otherwise.

1. Wipe the working surfaces and nondisposable items such as centrifuges, pipettes, and electrophoresis equipment and combs with the RNase decontamination solution to remove RNase contamination.
2. Label all tubes and columns required (Fig. 1).
3. Add 60 mL of 100% ethanol to Wash Buffer II (provided in the kit), then mix thoroughly.
4. Centrifuge the Phasemaker™ Tubes for 1 min at 16,000 × *g*.

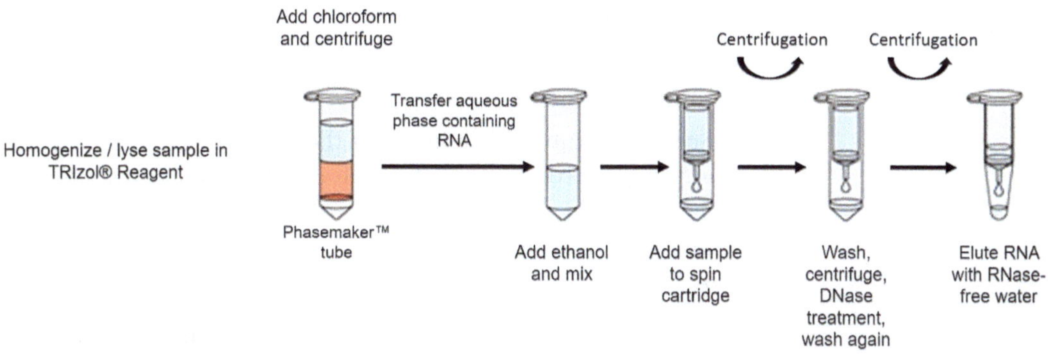

Fig. 1 Schematic representation of the silica-based purification protocol workflow using PureLink RNA Mini Kit in conjunction with TRIzol® Reagent and Phasemaker™ tubes

5. Cool down the centrifuge to 4 °C.
6. For cells growing in monolayer, remove the growth medium and add 1 mL of TRIzol™ reagent per 2 × 10^5–10^7 cells (equivalent to a 6-well plate well) directly to the culture dish to lyse the cells. Pipet the lysate up and down several times to homogenize (*see* **Notes 6** and 7).
7. At this point, samples can be stored at 4 °C overnight or at −20 °C for up to a year (*see* **Note 8**).
8. Transfer the samples (0.1–1.4 mL) to the Phasemaker™ Tubes.
9. Incubate 5 min at room temperature to permit complete dissociation of the nucleoproteins.
10. Add 0.2 mL of chloroform per each mL of TRIzol™ used during lysis, securely cap the tube. The total volume cannot exceed 1.7 mL.
11. Preventing the tube caps from opening with your fingers/hand palm, shake vigorously by hand 15–30 s (do not use vortex). The solution should become milky, if not shake for longer time. This step is very important, and the mixture should be as homogenous as possible.
12. Incubate for 2–3 min at room temperature. At this stage the phases will start to separate, avoid disturbing the tubes more than necessary.
13. Centrifuge the sample at 16,000 × *g* for 5 min at 4 °C. The mixture separates into a lower red phenol–chloroform, an interphase corresponding to the Phasemaker™ gel, and a colorless upper aqueous phase.
14. Remove carefully the tubes from the centrifuge (*see* **Note 9**). Warm up the centrifuge to room temperature.
15. Transfer 350 μL of the aqueous phase containing the RNA to a new tube (*see* **Note 10**). Aspirate the liquid from the top of the layer in way to avoid puncturing or touch the Phasemaker™ gel with the tip.
16. Add 350 μL of 70% ethanol and mix by pipet up and down 3–4 times (*see* **Note 11**).
17. Secure the tube caps and invert the tubes 20 times to disperse any visible precipitate that may form after adding the ethanol.
18. Transfer up to 700 μL of the sample to a spin cartridge placed in a 2 mL collection tube.
19. Centrifuge at 12,000 × *g* for 30 s.
20. Discard the flow-through, dry the collection tube briefly by inverting on a tissue paper, then reinsert the spin cartridge into the same collection tube (*see* **Note 12**).

21. Add 350 μL of Wash Buffer I. Centrifuge for 30 s at 12,000 × *g* and discard the flow-through, dry the collection tube briefly by inverting on a tissue paper, then reinsert the spin cartridge into the same collection tube.
22. Prepare the DNase master mix enough for all samples by mixing per sample: 8 μL of 10× DNase I Reaction Buffer, 10 μL of the resuspended DNase, and 62 μL of RNase-free water.
23. Add 80 μL of the DNase reaction mixture to the center of the column, without touching the filter, and incubate 15 min at room temperature.
24. Add 350 μL of Wash Buffer I. Centrifuge for 30 s at 12,000 × *g* and transfer the spin cartridge into a new collection tube.
25. Wash with 500 μL of Wash Buffer II (*see* **Note 13**). Centrifuge for 30 s at 12,000 × *g* and discard the flow-through, dry the collection tube briefly by inverting on a tissue paper, then reinsert the spin cartridge into the same collection tube.
26. Repeat **step 25** once.
27. Centrifuge at 12,000 × *g* for 2 min to dry the membrane. The membrane should be dry, if not repeat the centrifugation. Discard the collection tube and transfer the spin cartridge to the 1.5 mL recovery tube.
28. Add 30–40 μL of RNase free-water to the center of the spin cartridge (*see* **Note 14**).
29. Incubate 2–4 min at room temperature.
30. Centrifuge at 16,000 × *g* for 2 min.
31. Discard the spin column. The recovery tube contains the purified RNA and should be stored on ice if used within few hours or −80 °C for long-term storage (*see* **Note 15**).
32. Measure the RNA quantity and quality using 2 μL of the sample in a NanoDrop Microvolume Spectrophotometer. Use the same RNase free-water used for RNA elution as blank (*see* **Note 16**).
33. Measure the RNA integrity by running 200–500 ng of the purified RNA in a nondenaturing 1.2% (m/v) agarose gel in 1× TAE Buffer DEPC.
34. Prepare the agarose gel by adding 0.6 g of agarose in 50 mL of 1× TAE Buffer DEPC. Heat in the microwave at max potency. Mix the solution every 20–30 s to help dissolving agarose until no more "gelatine" particles are visible (be careful when stirring, since eruptive boiling can occur). Let cool down to 50 °C (when you can comfortably keep your hand on the flask, around 5 min at room temperature) and add 5 μL (1 μL per mL of gel) of SYBR® Safe DNA staining. Mix and pour into the

gel support containing the comb. Let cool down until firm (approximately 30 min, depending of the gel size).

35. Prepare the RNA samples by diluting **500** ng of RNA in a final volume of 10 μL of RNase free-water, heat to 70 °C for 1 min and cool down immediately on ice. Add 2 μL of 6× DNA Loading Dye and load all sample in the gel. Load 4 μL of the RNA ladder. Run the gel at 10 V/cm in cold room for 45 min and immediately analyze the bands with the gel imaging system (*see* **Note 17**).

3.2 cDNA Synthesis

This section describes all the steps required for the cDNA synthesis from 1 μg of total RNA in a final volume of **20** μL using the High-Capacity cDNA Reverse Transcription Kit (*see* **Note 18**). As in the previous section, always wear disposable gloves while handling reagents, RNA samples and tubes to prevent RNase contamination from the surface of the skin and change gloves frequently if contamination is detected.

Due to risk of cross-contamination, reactions should be set in an area where no PCR products have been handled.

1. Remove the RNA aliquots from −80 °C and the kit components from the −20 °C and allow them to de-frost on ice.
2. Prepare 10 μL RNA solutions containing 1 μg of total RNA in RNase free-water.
3. Heat the RNA solution at 65 °C for 5 min and immediately snap cold them on ice (*see* **Note 19**).
4. Briefly vortex and spin down all the kit components.
5. Prepare the 2× RT master mix. For 1 sample and 20 μL volume reaction: mix 3.2 μL of nuclease free-water; 2 μL of 10× RT Buffer; 0.8 μL of 25× dNTP Mix; 2 μL of 10× RT Random Primers; 1 μL of MultiScribe™ Reverse Transcriptase and 1 μL of RNase Inhibitor (*see* **Note 20**). Mix gently by pipetting up and down and keep on ice.
6. Prepare the 2× RT negative control master mix. For one sample and 20 μL volume reaction: mix 4.2 μL of nuclease free-water; 2 μL of 10× RT Buffer; 0.8 μL of 25× dNTP Mix; 2 μL of 10× RT Random Primers and 1 μL of RNase Inhibitor (*see* **Note 21**). Mix gently by pipetting up and down and keep on ice.
7. While keeping all tubes on ice, pipet **10** μL of the 2× master mix (RT or RT negative control) to the corresponding PCR tubes.
8. Pipet the 10 μL of the RNA solution to the respective PCR tube and pipet up and down 2–3 times to mix.
9. Close the tubes and briefly centrifuge the PCR tube to spin down the components and to eliminate any air bubbles.

10. Load the tubes on the PCR thermal cycler and start the program: 1 cycle of 10 min at 25 °C; 1 cycle of 120 min at 37 °C; 1 cycle of 5 min at 85 °C; 1 hold cycle at 4 °C.
11. Remove the tube samples from the thermal cycler. If performing the PCR in the same day, store them at 4 °C or on ice, otherwise cDNA should be stored immediately at −20 °C.

3.3 Polymerase Chain Reaction (PCR)

This section describes all the steps required for the PCR with the primers previously published for the detection of splice-forms from the *PCSK9* gene and the reference gene *HPRT* using the HotStar-Taq Plus DNA Polymerase kit. Also, for PCR, several DNA polymerases can be used (*see* **Note 22**).

As in the previous sections, always wear disposable gloves while handling reagents, cDNA samples and tubes to prevent DNase contamination and change gloves frequently if contamination is detected. Due to the risk of cross-contamination, reactions should be set in an area separate from that used for DNA preparation or PCR product analysis.

1. Thaw 10× PCR Buffer, dNTP mix, primer solutions, and 25 mM $MgCl_2$ at room temperature or on ice. Mix the solutions completely before use to avoid localized concentrations of salts.
2. Prepare a master mix containing all the components required for the PCR, except the cDNA. For 1 sample and 25 μL volume reaction: mix 16.2 μL of nuclease free-water; 2.5 μL of 10× PCR Buffer; 1.5 μL of 25 mM $MgCl_2$ solution; 0.5 μL of 10 mM dNTP mix; 0.8 μL of 5 μM Fw *PCSK9* primer; 0.8 μL of 5 μM Rv *PCSK9* primer; 0.8 μL of 5 μM Fw *HPRT* primer; 0.8 μL of 5 μM Rv *HPRT* primer, and 0.1 μL of HotStar Taq Plus DNA Polymerase (*see* **Note 20**).
3. Mix the master mix thoroughly and gently by pipetting up and down several times. Dispense 24 μL into PCR tube (*see* **Note 23**).
4. Dilute the cDNA sample 1:2 in nuclease free water and add 1 μL to the respective PCR tube containing the master mix (*see* **Note 24**). Mix by pipetting up and down and centrifuge briefly to remove any air bubbles.
5. Also prepare the negative controls, in which the cDNA sample is replaced by nuclease free-water and a control in which the RT was absent during cDNA conversion (*see* **steps 6–8** of Subheading 3.2 and **Notes 21** and **25**).
6. Place the tubes in the PCR thermal cycler and start the run using the following cycling program: 1 cycle of 5 min at 95 °C; a three-step cycling of 27 cycles of 30 s at 94 °C (denaturation),

30 s at 57 °C (annealing), and 45 s at 72 °C (extension); 1 cycle of 10 min at 72 °C followed by a hold cycle at 4 °C (*see* **Note 26**).

7. After amplification store samples overnight at 4 °C or at −20 °C for longer periods.

3.4 Agarose Gel Electrophoresis and Data Analysis

1. Prepare a 2% agarose gel in 1× TBE Buffer as described in **step 34** of Subheading 3.1 (*see* **Note 27**).
2. Prepare the samples by adding 5 μL of 6× DNA Loading Dye to the 25 μL of PCR product. Vortex and spin down.
3. In the first well load 4 μL of the DNA Ladder and in the remaining wells load 10 μL of the samples prepared in **step 2** of Subheading 3.4.
4. Run the gel at room temperature with a voltage of 5 V/cm (*see* **Note 17**) and until the blue dye reaches two-thirds of the gel.
5. Immediately after running, analyze the gel on the gel imaging system. Only three products should be amplified, two bands with 585 and 450 bp respectively, corresponding to the *PCSK9* isoforms and one band with 100 bp corresponding to the *HPRT* gene (Fig. 2). Take a picture of the gel but ensure that the image is not overexposed, and the bands are not saturated (*see* **Note 28**).
6. Proceed to the band intensity quantification. Using the Image J software or a gel doc software. Start by delimiting each of the bands using a rectangle. Insure that the same area is used to all the bands. Request the program to select a local background and retrieve the bands intensity.
7. Normalize all bands to the respective intensity of the *HPRT* product. This normalization is just required to correct for loading or cDNA or PCR efficacy adjustments. Normalization should be performed as follow:
   - Band 585 bp/Band *HPRT*.
   - Band 450 bp/Band *HPRT*.
   - (Band 585 bp + Band 450 bp)/Band *HPRT*.
8. Calculate the isoform proportion to each sample:

   Proportion of splice = Intensity band 450 bp corrected/(Intensity band 585 bp corrected + Intensity band 450 bp corrected).

   Proportion of wt = Intensity band 585 bp corrected/(Intensity band 585 bp corrected + Intensity band 450 bp corrected).
9. Calculate the % of the splice-form induced by the SSOs:

   % splice induced = Proportion of splice (SSOs treated sample)/Proportion of samples (untreated sample) × 100

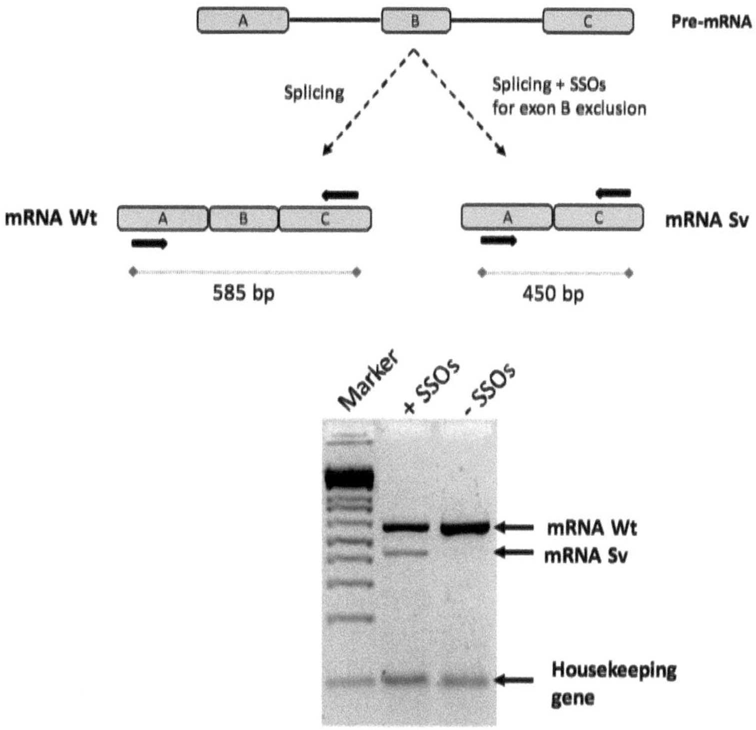

Fig. 2 *PCSK9* splice pattern modification by splice switching oligonucleotides (SSOs). Upper panel: A schematic representation of the putative mRNA products with the wild type mRNA (mRNA Wt) and the splice variant (mRNA Sv) induced by the SSO treatment. PCR primer localizations are indicated by arrows and the size of the PCR products are given below. The lower panel shows an agarose gel with the *PCSK9* PCR products together with the housekeeping gene

4 Notes

1. Since SSOs have high affinity to mRNA, the extraction protocol should be astringent enough to ensure that the SSO is released from the mRNA molecules, which can compromise the cDNA conversion and/or the PCR amplification. Thus, an acid guanidinium thiocyanate–phenol–chloroform extraction [24] would be preferential followed by a DNase treatment. This method in its traditional form, based on liquid–liquid extraction, can be quite tricky for untrained hands. Luckily, developments in the method allowed to combine the efficiency of the extraction using organic solvent, with a more robust phase separation together with a DNase treatment and cleanup in a silica column. This method is less time consuming and easy to perform without increasing the price per sample.
2. DNA contamination of the RNA sample compromises either RNA quantification (DNA and RNA absorb at the same

wavelength) or depending of the target region compromise further analysis by PCR by false positives. Thus, its removal by DNase treatment on the column should be performed. Dissolve the lyophilized PureLink® DNase by injection of 550 μL with a syringe of provided RNase-free water. Mix gently and do not vortex! Store at 4 °C. This will give ~3 U DNase/μL.

3. Use transparent 2 mL polypropylene disposable tubes when working with <2 mL volume of TRIzol™ reagent. For larger volumes use glass or polypropylene tubes, and ensure that the tubes can withstand centrifugation at 12,000 × *g*.

4. The primers should be ideally located at the exons upstream and downstream of the region (exon or intron) to be included or skipped by the SSOs (Fig. 2)

   This type of approach allows the amplification of all spliced mRNA species around the target sequence, granting the evaluation of the RNA species that could have been affected by the SSO binding at the specific target. Another advantage in this method is that both products can be amplified in the same reaction and from the same RNA sample, eliminating variability, which may occur if separate reactions would be performed. It is important that the PCR products, although of different sizes, do not differ significantly. A large size difference would result in unequal PCR product yields efficiencies. Small products tend to be more easily amplified compared to larger products (more than 1000 bp), which can give rise to biased data regarding product proportion [25]. For a good resolution on agarose gels, differences must be more than 30 bp for fragments below 300 bp and increasing with product size.

5. Together with the amplification of the target region, a housekeeping (or reference) gene should also be used as reference, not only for treatment effects evaluation, but also as control for the cDNA reaction efficiency and gel loading, allowing the possibility to normalize the data. Of course, when performing a PCR multiplex, primers should be checked during primer design in all combinations to avoid potential formation of primer cross-dimers. Moreover, melting temperatures need to be balanced for all primers to achieve an even performance. When choosing a reference gene, certain criteria must be taken in account. A good reference gene should be expressed at the same level as the target and its expression cannot be changed by the treatment, species in question or even tissue. A reference gene database with validated genes for specific species and diseases was compiled and can be used for better assessment [26]

6. Do not exceed the ratio of 10:1 between the volume of TRIzol from the TRIzol™ Plus RNA purification kit (mL) and the

mass of the sample (g), since lysis, homogenization, and RNAse inactivation will be decreased, compromising the extraction efficiency and sample quality. The maximum RNA binding capacity of the spin cartridge is ~1 mg, so if processed samples contain more than 1 mg total RNA, divide the sample into aliquots to give <1 mg total RNA and use a spin cartridge per aliquot. Clogging of the spin column will decrease the yield.

7. To lyse tissue samples a bead homogenizer, a mortar or a pestle homogenizer can be used. To use a bead homogenizer, transfer a 3 × 3 mm of snap frozen tissue to a cold 2 mL safe-cap polypropylene tube containing one 5 mm stainless bead and 1 mL of TRIzol™ reagent. Immediately proceed to the tissue disruption in the homogenizer. Run two times 25 s at 500 rpm. Between each run double check the lids to ensure that they remain properly closed. Centrifuge the lysates for 5 min at 12,000 × *g* at 4 °C and transfer the clear supernatant to the Phasemaker™ tubes.

   For cells growing in suspension: Pellet 1–2 × 10^7 cells by centrifugation at 300 × *g* for 5 min at room temperature. Remove the supernatant and add 0.75 mL of TRIzol™ reagent to the pellet. Pipet the lysate up and down several times to homogenize, and when no cells clumps are visible, transfer to the Phasemaker™ tubes.

8. In each case, I would recommend the transfer of the samples to polypropylene tubes before storage for safety purposes. Once stored, samples should be warm to room temperature before proceeding with the protocol.

9. The aqueous phase should be approximately 50% of the volume of the starting lysate, in this case, corresponding to 500 μL. Setting the pipette to, and collect, a lower volume will allow a more secure recovery. In this condition the amount of RNA recovered is in the order of 0.2–4 μg/μL, depending on the cell line or organ tissue. If recovering a larger volume of the aqueous phase, the ethanol volume (*see* **step 16** of Subheading 3.1) should be adjusted accordingly, to be the same volume as the aqueous solution collected.

10. When dealing with several samples it is recommended to prefill the tubes with the corresponding volume of ethanol to avoid keeping the aqueous phase more than necessary at room temperature.

11. The addition of ethanol allows the binding of the nucleic acids to the silica membrane. If the sample is from liver tissues, reduce the ethanol percentage to 50%. This will increase the RNA recovery yield from this type of tissues.

12. As mentioned in **Note 9**, if more than 350 μL of aqueous phase are collected, repeat **steps 18–20** of Subheading 3.1 until the entire sample has been processed.
13. Be sure that 60 mL of 100% ethanol where added to wash buffer II, as mentioned in **step 3** of Subheading 3.1
14. The volume provided in **step 28** of Subheading 3.1 is the minimum volume to be used for the column and corresponds to the RNA ratios mentioned in **Note 6**. When processing larger tissue samples, volumes up to 100 μL can be used. Sequential elutions with up to 3 × 100 μL can be performed, by repeating **steps 28–30** of Subheading 3.1. When performing sequential elutions collect always in the same tube.
15. Several cycles of frost–defrost can induce the degradation of RNA by hydrolysis, thus quantification of RNA should be performed immediately after isolation, to allow the preparation and freezing of working aliquots with approximately 5 μg of RNA. The remaining amount can be stored as stock for further use. This working aliquot will be further used for cDNA synthesis and RNA quality assessment using gel electrophoresis or a bioanalyzer.
16. An absorbance reading (OD) of 1 at 260 nm is equivalent to about 40 μg/mL of RNA. When measuring RNA in water a good quality sample give A_{260}/A_{280} and A_{260}/A_{230} absorbance ratios close to 2. Always pay attention to the variations in the absorbance spectra of your sample: an OD ratio A_{260}/A_{230} below 1 is characteristic of guanidine isothiocyanate contamination (peak at 230 nm) and should be avoided. This compound might have a deleterious effect on downstream enzymatic reactions. Phenol contaminations are indicated by a shift of the absorbance peak toward 270 nm. Protein contamination in the RNA sample decreases the values both at 260 and at 280 nm, thus decreasing the OD ratio A_{260}/A_{280} below 1.9.
17. For eukaryotic RNA the best way to evaluate RNA integrity, and possible RNA degradation is by measuring the proportion of the 18 s (~2000 bp) and 28 s (~5000 bp) ribosomal RNAS (rRNA). In an agarose gel stained with SYBR safe, the 28 s/18 s rRNA bands should have an intensity ratio around 2 for good quality RNA. Additionally, no smear should be visible below the 18 s rRNA band. A smeary sample indicates RNA degradation and the presence of DNA contamination is possible to see as material stuck in the well. The quick heating and snap cooling of the RNA samples prior to loading is required to unfold conformations that can interfere with the migration of the samples. Use as little loading dye as possible, or a loading dye without xylene cyanol since this dye comigrates with the

28 s rRNA, making it hard to estimate the correct 28 s/18 s ratio.

Running the gel at low voltage in the cold and for a minimal time reduces the risk for overheating, which can induce sample degradation during the gel run. A voltage of 10 v/cm means 10 v per each cm of space between the electrodes in an electrophoretic chamber, so if the chamber has 10 cm, then the gel should be run at 100 v.

18. Other RT enzymes are available in the market and can be used in the cDNA synthesis step, although protocol steps regarding reaction assembly and incubation conditions should be adapted to the manufacturer's instructions. The quantity of 1–2 μg is optimal for conversion of total RNA to cDNA, although lower quantities as 100 ng can also be used. The only drawback of lower quantities is that since cDNA is a 1:1 reaction, correct evaluation of the presence of low expressed RNAs can be difficult. Personally, I try never to go below 500 ng of total RNA, unless I have RNA samples that are very diluted and cannot be further precipitated and resuspended.
19. Heating the RNA at 65 °C allows to unfold most of the secondary structures of the RNA that can hamper the cDNA synthesis. The snap cool down avoids their reformation.
20. When preparing more than one sample calculate the volume of components needed to prepare the required number of reactions. Prepare the master mix and add 10% extra of the volumes required, mixing the components in the order specified. The order of the components is very important to ensure that all salts are in the correct concentration before the addition of the enzymes, while facilitating the dissolution of the enzyme (enzymes are maintained in glycerol rich-solutions).
21. The negative controls are important to assess that samples are free of DNA contamination. Random RNA samples should be selected, preferentially the ones with higher and lower yields of total mRNA. The same principles from **Note 20** should be applied.
22. For each new polymerase, primers should be optimized in terms of amplification temperature and the number of cycles, since different polymerases require different Mg^{2+} concentrations and this cation interferes with primer binding affinity.
23. Alternatively, a gently and short vortex and spin down can also be performed to mix the master mix, especially when several samples are being assembled. Due to the inactive state of HotStarTaq Plus DNA polymerase at room temperature, it is not necessary to keep the PCR tubes on ice to avoid nonspecific DNA synthesis.

24. On average, only 10–30% of the original RNA molecules are reverse-transcribed into cDNA. The expression level of the target RNA molecules and the relatively low efficiency of the reverse transcription reaction must be considered when calculating the appropriate amount of starting template for subsequent PCR. The volume of the RT reaction transferred should not exceed 10% of the total PCR volume.

    For a 25 μL reaction, for this kit, the DNA template should be less than 250 ng and the volume of template should never be more than 2.5 μL. When changing the template volume from the one indicated in **step 4** of Subheading 3.3, adjust the nuclease-free water and master mix volumes in **steps 2** and **3** of Subheading 3.3 accordingly.

25. The negative control is important to assess that reagents and RNA samples are not contaminated with DNA and thus shouldn't give any product. Additionally, they can also be used to determine the degree of primer dimer formation.

26. The initial cycle of 5 min at 95 °C is required to activate the polymerase while disrupts any primer–primer hybridization or cDNA secondary structures. Do not exceed the 5 min, which can compromise the polymerase activity.

    In the three-step cycling the annealing temperature is dependent of the primers and should be optimized before. This temperature should be the optimal to allow the primers to hybridize to the template and normally is 5 °C below the melting temperature (T_m) of the primer set. Regarding the extension step at 72 °C, the time of extension should be approximately 1 min/kb DNA. In the case described here, the PCR products are around 585 and 100 bp, so the 45 s are enough to allow the full extension of the larger products.

    The number of cycles is dependent on the starting material, the expression of the gene and should be determine beforehand. Since our intent is to use the bands intensity for quantification, it is important that the number of cycles corresponds to the linear amplification phase of the PCR reaction for both RNA isoforms. Normally the number of cycles should be comprehended between 25 and 35.

27. Alternatively, 0.5× TBE buffer can be used instead.

28. If additional products besides the expected ones are observed, this means that the PCR conditions are not optimized. Redo the optimization or design new primers. If the bands are saturated, run the PCR again with fewer cycles, to ensure that the PCR reaction does not reach a plateau.

References

1. Sterne-Weiler T, Sanford JR (2014) Exon identity crisis: disease-causing mutations that disrupt the splicing code. Genome Biol 15 (1):201–201. https://doi.org/10.1186/gb4150
2. Martinovich KM, Shaw NC, Kicic A, Schultz A, Fletcher S, Wilton SD, Stick SM (2018) The potential of antisense oligonucleotide therapies for inherited childhood lung diseases. Mol Cell Pediatr 5(1):3. https://doi.org/10.1186/s40348-018-0081-6
3. Havens MA, Hastings ML (2016) Splice-switching antisense oligonucleotides as therapeutic drugs. Nucleic Acids Res 44 (14):6549–6563. https://doi.org/10.1093/nar/gkw533
4. FDA grants accelerated approval to first drug for Duchenne muscular dystrophy. (19th September 2016)
5. FDA approves first drug for spinal muscular atrophy (23 December 2016)
6. Bestas B, Moreno PMD, Blomberg KEM, Mohammad DK, Saleh AF, Sutlu T, Nordin JZ, Guterstam P, Gustafsson MO, Kharazi S, Piątosa B, Roberts TC, Behlke MA, Wood MJA, Gait MJ, Lundin KE, El Andaloussi S, Månsson R, Berglöf A, Wengel J, Smith CIE (2014) Splice-correcting oligonucleotides restore BTK function in X-linked agammaglobulinemia model. J Clin Invest 124 (9):4067–4081. https://doi.org/10.1172/JCI76175
7. Rocha CSJ, Wiklander OPB, Larsson L, Moreno PMD, Parini P, Lundin KE, Smith CIE (2015) RNA therapeutics inactivate PCSK9 by inducing a unique intracellular retention form. J Mol Cell Cardiol 82:186–193. https://doi.org/10.1016/j.yjmcc.2015.03.009
8. van Pelt-Verkuil E, van Belkum A, Hays JP (2008) Principles and technical aspects of PCR amplification. doi:https://doi.org/10.1007/978-1-4020-6241-4
9. Hayward AL, Oefner PJ, Kainer DB, Hinojos CA, Doris PA (1999) 15- kinetics of competitive reverse transcriptase-PCR. In: Innis MA, Gelfand DH, Sninsky JJ (eds) PCR applications. Academic Press, San Diego, pp 231–261. https://doi.org/10.1016/B978-012372185-3/50016-X
10. Vandenbroucke II, Vandesompele J, Paepe AD, Messiaen L (2001) Quantification of splice variants using real-time PCR. Nucleic Acids Res 29(13):e68–e68. https://doi.org/10.1093/nar/29.13.e68
11. Dorak MT (2006) Real-time PCR. Taylor & Francis, London
12. Dheda K, Huggett JF, Bustin SA, Johnson MA, Rook G, Zumla A (2004) Validation of housekeeping genes for normalizing RNA expression in real-time PCR. Biotechniques 37(1):112–114, 116, 118-119. https://doi.org/10.2144/04371RR03
13. Forootan A, Sjoback R, Bjorkman J, Sjogreen B, Linz L, Kubista M (2017) Methods to determine limit of detection and limit of quantification in quantitative real-time PCR (qPCR). Biomol Detect Quantif 12:1–6. https://doi.org/10.1016/j.bdq.2017.04.001
14. Kolacsek O, Pergel E, Varga N, Apati A, Orban TI (2017) Ct shift: a novel and accurate real-time PCR quantification model for direct comparison of different nucleic acid sequences and its application for transposon quantifications. Gene 598:43–49. https://doi.org/10.1016/j.gene.2016.10.035
15. Schmittgen TD, Livak KJ (2008) Analyzing real-time PCR data by the comparative CT method. Nat Protoc 3(6):1101–1108. https://doi.org/10.1038/nprot.2008.73
16. Thornton B, Basu C (2011) Real-time PCR (qPCR) primer design using free online software. Biochem Mol Biol Educ 39(2):145–154. https://doi.org/10.1002/bmb.20461
17. Sun B, Tao L, Zheng YL (2014) Simultaneous quantification of alternatively spliced transcripts in a single droplet digital PCR reaction. BioTechniques 56(6):319–325. https://doi.org/10.2144/000114179
18. Verheul RC, van Deutekom JC, Datson NA (2016) Digital droplet PCR for the absolute quantification of exon skipping induced by antisense oligonucleotides in (pre-)clinical development for Duchenne muscular dystrophy. PLoS One 11(9):e0162467. https://doi.org/10.1371/journal.pone.0162467
19. Van Heetvelde M, Van Loocke W, Trypsteen W, Baert A, Vanderheyden K, Crombez B, Vandesompele J, De Leeneer K, Claes KBM (2017) Evaluation of relative quantification of alternatively spliced transcripts using droplet digital PCR. Biomol Detect Quantif 13:40–48. https://doi.org/10.1016/j.bdq.2017.09.001
20. Sun B, Zheng YL (2018) Simultaneous quantification of multiple alternatively spliced mRNA transcripts using droplet digital PCR. Methods Mol Biol 1768:387–400. https://doi.org/10.1007/978-1-4939-7778-9_22

21. Farrell RE (2010) Chapter 2 - RNA isolation strategies. In: Farrell RE (ed) RNA methodologies, 4th edn. Academic Press, San Diego, pp 45–80. https://doi.org/10.1016/B978-0-12-374727-3.00002-4
22. Untergasser A, Cutcutache I, Koressaar T, Ye J, Faircloth BC, Remm M, Rozen SG (2012) Primer3 – New capabilities and interfaces. Nucleic Acids Res 40(15):e115. https://doi.org/10.1093/nar/gks596
23. Lorenz TC (2012) Polymerase chain reaction: basic protocol plus troubleshooting and optimization strategies. J Vis Exp 63: e3998–e3998. https://doi.org/10.3791/3998
24. Chomczynski P, Sacchi N (1987) Single-step method of RNA isolation by acid guanidinium thiocyanate-phenol-chloroform extraction. Anal Biochem 162(1):156–159. https://doi.org/10.1006/abio.1987.9999
25. Shagin DA, Lukyanov KA, Vagner LL, Matz MV (1999) Regulation of average length of complex PCR product. Nucleic Acids Res 27 (18):e23
26. Sang J, Wang Z, Li M, Cao J, Niu G, Xia L, Zou D, Wang F, Xu X, Han X, Fan J, Yang Y, Zuo W, Zhang Y, Zhao W, Bao Y, Xiao J, Hu S, Hao L, Zhang Z (2018) ICG: a wiki-driven knowledgebase of internal control genes for RT-qPCR normalization. Nucleic Acids Res 46(D1):D121–D126. https://doi.org/10.1093/nar/gkx875

Chapter 5

Assessing Oligonucleotide Binding to Double-Stranded DNA

Negin Mozafari and Tea Umek

Abstract

Sequence-specific targeting of double-stranded DNA (dsDNA) using synthetic oligonucleotides (ONs) has been under investigation in different therapeutic approaches. Several methods can be used to evaluate ONs effect and binding capacity to their target sequence. Here we describe some of the methods, which have been frequently used for assessing ONs binding to dsDNA.

Key words Antigene oligonucleotides, EMSA, S1 nuclease assay, Restriction inhibition assay, BQQ-OP cleavage, CAA chemical probing

1 Introduction

Therapeutic oligonucleotides (ONs) are short nucleic acid polymers comprising nucleotide analogs [1]. They are typically between 8 and 50 nucleotides (nt) long and intended to regulate gene expression via different mechanisms. ONs bind in a sequence-specific manner to RNA and DNA. Depending on the ONs chemical modifications and nucleic acid target, different methods can be used to evaluate the ONs binding capacity. Most ON therapies are directed toward different RNA species including precursor messenger RNA (pre-mRNA) and mRNA. The principle of most RNA therapeutics so far is that they bind as complementary ONs to particular RNAs target through Watson–Crick base pair hybridization [2, 3]. The group of ONs directed against RNA are called antisense ONs (ASOs). Several modes of action have been proposed to modify gene expression at the RNA level: microRNAs, RNA interference (RNAi) [4], ASOs for splice switching, gapmers [1, 5], and steric blocking ONs [6].

On the other hand, ONs have also been developed to regulate gene expression at the transcriptional level. In this strategy ONs are evaluated as potential therapeutic reagents to modulate gene expression at the DNA level (antigene ONs), which is based as well on sequence-specific targeting using chemically modified

Olof Gissberg et al. (eds.), *Oligonucleotide-Based Therapies: Methods and Protocols*, Methods in Molecular Biology, vol. 2036, https://doi.org/10.1007/978-1-4939-9670-4_5, © Springer Science+Business Media, LLC, part of Springer Nature 2019

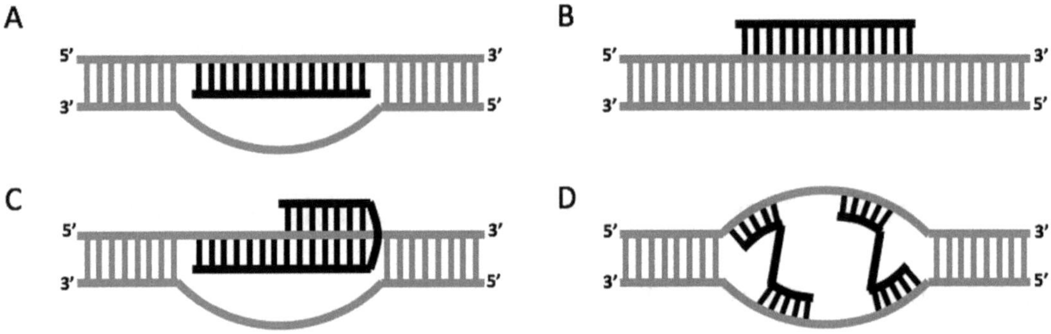

Fig. 1 Schematic illustration of antigene ON and principles of binding to dsDNA. (**a**) invasion of a single stranded ON. (**b**) binding of a triplex forming ON (TFO). (**c**) invasion of an ON with combined mode of binding as TFO and strand invasion. (**d**) zorro-LNA invasion. The DNA is in grey and the ONs are in black. Thicker horizontal lines represent the backbone and thinner vertical lines represent either Watson–Crick or Hoogsteen base pairing

ONs. The proposed mechanisms for targeting DNA with ONs include: (a) blocking of DNA-protein interactions via binding of triplex forming oligonucleotides (TFOs) [7] and formation of triplex structures through Hoogsteen or reverse Hoogsteen hydrogen bonds [8], (b) invasion of the DNA duplex to either facilitate or block gene expression [2], or (c) destabilizing disease-related non B-DNA structures [9, 10] (Fig. 1). Here we present these concepts briefly and provide protocols for some of the applications, which have been generally used to characterize ON–dsDNA complexes. Different enzymes have been used for assessing ONs binding in dsDNA, including DNaseI, S1 nuclease and restriction endonucleases. Moreover, chemical probing using DNA modifying chemical reagents have also been extensively examined.

Restriction endonucleases (restriction enzymes) have been used widely in a variety of molecular biology techniques. This group of enzymes originates from bacteria as a tool for protection against viral attacks. Restriction enzymes cleave DNA at a specific sequence, termed recognition site, and restriction endonucleases are classified into four groups. The most frequently used and studied class of restriction enzymes is the type IIs, which cleave DNA within or proximal to their recognition sites while other enzymes cleave at distant positions [8, 11, 12]. It has been shown that different ON constructs, such as TFOs and ONs with combined TFO binding and strand-invading mechanism, can inhibit DNA cleavage by restriction endonucleases [13, 14]. The ability of ONs to sterically block enzymatic digestion has been used as a method to evaluate binding of ONs to their dsDNA target sequences. The restriction site should be located within or proximal to the ONs target sequence. By hybridizing the ON to the dsDNA, the cleavage of DNA by a restriction enzyme is then blocked. This will lead

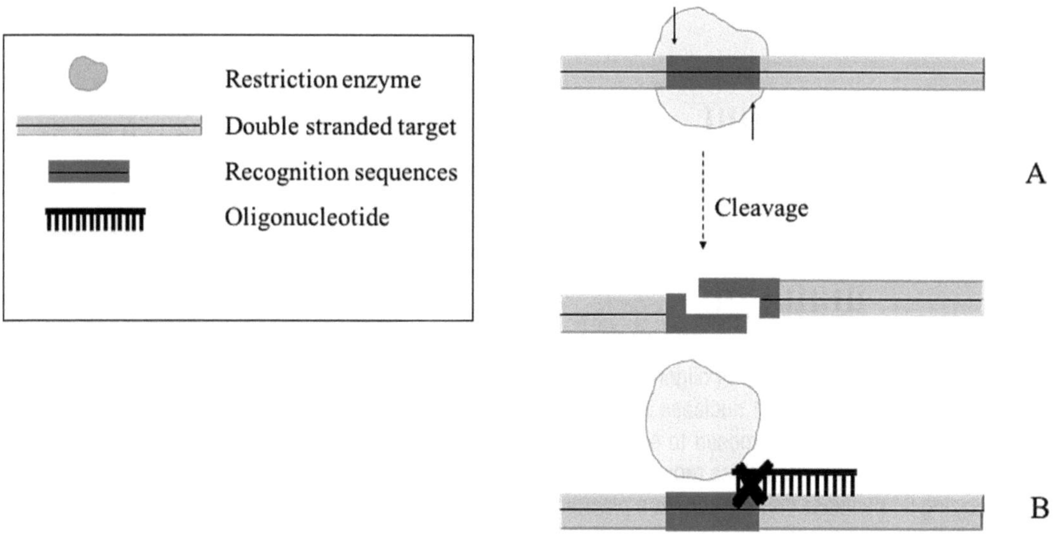

Fig. 2 Schematic illustration of the mechanism by which ONs block restriction enzyme cleavage. (**a**) the cleavage pattern in the absence of ONs (**b**) steric blocking of the restriction enzyme site in the presence of an ON

to a protection of the dsDNA target and thereby preventing cleavage at this location (Fig. 2).

S1 nuclease is an endonuclease, which recognizes and cleaves single-stranded DNA with high specificity [15, 16]. Invasion of a duplex DNA with an ON results in the formation of single-stranded regions at and around the binding site of the ON construct. The ability of S1 nuclease to recognize single-stranded regions can therefore be used as a method to evaluate the ONs binding and invading capacity. In this assay, the ON–dsDNA complex is digested with S1 nuclease creating linear and nicked plasmids at the site of invasion. As plasmid DNA exists mainly in three topologies: supercoiled, nicked (open circular) and linear [17], the ON strand- invading capacity can be quantified by comparing the ratio of linear/nicked plasmid to the remaining un-cleaved plasmid (Fig. 3).

Electrophoresis Mobility Shift Assay (EMSA) can also be used as a method for analyzing ON–dsDNA interactions [15, 18, 19]. It is based on the fact that the electrophoretic mobility of bound ON–dsDNA in a native polyacrylamide gel is retarded in comparison to the free DNA target. The change in mobility is due to conformational changes of the ON–dsDNA complex, as compared to the free dsDNA, and is not a result of a change in molecular mass, unless very small DNA fragments are analyzed. EMSA is a method, which detects both bound and unbound dsDNA at the same time, and it can be used for determining the relative binding affinity of different ON constructs under specific conditions. While the EMSA has many advantages, there are some limitations in this

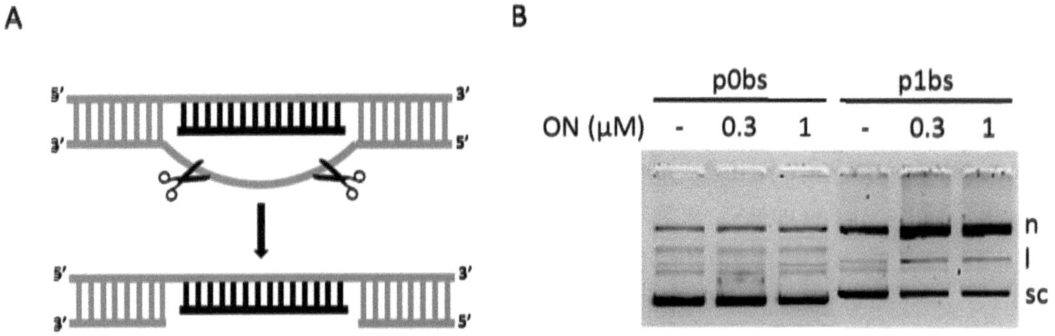

Fig. 3 Analyzing strand invasion of oligonucleotides (ONs) in a plasmid containing the correct target site. (**a**) A schematic illustration of the S1 nuclease assay. Upon strand invasion by an ON the DNA strand opposite to the target site is displaced and exposed to enzyme digestion (enzyme represented with scissors), resulting in a nicked plasmid. Short vertical lines represent Watson–Crick base pairing. (**b**) An example of gel electrophoresis analyzing S1 nuclease cleavage. *p1bs* a plasmid containing 1 target site for the ON, *p0bs* a plasmid lacking the binding site, used as a negative control, *N* nicked plasmid, *l* linearized plasmid, *sc* supercoiled plasmid

method. For instance, detailed information of the ON–dsDNA complex and the binding mode of the ONs needs to be evaluated by additional methods such as chemical probing and footprinting.

TFOs bind to dsDNA and form intermolecular triple helix (triplex) structures. TFO binding occurs in the major groove of the DNA duplex via Hoogsteen or reverse Hoogsteen hydrogen bonds between the bases, which requires stretches of polypurine: polypyrimidine regions [8, 20]. TFOs are commonly between 12 and 30 nts long [21, 22]. Formation of inter- and intramolecular triplex structures can be probed by triplex-specific DNA cleaving agents such as benzoquinoquinoxaline-1,10-phenanthroline (BQQ-OP) conjugates [23]. BQQ is a low molecular weight triplex specific intercalating agent [24, 25]. BQQ has been conjugated to 1,10-phenanthroline resulting in a dsDNA cleaving agent, which binds and acts specifically at the site of triplex formation [23]. The ability of BQQ-OP to probe for triplex formation has been shown for both intermolecular and intramolecular triple helix structures. BQQ-OP triplex-specific cleavage is performed in the presence Cu^{2+}, which chelates to the phenanthroline moiety, and 3-mercaptopropionic acid (MPA) as a reducing agent [23] (Fig. 4).

In chemical probing, analysis of ON–dsDNA complexes can be achieved with a resolution of a single nucleotide using denaturing polyacrylamide gel electrophoresis (PAGE), which enables the assessment of the precise binding location. Examples of commonly used chemical probing reagents are potassium permanganate (KMnO4) [26], dimethyl sulfate (DMS), and chloroacetaldehyde (CAA) [27]. CAA reacts with the exocyclic amino group in adenine and cytosine in single-stranded DNA and CAA modified ONs are not recognized by DNA polymerase [28]. Therefore, primer extension reactions using the CAA modified DNA strand as template can

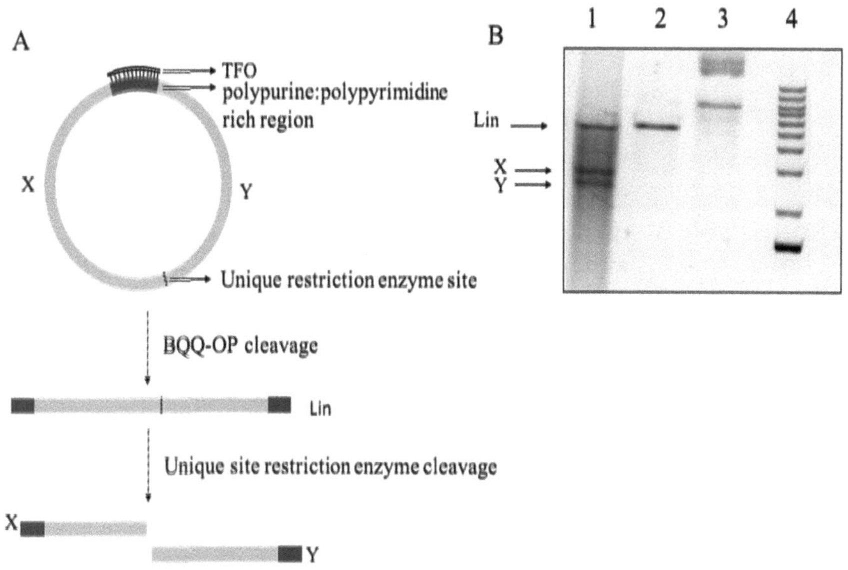

Fig. 4 Analyzing TFO binding to a polypurine:polypyrimidine region in a target plasmid using BQQ-OP cleavage of dsDNA. (**a**) schematic presentation of plasmid binding to a triplex forming oligonucleotide (TFO) and the fragments generated after BQQ-OP cleavage followed by restriction enzyme digestion at a unique site. (**b**) A typical gel for analyzing BQQ-OP cleavage: *Lane 1* triplex specific cleavage performed in presence of Cu^{2+} and MPA combined with restriction enzyme digestion. *Lane 2* Restriction enzyme digested (linearized) plasmid (Lin). *Lane 3* Supercoiled plasmid (SC) *Lane 4* 1 KB plus DNA ladder

be used to identify single-stranded sites. To this end, ^{32}P- or fluorescently labeled primers are used and DNA fragments can then visualized using PAGE and autoradiography [27] or capillary electrophoresis, respectively [29].

2 Materials

Prepare all solutions using ultrapure water. All reactions should be performed in low retention tubes as we have observed that ONs stick to the normal polypropylene tubes.

2.1 ON-Plasmid Hybridization

1. Maximum recovery or low binding 0.6 mL plastic tubes (*see* **Note 1**).
2. 10× Intranuclear buffer: 500 mM Tris–acetate (pH 7.4), 1.2 M KCl, 50 mM NaCl, 10 mM $Mg(OAc)_2$. Dissolve 12.1 g of Tris in 100 mL of water in a 250 mL glass bottle. Transfer 50 mL to another 250 mL glass bottle for further preparation and adjust the pH between 7.3 and 7.4 with a pH meter using acetic acid. Weigh 8.96 g of KCl and 0.29 g of NaCl and add them to the glass bottle. Make up to 100 mL

with deionized water. Sterile filter the buffer with 0.2 μM pore size. Store at room temperature.

3. Oligonucleotides at tenfold the preferred concentration (typically 10–100 μM), dissolve in nuclease-free water, aliquot and store at −20 °C (*see* **Notes 2** and **3**).
4. Plasmid DNA: 500 ng/μL purified high quality plasmid DNA (minimum 80% supercoiled fraction), diluted in nuclease-free water (*see* **Note 4**). Store at −20 °C (*see* **Note 5**).
5. Nuclease-free water.
6. Oven incubator.

2.2 EMSA and Restriction Enzyme Inhibition

1. ON-plasmid hybridization reaction: 100 ng plasmid/μL.
2. Oven incubator.
3. Restriction enzyme.
4. Restriction enzyme buffer (*see* **Note 6**).
5. Nuclease-free water.
6. Polyacrylamide and agarose gels and electrophoresis equipment (*see* Subheadings 2.5 and 2.6).
7. Ice.

2.3 S1 Nuclease Assay

1. Plasmid-ON hybridization reaction: 100 ng plasmid/μL.
2. 10× S1 Nuclease reaction buffer: 500 mM sodium acetate (pH 4.5), 2.8 M NaCl, 45 mM $ZnSO_4$. Supplied with the enzyme.
3. S1 nuclease.
4. 0.5 M Ethylenediaminetetraacetic acid (EDTA): 0.5 M EDTA pH 8.0. Prepare a 1000 mL glass bottle and add 900 mL of water. Add 186.12 g of EDTA and mix vigorously on a magnetic stirrer. Adjust the pH to 8.0 using NaOH pellets (approximately 20 g). Add water up to 1000 mL. Sterilize the solution by passing it through a 0.22 μm filter unit. Store at room temperature.
5. Nuclease-free water.
6. Timer.
7. Bucket of wet ice.
8. 0.9% agarose gel in 0.5× TBE buffer *see* Subheading 2.5.

2.4 BQQ-OP Triplex-Specific DNA Cleavage of DNA-ON Complexes

1. Plasmid-ON hybridization complex: 100 ng plasmid/μL.
2. 10× BQQ-OP reaction buffer: 100 mM sodium cacodylate, 1 M NaCl, 20 mM $MgCl_2$
3. Siliconized tubes.

4. BQQ-OP solution: 30 μM BQQ-OP in nuclease-free water. Prepare a fresh working solution for each experiment. Incubate the available stock solution in a dry heat incubator at 37 °C for 10–15 min. At the same time add the required volume of nuclease-free water to the siliconized tube and incubate for equal amount of time. When ready, pipet the required volume of BQQ-OP to the siliconized tube with nuclease-free water and incubate again for 15 min (*see* **Note 7**).
5. Copper(II) sulfate pentahydrate ($CuSO_4.5H_2O$) solution (*see* **Note 8**): 45 μM $CuSO_4$ in water. Prepare a fresh working solution for each experiment. First prepare a 0.1 M solution. Weigh 0.0249 g of $CuSO_4.5H_2O$, transfer it to a 1.5 mL microcentrifuge tube and dissolve it in 1 mL nuclease-free water by vortexing. Perform a serial dilution to achieve 45 μM final concentration.
6. 3-mercaptopropionic acid (MPA) solution: 20 mM. Prepare a fresh 20 mM working solution for each experiment. Remove ≥99% MPA from the fridge approximately 1 h before needed, to allow it to melt. Mix 1.74 μL of MPA and 998.26 μL of nuclease-free water in a 1.5 mL microcentrifuge tube (*see* **Note 9**)
7. PCR purification kit.
8. Restriction enzyme (*see* **Note 10**).
9. Nuclease-free water.
10. Oven incubator.
11. 0.7% agarose gel in 0.5× TBE buffer (*see* Subheading 2.5).

2.5 Agarose Gel Electrophoresis

1. EDTA: 0.5 M. For preparation *see* Subheading 2.3.
2. 50× Tris–acetic acid–EDTA (TAE) buffer: 2 M Tris, 1 M acetic acid, 50 mM EDTA, pH 8.0. Take 1000 mL glass bottle and add 800 mL of water. Add 242 g Tris base, 57.1 mL glacial acetic acid, and 100 mL 0.5 M EDTA, adjust the pH to 8.5 and fill to the final volume of 1 L. Store at room temperature.
3. 1× TAE buffer: Prepare by diluting 20 mL 50× TAE stock solution with 980 mL water.
4. 10× Tris–boric acid–EDTA (TBE) buffer: 1 M Tris, 0.9 M boric acid, 0.01 M EDTA. Take 1000 mL glass bottle and add 800 mL of water. Add 7.5 g of EDTA, 108 g of Tris base and 55 g of boric acid. Mix on a magnetic stirrer to dissolve the reagents. Adjust the pH to 8.2–8.4 using diluted HCl. Add water up to 1000 mL. Store at room temperature (*see* **Note 11**)
5. 0.5× TBE: Dilute 50 mL of 10× stock solution with water to 1 L.
6. Agarose in powder.

7. TE buffer: 10 mM Tris–HCl, pH 8.0, 1 mM EDTA.
8. Gel casting unit.
9. Horizontal gel electrophoresis unit.
10. 6× loading buffer: 30% (v/v) glycerol, 0.25% (w/v) xylene cyanol, nuclease-free water. Store at room temperature
11. DNA ladder ranging from 100 to 15,000 bp (0.5 μg/μL).
12. SYBR Gold Nucleic Acid Gel Stain (10,000× concentrated in DMSO).
13. Electrophoresis power supply.
14. Gel documentation equipment with quantification software.

2.6 Native Polyacrylamide Gel Electrophoresis

1. 40% acrylamide–bis-acrylamide(29:1): 29 mL 40% (w/v) acrylamide, 1 mL 2% (w/v) *N,N′*-methylbisacrylamide in water (*see* **Note 12**). Measure pH (should be 7.0 or less). Store the solution in dark at room temperature.
2. 10× Tris–borate–EDTA (TBE) buffer: *see* Subheading 2.5, **item 4**
3. 10% Ammonium persulfate (APS) solution (*see* **Note 13**)
4. *N,N,N′,N′*-tetramethylethylenediamine (TEMED) (*see* **Note 14**).
5. Mini gel casting unit with 1.0 mm spacers.
6. Vertical gel electrophoresis unit.
7. 6× loading buffer, *see* Subheading 2.5.
8. DNA ladder, *see* Subheading 2.5.
9. Intercalating dye, *see* Subheading 2.5.
10. Electrophoresis power supply.
11. Gel documentation equipment with quantification software.

2.7 Chemical Probing with Chloroacetaldehyde

2.7.1 Chloro-acetaldehyde (CAA) Reaction

1. Plasmid-ON hybridization complex: 100 ng plasmid/μL (*see* **Note 15**).
2. CAA solution: 8% CAA diluted in nuclease-free water. Prepare a fresh working solution for each experiment (*see* **Note 16**).
3. Plasmid DNA miniprep kit.
4. Oven incubator.

2.7.2 Enzymatic Restriction Digestion (Optional. Note 17)

1. CAA modified plasmid: 25 ng/μL.
2. Restriction enzyme with a unique site in the plasmid.
3. 10× Restriction enzyme buffer: supplied with the enzyme.
4. Dry block incubator.

2.7.3 Hydroxide Treatment and Neutralization (Optional. ***Note 18****)*

1. CAA modified plasmid: 25 ng/μL.
2. NaOH solution: 26 mM NaOH in nuclease-free water, diluted from a 0.1 M stock solution. For preparation (*see* **Note 19**).
3. 100 mM Tris–HCl buffer pH 7: For preparation (*see* **Note 20**).
4. Dry block incubator.

2.7.4 Primer Extension Reaction

Depending on the selected primer labeling, either capillary electrophoresis or PAGE and autoradiography should be used for analysis.

1. CAA-modified plasmids: 25 ng/μL (100 ng per reaction).
2. Filter tips.
3. Labeled forward or reverse primer: 100 nM (*see* **Notes 21–23**).
4. Taq polymerase: 10 U/μL (*see* **Note 24**).
5. Buffer supplied with the Taq polymerase.
6. 25 mM $MgCl_2$ (*see* **Note 25**)
7. Deoxynucleotide (dNTP) solution: 10 mM each of dATP, dTTP, dGTP, and dCTP (*see* **Note 26**).
8. Thermocycler.

2.7.5 Sequencing Ladder Preparation

1. Template for sequencing ladder: 100 ng of the target plasmid.
2. Restriction enzyme cutting upstream of the ON target site.
3. Restriction enzyme cutting downstream of the ON target site (*see* **Note 27**).
4. Restriction enzyme buffer (10×): supplied with the restriction enzymes.
5. Dideoxynucleotide solution (ddNTPs): 40.5 mM ddATP, 20.5 mM ddCTP, 10 mM ddGTP, and 24 mM ddTTP.
6. dNTP solution, *see* Subheading **2.7.4**, **item 6**,
7. Labeled forward or reverse primer: 100 nM (*see* **Notes 21** and **22**).
8. Taq polymerase: 10 U/μL (*see* **Note 24**).
9. Buffer supplied with the Taq polymerase.
10. Thermocycler.

3 Methods

Carry out all procedures at room temperature unless otherwise specified.

3.1 Plasmid ON-Hybridization

1. Mix 1 μL of 10× intranuclear buffer with 7 μL nuclease-free water in a 0.6 mL low retention tube.
2. Add 2 μL (1000 ng) of plasmid.

3. Add 1 μL of 10× ON. The final volume should be the same in all reactions (*see* **Notes 28–30**).
4. Mix and spin down (*see* **Note 31**).
5. Put the reactions at 37 °C and incubate during the desired time (normally 16–72 h) in the oven incubator (*see* **Note 32**).
6. Stop the hybridization by freezing the sample or immediately proceed to analysis.

3.2 EMSA and Restriction Inhibition

1. Mix 500 ng of prehybridized plasmid-ON, with 2 μL of 10× restriction buffer, and the amount of nuclease-free water required for a final volume of 20 μL, while still allowing for the volume of the restriction enzyme.
2. Add 10 U of restriction enzyme, to reach the total volume of 20 μL (*see* **Note 33**).
3. Incubate at 37 °C in the oven incubator for the defined incubation time.
4. Stop the reaction by freezing on ice. The samples can be kept at −20 °C.
5. Analyze an aliquot (250 ng) by native gel electrophoresis. Depending on the size of the fragment containing the ON target site, agarose gel electrophoresis, *see* Subheading 3.5, or polyacrylamide gel electrophoresis, *see* Subheading 3.6, can be used.
6. Determine the ON/dsDNA interaction (*see* **Notes 34–36**).

3.3 S1 Nuclease Assay

Perform this assay on wet ice. Keep all the reagents and the enzyme constantly on wet ice. When performing the assay with more than one sample *see* additional instructions in (*see* **Note 37**).

1. Dilute the 10× S1 Nuclease reaction buffer to 1× with nuclease-free water in a 0.6 mL tube.
2. Dilute S1 nuclease with 1× S1 reaction buffer to a concentration of 24 U/μL in another 0.6 mL tub, stored on ice (*see* **Note 38**).
3. Mix 1 μL of diluted S1 nuclease, 6.5 μL of nuclease-free water and 1 μL of 10× S1 nuclease buffer in a new 0.6 mL tube.
4. Add 2.5 μL of plasmid-ON hybridization solution and mix by pipetting (do not remove the tubes from ice).
5. Start timing immediately.
6. After exactly 6 min stop the reaction by adding 3 μL of 0.5 M EDTA. Mix by pipetting.
7. Vortex and spin down, and put the tube back on ice for 10 min to allow full inactivation of the enzyme.

8. Mix 1 μL of 6× loading buffer, 3.5 μL of TE buffer and 1.5 μL of reaction sample.
9. Run the samples on 0.9% agarose, in 0.5× TBE buffer, gel electrophoresis (*see* Subheading 3.6).
10. Visualize the separated DNA fragments in a gel documentation system with a quantification tool. Avoid saturation of the signal in any of the bands.
11. To determine the percentage of the ON invasion, calculate the ratio of nicked plasmid to the total plasmid amount in the sample and normalize it to the same ratio in the mock hybridized plasmid (plasmid incubation without added ON) (*see* **Note 39**).

3.4 BQQ-OP Triplex-Specific dsDNA Cleavage of DNA-ON Complexes

1. Add 2 μL of 10× BQQ-OP reaction buffer to 10 μL plasmid-ON complex (*see* **Notes 40** and **41**).
2. Prepare the BQQ-OP and $CuSO_4$ solutions.
3. Remove the MPA bottle from the fridge.
4. Mix 1 μL of 30 μM BQQ-OP solution with 1 μL of 45 μM $CuSO_4$ solution per reaction in a 0.6 mL siliconized microcentrifuge tube (*see* **Note 42**).
5. Mix by pipetting.
6. Incubate at room temperature for 15 min.
7. Add 2 μL of BQQ-OP/$CuSO_4$ mixture to the 0.6 mL siliconized microcentrifuge tube with plasmid-ON and buffer.
8. Mix by pipetting and spin down gently.
9. Incubate at room temperature for 45 min.
10. 10 min before completed time prepare the 20 mM MPA solution.
11. Add 2 μL of the 20 mM MPA solution to the mixture (prepared in **steps 1–9**).
12. Mix by pipetting and spin down (*see* **Note 43**).
13. Put the tube in a dry heat incubator and incubate at 37 °C during 3 h.
14. Purify the DNA using the PCR purification kit according to the manufacturer's protocol. Elute the DNA with 20 μL elution buffer (*see* **Note 44**).
15. Take 17 μL of the eluted sample (*see* **Note 45**) and digest using a restriction digestion enzyme that only cleaves at a unique site in the plasmid (*see* Subheading 3.2).
16. Mix 2 μL of 6× loading buffer, 4 μL of nuclease-free water and 6 μL of reaction sample (approximately 300 ng plasmid DNA).

17. Analyze the samples on 0.7% agarose in 0.5× TBE buffer (*see* Subheading 3.5).
18. ON binding, forming a triplex, will be indicated by a specific fragment pattern. The combined BQQ-OP and enzymatic restriction will result in two fragments, whose length depended on the plasmid size, the position of the ON target site and the enzyme restriction site (*see* Fig. 4).

3.5 Agarose Gel Electrophoresis

1. Weigh the appropriate amount of agarose in a 250-mL glass bottle and add 0.5× TBE buffer or 1× TAE buffer to give the desired percentage of the gel for the analysis (*see* **Note 46**).
2. Place the flask in a microwave oven and heat for 1–2 min with 20–60 s intervals. Swirl the flask gently at each interval in order to dissolve the agarose completely. Continue heating the agarose solution until the agarose is completely dissolved (*see* **Note 47**).
3. Cool the solution to 65 °C, for running unstained gels continue to **step 5**.
4. Add the SYBR Gold nucleic acid gel stain to 1× concentration (*see* **Note 48**).
5. Pour the appropriate volume of agarose solution into a gel tray, without creating bubbles. Place the well-forming comb and leave the gel at room temperature to polymerize.
6. Place the gel in horizontal electrophoresis equipment. Fill the electrophoresis device with 0.5× TBE running buffer until all the wells are covered with the buffer or until the maximum mark on the gel electrophoresis unit, and remove the comb.
7. Carefully pipet the samples, controls, and the corresponding DNA ladder into the wells (*see* **Note 49**).
8. Put the lid on the gel apparatus and connect the wires to the power supply. Run the gel at a constant voltage of maximum 10 V/cm (*see* **Note 50**). Check that the gel is running by controlling the current in the power supply.
9. Put the gel in the stain solution (*see* **Note 51**) or continue directly to analysis for gels already containing the DNA stain.
10. Capture an image of the gel in gel documentation equipment with 300 nm ultraviolet transilluminator (*see* **Note 52**).

3.6 Polyacrylamide Gel Electrophoresis

If using ready-made gels go directly to **step 8**.

1. All components should be cleaned with a suitable laboratory detergent and washed thoroughly with distilled water, and dried before use.
2. Assemble the gel glass plates with spacers and place it in the molding device.

3. Prepare 10% gel by mixing 5.2 mL water, 2 mL of 40% acrylamide/bis-acrylamide mixture 29:1 and 0.8 mL 10× TBE buffer.
4. Add 8 μL TEMED to the solution and mix gently in order to avoid air bubbles in the gel solution.
5. Add 80 μL 10% APS, mix and immediately pour the gel.
6. Insert the well forming comb immediately without forming air bubbles.
7. Let the gel polymerize for 15–30 min.
8. For ready-made gels, remove the gel from the plastic bag and remove the tape at the bottom of the gel.
9. Place the plates with the gel in the vertical electrophoresis apparatus and fill the chamber with 1× TBE buffer.
10. Remove the comb and rinse the wells by flushing with buffer using a pipette (*see* **Note 53**).
11. Pipet 5 volumes of the digested plasmid samples (250–500 ng) into a clean tube and add 1 volume of 6× loading buffer. Mix and spin down.
12. Carefully pipette the samples and DNA ladder in corresponding wells.
13. Run the gel at 125–150 V for 2–4 h (*see* **Notes 54** and **55**).
14. When the electrophoresis is completed open the glass plates, remove the power supply.
15. Put the gel in a suitable container and stain with 1× SYBR Gold nucleic acid gel stain in 1× TBE buffer (*see* **Note 51**).
16. Capture an image of the gel in a gel documentation equipment with 300 nm ultraviolet transilluminator (*see* **Note 52**).

3.7 Chemical Probing with Chloroacetaldehyde

3.7.1 CAA Modification of Supercoiled Plasmids (see Note 16)

1. Take 10 μL of plasmid-ON hybridization reaction.
2. Add 5 μL nuclease-free water and 5 μL of 8% CAA to give 2% final concentration in a final volume of 20 μL.
3. Briefly vortex and spin down.
4. Incubate the tube at 37 °C in an oven incubator during 30 min.
5. Purify the DNA using a plasmid DNA miniprep kit and use 20 μL for the elution.
6. Move on to Subheading 3.7.2 or directly to Subheading 3.7.4.

3.7.2 Restriction Enzyme Digestion (Optional. Note 17)

1. Take 15 μL of the isolated sample and transfer to a new tube.
2. Add 2.5 μL of the 10× restriction enzyme buffer and 5.5 μL of nuclease-free water.
3. Add 2 μL of the enzyme to cut approximately 1 μg of plasmid DNA in a final volume of 25 μL.

4. Briefly vortex and spin down.
5. Incubate for 1 h at 37 °C until DNA digestion is completed by the selected enzyme.
6. Move on to Subheading 3.7.3 or directly to Subheading 3.7.4.

3.7.3 Alkaline Treatment and Neutralization (Optional. Note 18)

1. Add 1 μL of 26 mM NaOH to the 25 μL of CAA treated plasmid.
2. Briefly vortex and spin down.
3. Incubate in a heat block during 30 min at 90 °C.
4. Cool to room temperature.
5. Add 4 μL of Tris–HCl buffer. The final volume should then be 30 μL. Proceed to Subheading 3.7.4.

3.7.4 Primer Extension Reaction

1. Prepare a master mix for all samples to be analyzed. For each sample add 11.7 μL nuclease-free water, 2.5 μL of Taq polymerase buffer, 5 μL of dNTPs, 1.25 μL labeled primer, and 0.6 μL of Taq polymerase (*see* **Notes 21**, **22**, and **56**).
2. Briefly vortex and spin down.
3. Aliquot 21 μL of the master mix in each PCR tube.
4. Add 4 μL of CAA-modified plasmid from Subheading 3.7.2 (or from Subheading 3.7.3). The final volume of the reaction is, thereby, 25 μL (*see* **Note 57**).
5. Briefly vortex and spin down.
6. Set the steps on a thermocycler according to the standard protocol for the Taq polymerase (*see* **Note 58**).
7. Analyze the samples on a 6% Urea PAGE electrophoresis sequencing gel if radiolabeled primers were used, or with capillary electrophoresis for fluorescently labeled primers.

3.7.5 Sequencing Ladder

1. To create a template for the sequencing ladder, digest the free target plasmid with restriction enzymes as in Subheading 3.7.2. The final concentration of the plasmid in the reaction should be 20 ng/μL.
2. Transfer 5 μL (100 ng) to a new tube.
3. Add 2.5 μL of Taq polymerase buffer, 5 μL of dNTPs, 1.25 μL labeled primer mix and 0.6 μL of Taq polymerase (*see* **Notes 21** and **22**).
4. Add 2.5 μL of the ddNTP mix.
5. Add 8.2 μL of nuclease-free water.
6. Vortex briefly and spin down.

7. Set the protocol steps on a thermocycler as for the primer extension reaction (*see* Subheading 3.5, **step 4**) (*see* **Notes 58** and **59**).
8. Analyze the samples on a 6% Urea PAGE electrophoresis sequencing gel if radiolabeled primers were used, or with capillary electrophoresis for fluorescently labeled primers.

4 Notes

1. ONs used in the experiments can stick to the tubes made of polypropylene. Low binding tubes with maximum recovery minimizes adhesion, which enables more accurate and reproducible results.
2. Heat up stock solution at 65 °C to prevent self-hybridization and make sure that the ON is fully solubilized. To avoid multiple freezing and thawing cycles that could cause degradation of the ON, prepare multiple aliquots at the same time.
3. It is recommended to use labeled ON in EMSA in order to facilitate subsequent analysis.
4. Plasmids can be isolated from bacterial cells with various techniques such as the classical phenol–chloroform extraction and plasmid isolation kits, which are commercially available. Plasmid DNA preparation kits without filters and vacuum suction induce less nicking of the plasmid DNA. Frequent freezing and thawing of the plasmid preparation can induce damage to the plasmid DNA as well. Dissolve the isolated plasmid in nuclease-free buffer or the buffer provided with the kit. To avoid repeated freeze-thawing prepare several small volume aliquots with plasmid at 500 ng/μL concentration.
5. The distance between the target site and the restriction site (s) differs for EMSA and restriction inhibition assays. In the restriction inhibition assay, the restriction site should be within or next to the target site. In EMSA the restriction site should be further away, in order not to be influenced by the bound ON. The sequence of ON/target site should be selected carefully e.g. TFOs bind to the major groove in a polypurine: polypyrimidine sequence.
6. Typically, restriction digestion buffers are supplied as 10× concentrated stocks, meaning that the stock need to be diluted tenfold in order to achieve the optimal salt concentrations for enzyme activity. As restriction enzymes are derived from different bacterial species, they are adjusted to perform in their native environment. Hence, the optimal reaction conditions vary for different enzymes. The enzyme manufacturers normally have different kinds of buffers. It is necessary to check

restriction enzyme buffer compatibility chart from the enzyme supplier to adjust the requirement for each digestion.

7. BQQ-OP is dissolved in DMSO. Store the stock solution at −20 °C.
8. $CuSO_4 \cdot 5H_2O$ is a blue powder with molar mass 249.68 g/mol. It turns white when it is hydrated. Keep in sealed container at room temperature.
9. MPA is corrosive and causes acute toxicity. Work in the fume hood with proper protection.
10. The enzyme should have a single target site to simplify consequent analysis.
11. After a while the stock solution might start to precipitate. To remove the particles, pass the buffer through a 0.22 μm filter unit.
12. It may be necessary to heat the solution in order to dissolve the acrylamide. Acrylamide is carcinogenic, neurotoxic and irritant. Work in the fume hood and wear protective gloves. Store at 4 °C. Due to the safety issues, it is recommended to purchase ready-made acrylamide gels and solutions instead of preparing your own.
13. Avoid repeated freeze–thaw cycles by making aliquots. Store at −20 °C and always use fresh aliquots when preparing acrylamide gels.
14. Store TEMED at 4 °C.
15. Use the concentration of the plasmid DNA to calculate the required volume. When the plasmid contains sequences that potentially form non-B-DNA structures it is recommended to perform the experiment using a linearized plasmid in order to avoid false positive result. Use an enzyme that does not cut within or in the vicinity of the target site.
16. Work in a fume hood with extra care. CAA is corrosive and causes acute toxicity, is hazardous to health and to aquatic environment. Store in cold, well-ventilated and dry place. The chemical can be supplied in concentrations ~50 wt.%.
17. Linearization of the plasmid contributes to a more efficient primer extension reaction and gives a better image quality on the gel.
18. If the polymerase used in the primer extension reaction reads through the modified A and C bases—the so-called ethenonucleotides—use NaOH treatment. The alkaline treatment transforms the etheno modified base into a pyrimidine open-ring structure, which efficiently stops the polymerase.
19. Dissolving NaOH in water involves exothermic reaction. Always add NaOH to water and not the opposite! Work in

fume hood with extreme care. Putting the container on ice cools down the reaction. To prepare the desired solution, weigh 4.0 g of NaOH. Prepare in a 1 L glass beaker and add 800 mL of water. Slowly add NaOH and mix on a magnetic stirrer until it dissolves. Fill the beaker with water to make 1 L. The stock solution can be stored at room temperature. To prepare 26 mM working solution dilute the 0.1 M stock solution in a 0.6 mL tube.

20. Prepare a 1 L glass bottle. Weigh 12.114 g of Tris and add it to the bottle. Pour 800 mL of deionized water and adjust the pH to 7 with diluted HCl. Fill the bottle with deionized water to make 1 L. Store at room temperature.
21. Fluorescently labeled primers are used when the analysis is done with capillary electrophoresis. ^{32}P-radiolabeled primers are used when analysis is done using autoradiography.
22. For ^{32}P-radiolabeled primers, label selected primer with T4 polynucleotide kinase according to the manufacturer's protocol. Purify the primer using a nucleotide removal kit and dilute with nuclease-free water to approximately 100 nM. Store at −20 °C.

    (Working with radioactivity requires specific protection equipment and permission from the local irradiation control organization. Work behind Plexiglas screen, keep solutions in a Plexiglas chamber, and use filter tips for labeled radioactive samples.)
23. The positions of the selected primer should be between 20 and 30 bp away from the target site to achieve satisfactory resolution of the bands on the PAGE gel.
24. We use at least 3 units per reaction but the number of units needed could differ depending on the manufacturer.
25. Mg^{2+} is a cofactor for the polymerase. Increasing its concentration improves enzyme's activity. Adding too much will result in errors in copying. Insufficient amount results in no visible PCR product.
26. Depending on the supplier, the dNTPs are provided separately or already premixed. If supplied separately, mix them according to manufacturer's protocol and then dilute to 10 mM. dNTPs are sensitive to freezing and thawing cycles. After preparing the stock of 10 mM divide it to several smaller aliquots and store at −20 °C.
27. Both enzymes should work in identical buffer conditions.
28. The kinetic of the hybridization might change depending on the volume of the reaction. Keep the volumes constant for all experiments.

29. For restriction inhibition and EMSA, it is of importance to include a control plasmid DNA containing the restriction site but not the ON target sequence to verify the activity of the restriction enzyme.
30. For the BQQ-OP cleavage assay, the hybridization reaction can also be performed in 2× BQQ-OP reaction buffer used in Subheading 3.4.
31. To avoid nicking of the supercoiled plasmid do not vortex, mix by pipetting or by tapping on the tube.
32. The incubation time depends on the rate of ON binding to the DNA target.
33. Do not use more restriction enzyme than 10% of the final volume of the reaction, this is due to the presence of glycerol as an antifreeze reagent in the enzyme's storage buffer. Glycerol can inhibit the digestion reaction.
34. The transition of free dsDNA into bound DNA can be analyzed using fixed incubation time and variable ON concentrations. In this assay, following ON and plasmid hybridization, the restriction enzyme digestion is performed in a way to obtain DNA fragments containing ONs bound to their target sequence.
35. In EMSA, calculate the ratio of bound (shifted) to the total DNA in the sample and normalize it to the same ratio in the mock hybridized plasmid.
36. For the restriction inhibition assay, calculate the ratio of the new undigested fragment to the sum of the fully digested and the new undigested fragment in the sample. The mock hybridized plasmid control should only display fully digested DNA.
37. When performing the assay on more than one sample, start the timing immediately after adding the first sample to the enzyme buffer mix. After 6 min, stop the reaction with EDTA in the same order as adding the samples. Make sure that the time needed for adding the samples is the same as when adding the EDTA.
38. Plasmid prehybridized with ON is digested with 24 units of S1 nuclease. The enzyme is supplied in different concentrations depending on the supplier and the batch. In our experiments, we use S1 nuclease from Promega. When using enzyme from different suppliers the enzyme concentration should be titrated in order to assure that the enzyme does not nick or cut the un-hybridized plasmid.
39. To correctly determine the strand invasion, it is important to include a mock-hybridized control in the experiment. The % of nicked and linear plasmids in this control will show how much damage that has been induced only by the incubation at 37 °C.

Longer incubation time can induce higher spontaneous nicking. A control plasmid without the binding site should also be incubated with the ONs as a control for the specificity of the ON hybridization.

40. If you have prepared the hybridization in 2× BQQ-OP reaction buffer you can skip this step and substitute the 2 μL with water.
41. As controls use the plasmid treated under the same conditions without the addition of BQQ-OP and restriction enzyme (supercoiled control); and the plasmid digested only with restriction enzyme (linearized control) but with no BQQ-OP.
42. If having more than one sample make a master mix. Prepare 10% more to compensate for the pipetting error.
43. We have observed that the PCR purification kit removes the BQQ-OP-Cu^{2+} and MPA better than the plasmid miniprep kit used in previous publications [10, 23]. The samples can be stored after the purification at −20 °C and still give the same results. With the miniprep kit certain amount of the reagents remains in the solution leading to unspecific cleavage or total degradation of the plasmid.
44. If you have less than 17 μL fill up with nuclease-free water.
45. The volume of the flask must be 2.5–4 times of the volume of the gel solution. Select buffer depending on the size of the fragments. TAE gives better resolution for larger fragments, while TBE is better for shorter fragments. The agarose concentration depends on the size of fragments to be electrophoresed. To separate larger fragments (4–12 kb), 0.6–0.8% agarose is used. For medium sized fragments (500 bp–4 kb) 0.8–1% and for shorter fragments (100–500 bp), 1–1.5% agarose can be used.
46. If you prepare the agarose gel solution in advance store it in an oven incubator set at 65 °C. You can store the gel 1–2 weeks or until it turns yellow.
47. For the in-gel stain method, cool the agarose to 65 °C and add the gel stain to achieve the final 1× concentration. Mix carefully and directly pour the solution into the gel tray.
48. In the S1 assay, plasmid control samples in supercoiled, linear and nicked state should be included, each in separate wells. This will allow determination of the corresponding bands in the samples.
49. Voltage and time depend on the gel size and the size of and difference between the fragments to be separated.
50. To stain the gel after electrophoresis, add the nucleic acid gel stain to a fresh running buffer to achieve a 1× final

concentation. After electrophoresis place the gel in a staining container such as a petri dish, and soak the gel in staining solution for 10–20 min (depending on the thickness of the gel).

51. Gels stained with SYBR Gold can also be visualized with blue-light transilluminators and laser scanners with 495 nm maximum visible light excitation.
52. The gel begins to polymerize after adding the APS to the solution. It is important not to move or disturb the gel during polymerization. Leave a small amount of gel in the mixing tube. This can be used to check that the polymerization has occurred properly.
53. It is better to perform a prerun at 5 V for 10 min.
54. The running time depends on different parameters including the percentage and the size of the gel. Run the gel until the dye indicating the smaller-size fragment reaches the bottom of the gel.
55. If needed also include $MgCl_2$. Compensate by removing the corresponding volume of nuclease-free water. Prepare a master mix for all samples and add 10% extra to compensate for loss during pipetting.
56. If you include the steps in Subheadings 3.7.2 and 3.7.3 recalculate the volume needed in order to have approximately 100 ng. Compensate by removing the corresponding volume of nuclease-free water.
57. The annealing temperature depends on the Tm of the primers when they bind to single-stranded DNA. For GC rich sequences a longer denaturing time is necessary. The extension time depends on the size of the amplicon. Usually 1 min/b applies.
58. If using ^{32}P-labeled primers, after finishing, check all laboratory areas and the thermocycler for radioactive contaminations.

Acknowledgments

This work was supported by the European Union's Horizon 2020 under the Marie Skłodowska-Curie grant agreement No 721613, the Swedish Research Council, the Stockholm County Council, Hjärnfonden, and Vinnova/SweLife.

References

1. Smith CIE, Zain R (2019) Therapeutic oligonucleotides: state of the art. Annu Rev Pharmacol Toxicol 59:605–630. https://doi.org/10.1146/annurev-pharmtox-010818-021050
2. Lundin KE, Gissberg O, Smith CI (2015) Oligonucleotide therapies: the past and the present. Hum Gene Ther 26(8):475–485. https://doi.org/10.1089/hum.2015.070. Epub 2015 Aug 1083
3. Crooke ST (2004) Antisense strategies. Curr Mol Med 4(5):465–487
4. Davidson BL, McCray PB Jr (2011) Current prospects for RNA interference-based therapies. Nat Rev Genet 12(5):329–340. https://doi.org/10.1038/nrg2968
5. Goodchild J (2011) Therapeutic oligonucleotides. Methods Mol Biol 764:1–15. https://doi.org/10.1007/1978-1001-61779-61188-61778_61771
6. Kole R, Krainer AR, Altman S (2012) RNA therapeutics: beyond RNA interference and antisense oligonucleotides. Nat Rev Drug Discov 11(2):125–140. https://doi.org/10.1038/nrd3625
7. Moser HE, Dervan PB (1987) Sequence-specific cleavage of double helical DNA by triple helix formation. Science 238 (4827):645–650
8. Pauling L, Corey RB (1953) A proposed structure for the nucleic acids. Proc Natl Acad Sci U S A 39(2):84–97
9. Bacolla A, Wells RD (2009) Non-B DNA conformations as determinants of mutagenesis and human disease. Mol Carcinog 48(4):273–285. https://doi.org/10.1002/mc.20507
10. Bergquist H, Rocha CS, Alvarez-Asencio R, Nguyen CH, Rutland MW, Smith CI, Good L, Nielsen PE, Zain R (2016) Disruption of higher order DNA structures in Friedreich's ataxia (GAA)n repeats by PNA or LNA targeting. PLoS One 11(11):e0165788. https://doi.org/10.1371/journal.pone.0165788
11. Loenen WA, Dryden DT, Raleigh EA, Wilson GG, Murray NE (2014) Highlights of the DNA cutters: a short history of the restriction enzymes. Nucleic Acids Res 42(1):3–19. https://doi.org/10.1093/nar/gkt990
12. Pingoud A, Jeltsch A (2001) Structure and function of type II restriction endonucleases. Nucleic Acids Res 29(18):3705–3727
13. Nielsen PE, Egholm M, Berg RH, Buchardt O (1993) Sequence specific inhibition of DNA restriction enzyme cleavage by PNA. Nucleic Acids Res 21(2):197–200
14. Zaghloul EM, Gissberg O, Moreno PMD, Siggens L, Hallbrink M, Jorgensen AS, Ekwall K, Zain R, Wengel J, Lundin KE, Smith CIE (2017) CTG repeat-targeting oligonucleotides for down-regulating Huntingtin expression. Nucleic Acids Res 45 (9):5153–5169. https://doi.org/10.1093/nar/gkx111
15. Vogt VM (1973) Purification and further properties of single-strand-specific nuclease from Aspergillus oryzae. Eur J Biochem 33 (1):192–200
16. Evans T, Efstratiadis A (1986) Sequence-dependent S1 nuclease hypersensitivity of a heteronomous DNA duplex. J Biol Chem 261 (31):14771–14780
17. Balagurumoorthy P, Adelstein SJ, Kassis AI (2008) Method to eliminate linear DNA from mixture containing nicked circular, supercoiled, and linear plasmid DNA. Anal Biochem 381(1):172–174. https://doi.org/10.1016/j.ab.2008.06.037
18. Pabon-Martinez YV, Xu Y, Villa A, Lundin KE, Geny S, Nguyen CH, Pedersen EB, Jorgensen PT, Wengel J, Nilsson L, Smith CIE, Zain R (2017) LNA effects on DNA binding and conformation: from single strand to duplex and triplex structures. Sci Rep 7(1):11043. https://doi.org/10.1038/s41598-017-09147-8
19. Hartono YD, Pabon-Martinez YV, Uyar A, Wengel J, Lundin KE, Zain R, Smith CIE, Nilsson L, Villa A (2017) Role of pseudoisocytidine tautomerization in triplex-forming oligonucleotides: in silico and in vitro studies. ACS Omega 2(5):2165–2177. https://doi.org/10.1021/acsomega.7b00347
20. Helene C (1991) The anti-gene strategy: control of gene expression by triplex-forming-oligonucleotides. Anticancer Drug Des 6 (6):569–584
21. Knauert MP, Glazer PM (2001) Triplex forming oligonucleotides: sequence-specific tools for gene targeting. Hum Mol Genet 10 (20):2243–2251
22. Duca M, Vekhoff P, Oussedik K, Halby L, Arimondo PB (2008) The triple helix: 50 years later, the outcome. Nucleic Acids Res 36 (16):5123–5138. https://doi.org/10.1093/nar/gkn493
23. Zaid A, Sun JS, Nguyen CH, Bisagni E, Garestier T, Grierson DS, Zain R (2004) Triple-helix directed cleavage of double-stranded DNA by benzoquinoquinoxaline-1,10-phenanthroline conjugates.

Chembiochem 5(11):1550–1557. https://doi.org/10.1002/cbic.200400074

24. Escude C, Nguyen CH, Kukreti S, Janin Y, Sun JS, Bisagni E, Garestier T, Helene C (1998) Rational design of a triple helix-specific intercalating ligand. Proc Natl Acad Sci U S A 95 (7):3591–3596
25. Zain R, Marchand C, Sun J, Nguyen CH, Bisagni E, Garestier T, Helene C (1999) Design of a triple-helix-specific cleaving reagent. Chem Biol 6(11):771–777
26. Bentin T, Larsen HJ, Nielsen PE (2003) Combined triplex/duplex invasion of double-stranded DNA by "tail-clamp" peptide nucleic acid. Biochemistry 42(47):13987–13995. https://doi.org/10.1021/bi0351918
27. Moreno PM, Geny S, Pabon YV, Bergquist H, Zaghloul EM, Rocha CS, Oprea II, Bestas B, Andaloussi SE, Jorgensen PT, Pedersen EB, Lundin KE, Zain R, Wengel J, Smith CI (2013) Development of bis-locked nucleic acid (bisLNA) oligonucleotides for efficient invasion of supercoiled duplex DNA. Nucleic Acids Res 41(5):3257–3273. https://doi.org/10.1093/nar/gkt007
28. Kuśmierek JT, Singer B (1982) Chloroacetaldehyde-treated ribo- and deoxyribopolynucleotides. 1. Reaction products. Biochemistry 21(22):5717. https://doi.org/10.1021/bi00265a050
29. Zianni M, Tessanne K, Merighi M, Laguna R, Tabita FR (2006) Identification of the DNA bases of a DNase I footprint by the use of dye primer sequencing on an automated capillary DNA analysis instrument. J Biomol Tech 17 (2):103

Chapter 6

Modeling and Simulation of Oligonucleotide Hybrids: Outlining a Strategy

Lennart Nilsson and Alessandra Villa

Abstract

Molecular dynamics simulations with a state-of-the-art force field provide an atomistic detailed description of the structural and thermodynamic features of biomolecules. Effects of chemical modifications and of the environment such as sequence, solvent, and ionic strength can explicitly be taken into account. Molecular simulation techniques can also provide insight in change in binding affinity, in protonation (pK_a shift) and tautomeric propensity due to changes in the environment or in the molecular system. The quality and reliability of a simulation depend on the quality of the force field and on the reproducibility of the data, and validation depends on the availability of suitable experimental data. Here, we describe the workflow to investigate oligonucleotide hybrids using molecular simulation including hardware and software information.

Key words Molecular dynamics simulation, Force fields, Structural analysis, Free energy calculation, pK_a shift and tautomerism

1 Introduction

Oligonucleotide hybridization plays an important role in medical applications [1]. To be effective oligonucleotides need to bind a DNA or RNA target sequence with high affinity and specificity under physiological conditions. For instance, they can bind a target using Watson–Crick base pairing, or as a third strand in the major groove of a target duplex, forming a triple helix. To competitively bind an oligonucleotide to a target, the binding affinity needs to be higher than it is for the natural competitor. For example in the case of strand invasion, the newly designed oligonucleotide should bind a DNA strand in Watson–Crick manner with higher affinity than that of the complementary strand.

The design of such oligonucleotides is usually achieved by using nonnatural nucleotides, with a modified backbone, sugar, and/or base. Examples are backbone modifications such as peptide nucleic acid (PNA) [2], which make the backbone uncharged;

Olof Gissberg et al. (eds.), *Oligonucleotide-Based Therapies: Methods and Protocols*, Methods in Molecular Biology, vol. 2036, https://doi.org/10.1007/978-1-4939-9670-4_6,

sugar modifications, such as locked nucleic acid (LNA) [3, 4], which restrict the conformational flexibility of the sugar; base modifications, such as methylation [5], which increase binding affinity or base analogs such as pseudoisocytidine [6], which has a tautomer having hydrogen bond donors/acceptors as a protonated cytidine at physiological pH.

Modifications in DNA systems influence both molecular structure and thermodynamics, and can affect the protonation and tautomeric propensity of the bases. For example, LNA sugar and cytidine methylation affect helical structure, third-strand binding affinity, and pK_a [7, 8].

Molecular dynamics (MD) simulations using an up-to-date force field have been shown to be a powerful tools to provide structural properties at the molecular level and to be complementary to experiments [9–12]. For example, MD simulations have been successfully used to investigate the conformational change due to sugar and base modification in DNA duplexes and triple helices [13–17]. Simulations have also been used to study structural change upon binding [14] and to predict the change in binding affinity and/or solubility due to change in the targeting oligonucleotide [18, 19].

Molecular simulation methods, primarily λ-dynamics [20, 21], can be used to describe the change between protonation and/or tautomeric states. Protonation and tautomeric equilibria are influenced by chemical and physical factors including solvent, ion concentration, and biomolecular environment (i.e., sequence and/or neighboring residues). An accurate prediction should account for the small energy differences that cause shifts in the tautomeric equilibrium and the need to sample different conformational states accessible to the biomolecule. The λ-dynamics method with an explicit description of the solvent [22] addresses these issues by enabling the direct coupling between protonation processes and conformational dynamics. Moreover, the method accuracy can be improved through a fine calibration of the force field.

An alternative approach to λ-dynamics to evaluate protonation equilibrium (accounting for physicochemical factors that affect the protonation equilibrium such as solvent, ions, and neighboring residues) is the multiple pH regime method [13, 23]. Here a conformational ensemble is generated by MD simulations for each protonation state, and the snapshots are used to calculate the degree of protonation of the base of interest as a function of pH, by means of a continuum electrostatic model and then making an averaged over the snapshots.

A schematic workflow for setting up molecular dynamics simulation for oligonucleotide hybrids is shown in Fig. 1 and described in Subheadings 3.1–3.3. According to the questions to address, diverse approaches are proposed:

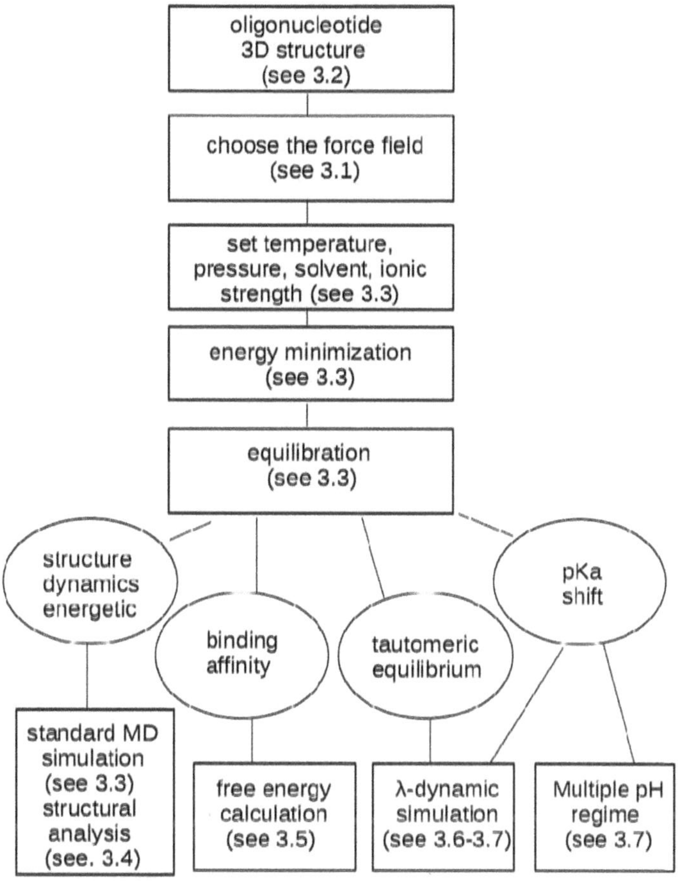

Fig. 1 Schematic workflow for setting up molecular simulations

- To investigate structural features, *see* Subheading 3.4;
- To investigate change in binding affinity, *see* Subheading 3.5;
- To investigate the effect of environment on base tautomerism, *see* Subheading 3.6;
- To investigate the base pK_a shift due to the environment, *see* Subheading 3.7.

For the principles behind molecular dynamics techniques and analysis *see* refs. [24, 25].

2 Materials

For molecular dynamics simulations of nucleic acids modern programs such as AMBER [26], CHARMM [27], GROMACS [28, 29], and NAMD [30] can be run efficiently using multiple central processing unit (CPU) cores in parallel on commodity hardware either in a single computer or on multiple computers in a cluster. Memory requirements are modest but the speed of the simulation depends directly on the speed of the CPU. If multiple computers are used in a cluster the communication hardware is critical, and it should provide both high bandwidth and low latency since MD simulations need to communicate a mix of short and long messages/data packages.

Today graphical processing units (GPUs) have become the workhorse of classical MD simulations. GPUs contain a large number (several thousand) of processing units and are very efficient. Simulations typically run 30–40 times faster on a GPU, which costs <$1000, compared to running the same simulations on 8–16 cores on a workstation; for example, a ~20,000-atom system, such as a dodecamer DNA duplex in a cubic water box with 6 nm side length, can be simulated for ~200 ns/day on an NVIDIA GEFORCE GTX1080TI GPU. The time it takes to simulate 1 ns of a system on a single GPU is roughly inversely proportional to the number of atoms in the system, so a 200,000 atom system can be simulated for ~20 ns/day. *See* https://www.charmm.org/charmm/program/performance/ for some recent benchmarks of various system sizes.

The amount of disk-space (M bytes) required to store a coordinate trajectory is proportional to the overall size of the simulation:

$$M = T \times F \times N \times 3 \times P$$

Here T is the length of the simulation (ns), F is the frequency of saving coordinate snaphosts (number of coordinate sets saved during 1 ns), N is the number of particles (atoms) in the system, 3 are the three Cartesian coordinates, and P is the number of bytes of disk-space required to store one number (one coordinate); storing a 1 μs trajectory sampled every 10 ps for a system of 20,000 atoms, using a single precision number representation (4 bytes/number), requires ca 25 GB disk space.

3 Methods

3.1 Molecular Model: Force Field

The most commonly used force fields for all-atom simulations of nucleic acids are CHARMM36 [31] and some of the recent AMBER force field variants, in particular the bsc1 [32] and OL15 [33] modifications; recent assessments of force fields have been presented in [34–36]. Standard DNA and RNA oligonucleotides, as well as a large number of naturally occurring modified nucleotides [37, 38], and even synthetic modifications can be treated with these force fields. Force fields should not be mixed—the whole system should be treated using the same force field. If the system contains functional groups for which no parameters exist, the user can develop the missing parameter using the same protocols as were used for the parent force field (AMBER or CHARMM) (*see* **Note 1**). There are also webservers, which can be used to obtain missing parameters, although the resulting parameters may not be as good as parameters in a carefully optimized force field [39, 40].

These are additive force fields, with fixed point charges. Polarizable force fields [41], which allow the charge distribution to change, are under development and have not yet been put to regular use.

There are a number of water models to choose from. The most commonly used water models are TIP3P [42], which is the model that is used in the development of the CHARMM force field, and SPC/E [43]. Ions can interact quite specifically with DNA structures, in particular in the grooves and with the phosphate groups. Divalent ions such as Mg^{2+} can be difficult to treat properly with a classical force field [44], and these ions must be properly coordinated and their positions must be carefully equilibrated.

3.2 Setting Up the Molecular System

A three dimensional structure for the oligonucleotide system is needed. The starting structure for oligonucleotide systems can be taken from experimentally resolved structures. Experimental techniques such as X-ray crystallography, nuclear magnetic resonance (NMR) experiment, and cryo-electron microscopy provide high-resolution three-dimensional structures (*see* **Note 2**) and the resolved structures are deposited in the RCSB PDB data bank (www.rcsb.org) [45]. Alternatively, if no experimental structure is available, one can build a starting structure using software like NAB [46] and/or 3DNA web server [47].

1. Find in the database or generate the oligonucleotide structure with the selected sequence, then introduce the chemical modification manually and add an eventually extra oligonucleotide strand applying a restraint potential on the hydrogen bond distance during the initial energy minimization and equilibration (*see* Subheading 3.3, **step 2**) to locate the new strand in the desired position.
2. Locate the oligonucleotide structure in a box and solvate it. Diverse type of boxes are available, the most common used are cubic, truncated octahedron and/or rhombic dodecahedron (*see* **Note 3**). To solvate the structure a preequilibrated solvent molecular box is used. To mimic physiological conditions, water is used as solvent and ions are added to neutralize the system and to achieve the desired ions concentration. Commonly a salt concentration of 0.15 M NaCl is used. For water, the most used models are TIP3P [42] and SPC/E [43] (*see* **Note 4**).

3.3 Setting Up the Molecular Simulation

1. Define a cutoff for short-range nonbonded interactions and a treatment for long range interactions in line with the force field and apply periodic boundary conditions to eliminate boundary effects (*see* **Note 5**).
2. Energy minimize the system using steepest descent and/or adopted-basis Newton–Raphson methods. A harmonic restraint using a force constant of 10 kcal/mol Å^2 can be applied on the backbone atom positions and on the distances of base pair hydrogen bonds, to avoid structural distortions due to the nonoptimal position of solvent molecules and ions in the starting structure.
3. Perform molecular dynamics simulations in a thermodynamic ensemble. The most common ones are the canonical (NVT, constant number of particles, volume, and temperature) or isothermal-isobaric (NPT, constant number of particles, pressure, and temperature) ensembles. To maintain the temperature and/or the pressure constant, a thermostat and/or a barostat is applied and a reference temperature (e.g., 298 K) and/or pressure (e.g., 1 atm) is defined (*see* for details [24, 25]).
4. In MD simulation, the molecular system evolves in time by numerically integrating Newton's equation of motion. The leapfrog integrator is normally used with an integration time-step of 2 fs. For oligonucleotide systems, SHAKE [48] or LINCS [49] algorithm has to be applied to constrain bonds involving hydrogens, when a time step of 2 fs is used.
5. Equilibrate the molecular system (*see* **Note 6**). During this phase, thermodynamics and structural properties stabilize. The equilibration time varies depending on the system starting conditions. For small B-DNA helices (10-mer), a 10 ns equilibration is normally enough. Properties to monitor during the equilibration phase are thermodynamic quantities such as energy, temperature and pressure and structural properties.
6. After the equilibration phase, the production runs are performed. The length of production phase depends on the properties of interest, different properties have different relaxation time (*see* **Note 7**).

3.4 Structural Analysis

A simulation study should always be performed with specific questions concerning the system in mind. Important structure-related properties for DNA are hydrogen bonding patterns (Watson–Crick or Hoogsteen), groove widths, base pair and base pair step geometries, which are usually described using helicoidal parameters [46, 50, 51]. For flexible systems it is most useful to present distributions of the structural parameters. Recently a robust method to characterize DNA curvature has been presented [52].

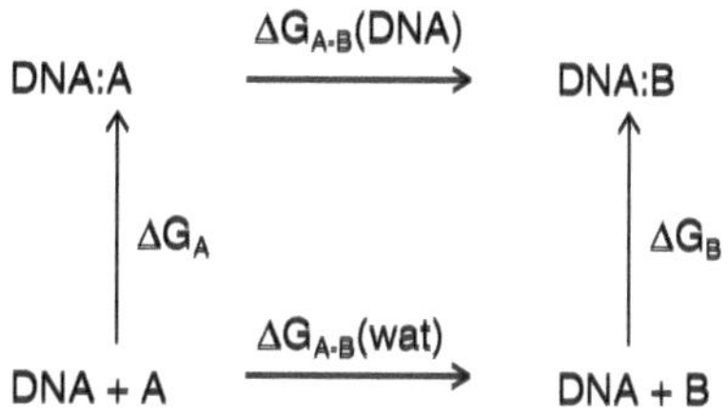

Fig. 2 Thermodynamics cycle for the binding ligand A and B to DNA duplex. The relative binding affinity of ligand B and A is ΔG_B-ΔG_A = $\Delta G_{A\text{-}B}$(DNA) − $\Delta G_{A\text{-}B}$(wat) where $\Delta G_{A\text{-}B}$(DNA) is the free energy difference of the two ligands in complex with DNA and $\Delta G_{A\text{-}B}$(wat) is the free energy difference of the two ligands in solutions (*see* **Note 8**)

Root-mean-square deviations (RMSD) from the starting structure, or between structural variants (different conformations), can also be useful as a simple, overall measure of the structural integrity of the system or of the similarity between two conformations. RMSD can also be analyzed for parts of the system.

Dynamical properties can be quite easily analyzed from a simulation. Root-mean-square fluctuations can be compared with temperature factors (B-factors) from X-ray crystallographic structure, or dipolar relaxation order parameters can be computed and compared with data from NMR experiments.

3.5 Setting Up Free Energy Calculations

1. Define a thermodynamics cycle for binding ligand A and B to DNA duplex (Fig. 2).
2. Calculate $\Delta G_{A\text{-}B}$ by transforming the atoms in ligand A in the atoms in the ligand B (*see* **Note 9**) in water and in complex with DNA. Among the diverse methods available to calculate the free energy differences, $\Delta G_{A\text{-}B}$, Bennett Acceptance Ratio (BAR) method (*see* [53] for details) has been shown to be very efficient [54]. A coupling parameter λ ($\lambda \in [0, 1]$) represents the alchemical states. Calculation has been performed at diverse values of parameter λ. The number and the length of *λ-windows* vary accounting to the type of transformations. For example for the transformation from methyl-cytosine to cytosine in water solution ($\Delta G_{A\text{-}B}$(wat) in Fig. 2) 11 *λ-windows* of 10 ns give an accuracy in the order of 0.1 kcal/mol (using 5 replicas) [18] (*see* **Note 9**).

3.6 Setting Up Calculation to Evaluate Tautomer Propensity

1. Use λ-dynamics simulation [20] to calculate the tautomeric propensity of a nucleobase/nucleotide in the oligonucleotide system. For convenience, we used, as example, two tautomeric states, labelled H1 and H3, of the cytidine analog pseudoisocytidine (Fig. 3).
2. Define a model compound (*see* **Note 10**) and the corresponding tautomeric states.

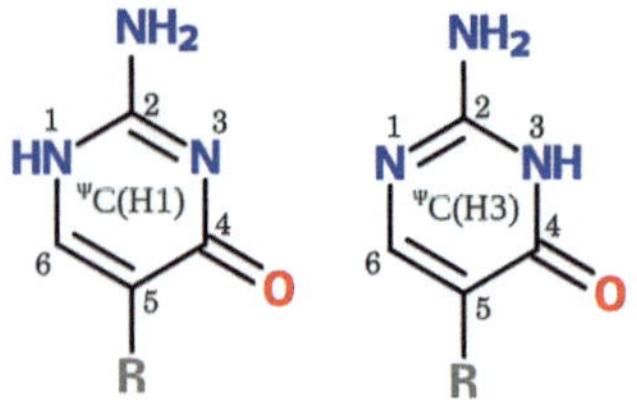

Fig. 3 Tautomeric states for pseudoisocytidine (H1 and H3)

3. Associate a continuous variable λ ($\lambda \in [0, 1]$) to each tautomeric state: the tautomeric states H1 and H3 are described by λ_{H1} and λ_{H3}, respectively.
4. Calculate free energy (*see* Subheading 3.5) for transforming tautomer H1 into H3 for the model compound in solution, $\Delta G_{H1 \to H3} = \Delta G_{model}$ (*see* **Note 11**).
5. Calibrate the force constant, k_{bias}, of the harmonic biasing potentials, to increase transitions between the physical end states (*see* **Note 12**).
6. Perform λ-dynamics simulation [20] for oligonucleotides containing the tautomeric nucleotide or nucleotides, using the above settings. For small oligonucleotides (i.e., 7-mer DNA triplexes) five independent replicas of around 40 ns each give a standard error of the mean < 10% for the tautomeric propensity of a nucleobase [55]. Only $0.8 \le \lambda \le 1$ values are considered as a physical end state for population counting.

3.7 Setting Up Calculation to Evaluate pK_a Shift

Constant pH molecular dynamics, in the framework of multisite λ-dynamics (CPHMD$^{MS\lambda D}$) [21] and multiple pH regime method [23] can be used to calculate pK_a shift due to the effect of the environment.

3.7.1 Setting Up Constant pH Molecular Dynamics Simulations

1. Define a model compound (*see* **Note 13**) and the corresponding protonation states. As example, Fig. 4 reports two protonation states for the cytidine.
2. Associate a continuous variables λ ($\lambda \in [0, 1]$) to each protonation state of the nucleoside: the deprotonated states are described by λ_{deprot} and λ_{prot}, respectively.
3. Calculate free energy (*see* Subheading 3.5) of protonation for the model compound in solution, ΔG_{model} (*see* **Note 14**).
4. Calibrate the force constant, k_{bias}, of the harmonic biasing potentials, to increase transitions between the physical end states (*see* **Note 12**).
5. Perform constant pH simulations at diverse titration points in parallel (pH replica exchange). For example to evaluate the titration curve for cytidine (experimental cytosine pK_a is around 4.4) in 5-mer DNA triplex, the titration points

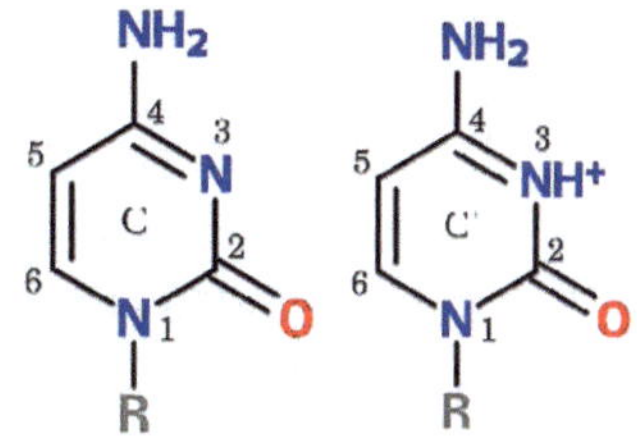

Fig. 4 Two protonation states of the cytidine, C and C^{+}

at pH = 3, 4, ... 12 can be used. Five independent pH-exchange-replica runs of around 20 ns each give an standard error of the pK_a mean of 0.1–0.2 pH unit [13].

6. Calculate pK_a, using the fraction of protonated state, S_{pro}, at each titration point and fitting to the Henderson-Hasselbalch equation: $S_{\text{pro}} = 1 - \frac{1}{1+10^{-n(\text{pH}-\text{p}K_a)}}$, where n is the Hill coefficient and indicates the degree of cooperativity between titratable groups. Only $0.8 \leq \lambda \leq 1$ values are considered as a physical end state for population counting.

3.7.2 Setting Up Multiple pH Regime Simulations

1. Perform at least two standard MD simulations (*see* Subheading 3.3) for the oligonucleotide system to generate the conformational ensemble for each protonated state or deprotonated state, and collect snapshots at equal time intervals. For 10-mer helical oligonucleotides, the conformational ensembles can be collected every 100 ps from 100 ns MD simulation.
2. Apply the multiple pH regime method [23] to the protonated and deprotonated ensembles using a relative dielectric constant of 80 for the solvent and 4 for the oligonucleotide moiety (*see* **Note 15**).
3. Calculate the final titration curves by averaging over the ensembles for each system. The pK_a values can be extracted from the titration curves as the value of pH where the corresponding site is half protonated.

4 Notes

1. Force field parameters cannot be transferred between force fields, new parameters should be parameterized in line with the force field philosophy (*see* Subheading 3.1).
2. Since the hydrogen positions are not always resolved in experimental structures, hydrogen atoms have to be manually added to the structure accounting for protonation and tautomerization state of the functional group at the selected pH (*see* Subheading 3.2).

3. The box dimension should be carefully chosen to avoid artifacts. The shortest distance between a box edge and the solute should be larger than half of the cutoff used to define nonbonded interactions (*see* Subheading 3.3). For example, when a nonbonded cutoff of 12 Å is used, it is good to use a distance between box edge and the solute of at least 8 Å. The distance should also take into account solute conformational rearrangements (extended conformations). Among the three most used box types, the rhombic dodecahedron allows a reduction of around 29% of CPU-time compared to a cubic box when simulating a spherical or flexible molecule in solvent (*see* Subheading 3.2).
4. It is of fundamental importance that the solvent and the ion models are compatible with the force field used to describe the oligonucleotides. Note also that deficiencies of the solvent or ion model in describing kinetic, thermodynamics and structure properties may affect the oligonucleotide simulations and should be taken into account in the analysis of the simulation data (*see* Subheading 3.2).
5. Correct treatment of boundary effects is important since it allows the evaluation of macroscopic properties from a simulation of one or a few biomolecules in solution (for principles behind molecular simulations *see* [24, 25]). In the simulation, a box is surrounded by images (e.g., 26 images for a cubic system), in this way the molecules experience forces as they were in a bulk fluid (no wall), but they should not experience the force generated by themselves. For this reason the distance between box edge and the solute should be larger than half of the cutoff used for nonbonded interactions (*see* Subheading 3.3 and **Note 3**).
6. A highly charged system or high ionic strength may require a preequilibration where a harmonic restraint using a force constant of 10 kcal/mol·Å^2 is applied on the oligonucleotide heavy atom positions, to allow the relaxation of water molecules and ion positions (*see* Subheading 3.3).
7. To check the reproducibility and to estimate statistical error of simulation data, at least three independent replicas have to be performed (*see* Subheading 3.3).
8. The energy changes $\Delta G_{\text{A-B}}$(DNA) and $\Delta G_{\text{A-B}}$(wat) do not correspond to any transformation that can be performed experimentally (*see* Fig. 2 in Subheading 3.5).
9. Each particle of initial state (state A) should have a correspondence in the final state (state B). The atoms that are unique in one state are defined as dummies (zero nonbonded interactions) in the other state. Problematic cases are when the free energy calculation requires the breaking of covalent bond. To

address these cases, an ad hoc protocol should be developed. An example is the transformation from DNA to LNA nucleosides that requires the breaking of the bridging group across the deoxyribose ring [18] (*see* Subheading 3.5).

10. Model system is a nucleobase or nucleoside in aqueous solution for which experimental data or prediction on the protonation propensity is available. The model system is used to calculate ΔG_{model} and k_{bias} (*see* Subheading 3.6).
11. ΔG_{model} flattens the potential energy surface such that the two tautomeric states of the model system in solution are equipopulated as the free energy between the two states becomes zero. If the tautomeric ratio of the model is 1:1, the state population obtained from the simulation can be used directly, as in the case of the pseudoisocytidine where tautomeric ratio $^{\Psi}$C(H1):$^{\Psi}$C(H3) for the model system is 1:1 at physiological conditions [55]. In other cases, the obtained population should be corrected to account for the fact that the tautomer population is not 1:1 at the simulated condition (*see* Subheading 3.6).
12. The value of k_{bias} is calibrated by performing λ-dynamics simulation for the model system at various k_{bias} values and looking at the fraction of physical end states in the trajectory (FPL, fraction physical ligand) and at the frequency of transitions between the two tautomeric states (transition rate, ns^{-1}). An optimal value of k_{bias} has to yield a high transition rate and simultaneously maintain high FPL (above 0.8) [21] (*see* Subheadings 3.6 and 3.7.1).
13. The model system is a nucleobase or nucleoside in aqueous solution for which experimental or predicted pK_a data are available. In a study on cytidine pK_a shift in DNA triplex, we observed that deoxyribocytosine 5′-monophosphate in aqueous solution was a better model compound than the corresponding base [13]. The model system is used to calculate ΔG_{model} and k_{bias} (*see* Subheading 3.7.1).
14. ΔG_{model} flattens the potential energy surface such that the two protonation states of the nucleoside in solution are equipopulated as the free energy between the two states becomes zero ($pH = pK_{ref}$). A term $\ln(10)k_B T(pK_{ref} - pH)$ adds an offset when $pH \neq pK_{ref}$, where pK_{ref} is the experimentally measured pK_a of the model compound (*see* Subheading 3.7.1).
15. The charge and the position of the mobile ions have to be explicitly included in the ensemble configurations. Thus, the electrostatic interactions involving the ions are directly calculated with the assumption that the ions positions on average obey the Boltzmann distribution (*see* Subheading 3.7.2).

References

1. Lundin KE, Gissberg O, Smith CIE (2015) Oligonucleotide therapies: the past and the present. Hum Gene Ther 26(8):475–485. https://doi.org/10.1089/hum.2015.070
2. Kuhn H, Demidov VV, Nielsen PE, Frank-Kamenetskii MD (1999) An experimental study of mechanism and specificity of peptide nucleic acid (PNA) binding to duplex DNA 1 1Edited by I. Tinoco. J Mol Biol 286 (5):1337–1345
3. Obika S, Nanbu D, Hari Y, Morio K-I, In Y, Ishida T, Imanishi T (1997) Synthesis of 2′-O, 4′-C-methyleneuridine and -cytidine. Novel bicyclic nucleosides having a fixed C 3,-endo sugar puckering. Tetrahedron Lett 38 (50):8735–8738. https://doi.org/10.1016/S0040-4039(97)10322-7
4. Koshkin AA, Singh SK, Nielsen P, Rajwanshi VK, Kumar R, Meldgaard M, Olsen CE, Wengel J (1998) LNA (locked nucleic acids): synthesis of the adenine, cytosine, guanine, 5-methylcytosine, thymine and uracil bicyclonucleoside monomers, oligomerisation, and unprecedented nucleic acid recognition. Tetrahedron 54(14):3607–3630. https://doi.org/10.1016/S0040-4020(98)00094-5
5. Lee JS, Woodsworth ML, Latimer LJ, Morgan AR (1984) Poly(pyrimidine). Poly(purine) synthetic DNAs containing 5-methylcytosine form stable triplexes at neutral pH. Nucleic Acids Res 12(16):6603–6614. https://doi.org/10.1093/nar/12.16.6603
6. Ono A, Ts'o POP, Kan LS (1991) Triplex formation of oligonucleotides containing 2′-O-methylpseudoisocytidine in substitution for 2′-deoxycytidine. J Am Chem Soc 113:4032–4033. https://doi.org/10.1021/ja00010a077
7. Sun B-W, Babu BR, Sørensen MD, Zakrzewska K, Wengel J, Sun J-S (2004) Sequence and pH effects of LNA-containing triple helix-forming oligonucleotides: physical chemistry, biochemistry, and modeling studies. Biochemistry 43 (14):4160–4169. https://doi.org/10.1021/bi036064e
8. Petersen M, Bondensgaard K, Wengel J, Jacobsen JP (2002) Locked nucleic acid (LNA) recognition of RNA: NMR solution structures of LNA: RNA hybrids. J Am Chem Soc 124 (21):5974–5982. https://doi.org/10.1021/ja012288d
9. Karplus M, Lavery R (2014) Significance of molecular dynamics simulations for life sciences. Isr J Chem 54(8–9):1042–1051. https://doi.org/10.1002/ijch.201400074
10. Cheatham TE, Case DA (2013) Twenty-five years of nucleic acid simulations. Biopolymers 99(12):969–977. https://doi.org/10.1002/bip.22331
11. Pérez A, Luque FJ, Orozco M (2012) Frontiers in molecular dynamics simulations of DNA. Acc Chem Res 45(2):196–205. https://doi.org/10.1021/ar2001217
12. Foloppe N, Guéroult M, Hartmann B (2013) Simulating DNA by molecular dynamics: aims, methods, and validation. In: Monticelli L, Salonen E (eds) Biomolecular simulations: methods and protocols. Humana Press, Totowa, NJ, pp 445–468. https://doi.org/10.1007/978-1-62703-017-5_17
13. Hartono YD, Xu Y, Karshikoff A, Nilsson L, Villa A (2018) Modeling pK shift in DNA triplexes containing locked nucleic acids. J Chem Inf Model 58(4):773–783. https://doi.org/10.1021/acs.jcim.7b00741
14. Pabon-Martinez YV, Xu Y, Villa A, Lundin KE, Geny S, Nguyen C-H, Pedersen EB, Jørgensen PT, Wengel J, Nilsson L, Smith CIE, Zain R (2017) LNA effects on DNA binding and conformation: from single strand to duplex and triplex structures. Sci Rep 7(1):11043. https://doi.org/10.1038/s41598-017-09147-8
15. Yildirim I, Kierzek E, Kierzek R, Schatz GC (2014) Interplay of LNA and 2′-O-methyl RNA in the structure and thermodynamics of RNA hybrid systems: a molecular dynamics study using the revised AMBER force field and comparison with experimental results. J Phys Chem B 118(49):14177–14187. https://doi.org/10.1021/jp506703g
16. Suresh G, Priyakumar UD (2013) Structures, dynamics, and stabilities of fully modified locked nucleic acid (β-d-LNA and α-l-LNA) duplexes in comparison to pure DNA and RNA duplexes. J Phys Chem B 117 (18):5556–5564. https://doi.org/10.1021/jp4016068
17. Suresh G, Priyakumar UD (2014) Atomistic investigation of the effect of incremental modification of deoxyribose sugars by locked nucleic acid (β-d-LNA and α-l-LNA) moieties on the structures and thermodynamics of DNA–RNA hybrid duplexes. J Phys Chem B 118(22):5853–5863. https://doi.org/10.1021/jp5014779
18. Xu Y, Villa A, Nilsson L (2017) The free energy of locking a ring: changing a deoxyribonucleoside to a locked nucleic acid. J Comput Chem 38(15):1147–1157. https://doi.org/10.1002/jcc.24692

19. Allnér O, Nilsson L (2011) Nucleotide modifications and tRNA anticodon-mRNA codon interactions on the ribosome. RNA 17 (12):2177–2188. https://doi.org/10.1261/rna.029231.111
20. Khandogin J, Brooks CL (2005) Constant pH molecular dynamics with proton tautomerism. Biophys J 89:141–157. https://doi.org/10.1529/biophysj.105.061341
21. Goh GB, Knight JL, Brooks CL (2012) Constant pH molecular dynamics simulations of nucleic acids in explicit solvent. J Chem Theory Comput 8:36–46. https://doi.org/10.1021/ct2006314
22. Wallace JA, Shen JK (2009) Predicting pKa values with continuous constant pH molecular dynamics. Methods Enzymol 466:455–475. https://doi.org/10.1016/S0076-6879(09)66019-5
23. Nilsson L, Karshikoff A (2011) Multiple pH regime molecular dynamics simulation for pK calculations. PLoS One 6(5):e20116. https://doi.org/10.1371/journal.pone.0020116
24. Leach AR (2001) Molecular modeling: principles and applications, 2nd edn. Pearson Education Limited, London
25. Schlick T (2010) In: Antman SS, Marsden JE, Sirovich L (eds) Molecular modeling and simulation: an interdisciplinary guide, Interdisciplinary applied mathematics, vol 21. Springer, New York
26. Case DA, Cheatham TE III, Darden T, Gohlke H, Luo R, Merz KM Jr, Onufriev A, Simmerling C, Wang B, Woods RJ (2005) The AMBER biomolecular simulation programs. J Comput Chem 26(16):1668–1688. https://doi.org/10.1002/jcc.20290
27. Brooks BR, Brooks CL 3rd, Mackerell AD Jr, Nilsson L, Petrella RJ, Roux B, Won Y, Archontis G, Bartels C, Boresch S, Caflisch A, Caves L, Cui Q, Dinner AR, Feig M, Fischer S, Gao J, Hodoscek M, Im W, Kuczera K, Lazaridis T, Ma J, Ovchinnikov V, Paci E, Pastor RW, Post CB, Pu JZ, Schaefer M, Tidor B, Venable RM, Woodcock HL, Wu X, Yang W, York DM, Karplus M (2009) CHARMM: the biomolecular simulation program. J Comput Chem 30 (10):1545–1614. https://doi.org/10.1002/jcc.21287
28. Hess B, Kutzner C, van der Spoel D, Lindahl E (2008) GROMACS 4: algorithms for highly efficient, load-balanced, and scalable molecular simulation. J Chem Theory Comput 4 (3):435–447. https://doi.org/10.1021/ct700301q
29. Abraham MJ, Murtola T, Schulz R, Páll S, Smith JC, Hess B, Lindahl E (2015) GROMACS: High performance molecular simulations through multi-level parallelism from laptops to supercomputers. SoftwareX 1 (2):19–25. https://doi.org/10.1016/j.softx.2015.06.001
30. Phillips JC, Braun R, Wang W, Gumbart J, Tajkhorshid E, Villa E, Chipot C, Skeel RD, Kalé L, Schulten K (2005) Scalable molecular dynamics with NAMD. J Comput Chem 26 (16):1781–1802. https://doi.org/10.1002/jcc.20289
31. Hart K, Foloppe N, Baker CM, Denning EJ, Nilsson L, MacKerell AD (2011) Optimization of the CHARMM additive force field for DNA: improved treatment of the BI/BII conformational equilibrium. J Chem Theory Comput 8 (1):348–362. https://doi.org/10.1021/ct200723y
32. Ivani I, Dans PD, Noy A, Perez A, Faustino I, Hospital A, Walther J, Andrio P, Goni R, Balaceanu A, Portella G, Battistini F, Gelpi JL, Gonzalez C, Vendruscolo M, Laughton CA, Harris SA, Case DA, Orozco M (2016) Parmbsc1: a refined force field for DNA simulations. Nat Methods 13(1):55–58. https://doi.org/10.1038/nmeth.3658
33. Zgarbová M, Šponer J, Otyepka M, Cheatham TE, Galindo-Murillo R, Jurečka P (2015) Refinement of the sugar–phosphate backbone torsion beta for AMBER force fields improves the description of Z- and B-DNA. J Chem Theory Comput 11(12):5723–5736. https://doi.org/10.1021/acs.jctc.5b00716
34. Galindo-Murillo R, Robertson JC, Zgarbová M, Šponer J, Otyepka M, Jurečka P, Cheatham TE (2016) Assessing the current state of Amber force field modifications for DNA. J Chem Theory Comput 12(8):4114–4127. https://doi.org/10.1021/acs.jctc.6b00186
35. Dans PD, Ivani I, Hospital A, Portella G, González C, Orozco M (2017) How accurate are accurate force-fields for B-DNA? Nucleic Acids Res 45(7):4217–4230. https://doi.org/10.1093/nar/gkw1355
36. Ben Imeddourene A, Elbahnsi A, Guéroult M, Oguey C, Foloppe N, Hartmann B (2015) Simulations meet experiment to reveal new insights into DNA intrinsic mechanics. PLoS Comput Biol 11(12):e1004631. https://doi.org/10.1371/journal.pcbi.1004631
37. Aduri R, Psciuk BT, Saro P, Taniga H, Schlegel HB, SantaLucia J (2007) AMBER force field parameters for the naturally occurring modified nucleosides in RNA. J Chem Theory Comput 3(4):1464–1475. https://doi.org/10.1021/ct600329w
38. Xu Y, Vanommeslaeghe K, Aleksandrov A, MacKerell AD Jr, Nilsson L (2016) Additive

CHARMM force field for naturally occurring modified ribonucleotides. J Comput Chem 37 (10):896–912. https://doi.org/10.1002/jcc.24307

39. Vanommeslaeghe K, MacKerell AD (2012) Automation of the CHARMM general force field (CGenFF) I: bond perception and atom typing. J Chem Inf Model 52(12):3144–3154. https://doi.org/10.1021/ci300363c

40. Vanommeslaeghe K, Raman EP, MacKerell AD (2012) Automation of the CHARMM general force field (CGenFF) II: assignment of bonded parameters and partial atomic charges. J Chem Inf Model 52(12):3155–3168. https://doi.org/10.1021/ci3003649

41. Savelyev A, MacKerell AD (2014) All- atom polarizable force field for DNA based on the classical Drude oscillator model. J Comput Chem 35(16):1219–1239. https://doi.org/10.1002/jcc.23611

42. Jorgensen WL, Chandrasekhar J, Madura JD, Impey RW, Klein ML (1983) Comparison of simple potential functions for simulating liquid water. J Chem Phys 79(2):926–935. https://doi.org/10.1063/1.445869

43. Berendsen HJC, Grigera JR, Straatsma TP (1987) The missing term in effective pair potentials. J Phys Chem 91(24):6269–6271. https://doi.org/10.1021/j100308a038

44. Allnér O, Nilsson L, Villa A (2012) Magnesium ion–water coordination and exchange in biomolecular simulations. J Chem Theory Comput 8:1493–1502. https://doi.org/10.1021/ct3000734

45. Berman HM, Westbrook J, Feng Z, Gilliland G, Bhat TN, Weissig H, Shindyalov IN, Bourne PE (2000) The Protein Data Bank. Nucleic Acids Res 28(1):235–242. https://doi.org/10.1093/nar/28.1.235

46. Macke TJ, Case DA (1997) Modeling unusual nucleic acid structures. In: Molecular modeling of nucleic acids, vol 682. ACS symposium series, vol 682. American Chemical Society, pp 379–393. https://doi.org/10.1021/bk-1998-0682.ch024

47. Zheng GH, Lu XJ, Olson WK (2009) Web 3DNA-a web server for the analysis, reconstruction, and visualization of three-dimensional nucleic-acid structures. Nucleic Acids Res 37:W240–W246. https://doi.org/10.1093/Nar/Gkp358

48. Ryckaert JP, Ciccotti G, Berendsen HJC (1977) Numerical-integration of Cartesian equations of motion of a system with constraints - molecular-dynamics of N-alkanes. J Comput Phys 23(3):327–341. https://doi.org/10.1016/0021-9991(77)90098-5

49. Hess B, Bekker H, Berendsen HJC, Fraaije JGEM (1998) LINCS: a linear constraint solver for molecular simulations. J Comput Chem 18(12):1463–1472. https://doi.org/10.1002/(sici)1096-987x(199709)18:12<1463::aid-jcc4>3.0.co;2-h

50. Lavery R, Moakher M, Maddocks JH, Petkeviciute D, Zakrzewska K (2009) Conformational analysis of nucleic acids revisited: curves+. Nucleic Acids Res 37(17):5917–5929. https://doi.org/10.1093/nar/gkp608

51. Lu XJ, Olson WK (2003) 3DNA: a software package for the analysis, rebuilding and visualization of three-dimensional nucleic acid structures. Nucleic Acids Res 31(17):5108–5121. https://doi.org/10.1093/nar/gkg680

52. Pasi M, Zakrzewska K, Maddocks JH, Lavery R (2017) Analyzing DNA curvature and its impact on the ionic environment: application to molecular dynamics simulations of minicircles. Nucleic Acids Res 45(7):4269–4277. https://doi.org/10.1093/nar/gkx092

53. Bennett CH (1976) Efficient estimation of free energy differences from Monte Carlo data. J Comput Phys 22:245–268. https://doi.org/10.1016/0021-9991(76)90078-4

54. Bruckner S, Boresch S (2011) Efficiency of alchemical free energy simulations. I. A practical comparison of the exponential formula, thermodynamic integration, and Bennett's acceptance ratio method. J Comput Chem 32 (7):1303–1319. https://doi.org/10.1002/jcc.21713

55. Hartono YD, Pabon-Martinez YV, Uyar A, Wengel J, Lundin KE, Zain R, Smith CIE, Nilsson L, Villa A (2017) Role of pseudoisocytidine tautomerization in triplex-forming oligonucleotides: in silico and in vitro studies. ACS Omega 2(5):2165–2177. https://doi.org/10.1021/acsomega.7b00347

Chapter 7

Characterization of Peptide–Oligonucleotide Complexes Using Electron Microscopy, Dynamic Light Scattering, and Protease Resistance Assay

Kärt Padari, Ly Porosk, Piret Arukuusk, and Margus Pooga

Abstract

Cationic peptides designed for cellular delivery of nucleic acid molecules form noncovalent nanocomplexes with negatively charged oligonucleotides (ON). The electrostatically associated complexes are further compacted by hydrophobic interactions yielding nanoparticles (NP) of homogeneous shape and size that are efficiently taken up by cells. The shape and size of NP often correlate with the biological activity of delivered ON inside cells; and the stability and accessibility of NP in biological fluids govern its circulation in organism and the cellular uptake. Therefore, here we provide protocols for characterizing the shape and size and surface charge of peptide/ON NP by negative staining transmission electron microscopy (TEM) and dynamic light scattering (DLS) respectively, and analysis of NP stability against proteolytic degradation.

Key words Nucleic acid delivery, Peptide–nucleic acid nanocomplexes, CPP–oligonucleotide nanoparticles, Negative staining TEM, CPP nanoparticle DLS, Protease resistance assay, Oligonucleotide therapeutics

1 Introduction

Oligonucleotides (ON) are highly attractive as therapeutically applicable molecules for correcting the expression of abnormally expressed genes [1–3]. The activity of the majority of gene expression-regulating ON is based on specific pairing with the complementary target sequence on mRNA or pre-mRNA, thereby triggering its degradation or interfering with its processing, making the ON-mediated gene modulation highly specific [4]. The straightforward principles of complementarity also facilitate design of targeting ON. However, the high molecular mass, negative charge and hydrophilicity render ON almost impermeable to biological membranes excluding the application of naked unmodified oligonucleotides in vivo [5]. For gaining their activity inside cells, various delivery vehicles have been utilized to translocate ON into cell cytoplasm and nucleus [6, 7]. In parallel with cationic

Olof Gissberg et al. (eds.), *Oligonucleotide-Based Therapies: Methods and Protocols*, Methods in Molecular Biology, vol. 2036, https://doi.org/10.1007/978-1-4939-9670-4_7,

polymers and lipids, the so-called cell-penetrating peptides (CPP), cationic sequences of 4–30 amino acids [8], have found wide application in transduction of ON to cell interior during the last decade [1]. Initially, the ON cargo was coupled to a CPP via a covalent bond and this is the preferred method for charge neutral ON so far [9]. However, noncovalent complexes assembled based on the electrostatic interaction of anionic ON with positively charged carrier peptides, have recently gained popularity due to higher efficiency and easy preparation [10]. Among CPPs, the peptides from the PepFect and NickFect family [11], designed for cellular delivery of nucleic acids, have been successfully applied for transduction of plasmid DNA [12], splicing switching ON [13], siRNA [14], miRNA [15], and antisense ONs into cells.

The structure of lipid nanoparticles (LNP) used for ON delivery has been thoroughly analyzed using a battery of complementary techniques like dynamic light scattering (DLS), transmission electron microscopy (TEM), nuclear magnetic resonance (NMR), fluorescence resonant energy transfer (FRET), protection against nucleases, molecular modeling, and others [4]. Electrostatically assembled ON-CPP complexes, in contrary, have been less extensively characterized; typically only by DLS, and the knowledge about the morphology and resistance to degradative enzymes is rather fragmentary [16]. TEM is the commonly used technique for characterizing the morphology of nanoparticles (NP) and both the size and shape of NP are known to correlate with their ability to translocate ON into cells [17] and with induced biological effects [18]. Due to rapid freezing of specimen cryo-TEM captures the morphology of NP in solution, and is the most relevant and preferred method in case of unstable and soft gel-like nanoparticles. However, the negative staining TEM [19] is still most often used for analysing the morphology of NP so far, since it yields identical results with cryo-TEM in majority of cases, and is more commonly available [10].

In negative staining procedure, the small particles in biological sample are adsorbed on an electron transparent sample support (EM grid) and a contrasting agent is applied to form a thin film of heavy metal salts. Higher absorption of electrons by metal atoms, like uranium or tungsten, compared to biological material reveals the structural details of particles, which in the transmission electron microscope appear white on a dark background (Fig. 1) [19].

The size and polydispersity of NP in solution is most commonly measured by DLS in a quantitative manner. NP in solution can be regarded as a colloidal dispersion system where molecules undergo random Brownian motion. Smaller particles move faster than larger particles, and when exposed to monochromatic light they will scatter light differently depending on their speed. The fluctuations in the intensity of scattered laser light is measured as a function of time by a fast photon counter, and is further used to calculate the

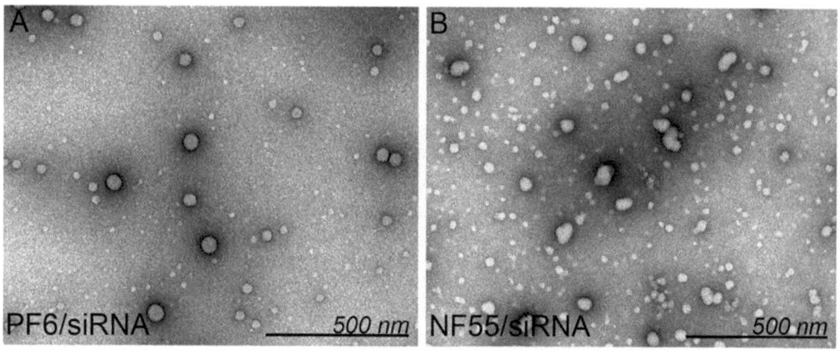

Fig. 1 TEM images of CPP–siRNA nanoparticles visualized by negative staining. The nanoparticles of CPP–siRNA formed by complexing of PepFect 6 at molecular ratio (MR)10 (**a**) or NickFect 55 (NF55) at MR 30 (**b**) with siRNA in water, and stained on grid with 2% aqueous uranyl acetate solution. The images were recorded using FEI Tecnai G2 Spirit BioTWIN electron microscope with Orius SC1000 camera at 120 kV accelerating voltage. Scale bars: 500 nm

particle hydrodynamic radius by the DLS apparatus software (Fig. 2). The homogeneity of NPs is characterized by the polydispersity index, which values lower than 0.05 describe monodisperse particles, whereas values over 0.7 indicate that the sample has a very broad size distribution [20].

Charged NP suspended in a solution attracts counter-ions to their surface and so electrical double layer will form around the particle. The electrical potential at the interface of the particle surface and the diffuse layer surrounding it is known as ζ potential; which can be calculated from the electrophoretic mobility of the particles in an applied electric field, and is deduced from the intensity fluctuation of scattered light from NP [21]. The Zeta potential correlates with the surface charge of the particle in a current medium [22] and is a highly essential characteristic for understanding of the NP-behavior in bio-relevant media.

The stability of NP in extracellular and intracellular environment is crucial for the functionality of the encapsulated ON molecule, which has to reach its target site in cells in an intact form. Both the ONs and the CPPs, if unmodified, are quickly degraded by hydrolytic enzymes present in culture media, in biological fluids and in cells. However, condensation of ON by CPPs to NP increases their stability, and might rescue the biological effect of the nucleic acid. The stability of such NP mostly depends on the resistance of delivery vector, so we introduced a protease protection assay (PPA) [23], in order to test and compare the stability of nanoparticles in vitro before proceeding with in vivo studies.

We harness in our assay a serine protease, Proteinase K that is routinely used for digestion of proteins. We consider Proteinase K particularly suitable, since it has a rather broad specificity by cleaving the peptide bonds adjacent to the carboxyl group of aliphatic and aromatic amino acids [24]. Furthermore, commercially

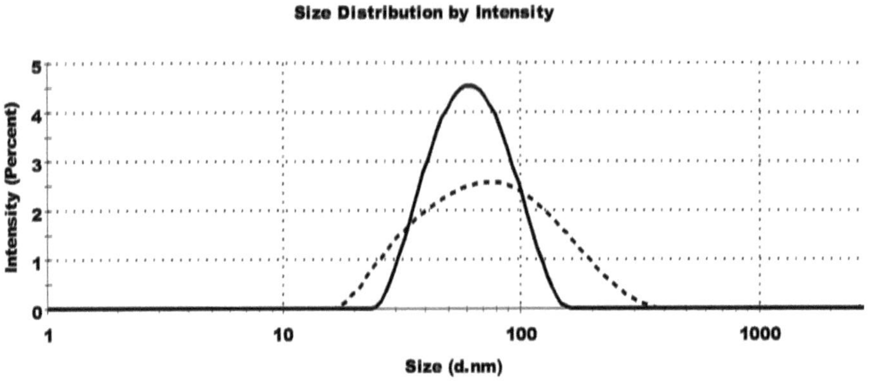

Fig. 2 DLS analysis of CPP–siRNA nanoparticles. The nanoparticles of CPP–siRNA formed by complexing of PepFect 6 (PF6) or NickFect 55 (NF55) at molecular ratio 30 with siRNA in water. Dynamic light scattering from 150 μl of complexes solution in ZEN0118 cuvette was measured with Malvern Zetasizer Nano ZS in three consecutive runs. Particles size distribution of PF6–siRNA complexes (solid line) and NF55–siRNA complexes (dotted line) are presented on the graph in percentages of the total scattered light intensity

available proteinase K from *Tritirachium album* has an optimal activity in the biologically relevant pH range (pH 6.5–7.5), it remains active at high temperature, and even in the presence of denaturing components (e.g., urea, SDS) and metal chelating agents (e.g., EDTA).

The PPA assay is based on dyes that upon intercalation in nucleic acid molecules emit fluorescent signals, depending on the accessibility of the ONs. In stable NP, only a negligible fraction of siRNA is accessible. However, upon digestion of NP by added enzyme, the accessibility of ONs increases, yielding increased fluorescence signal, allowing estimation of the stability of the NPs (Fig. 3).

2 Materials

Prepare all solutions using ultrapure water of MilliQ quality with resistance of 18 MΩ-cm at 25 °C and analytical grade reagents if not stated otherwise. Prepare and store all reagents at room temperature (unless indicated otherwise). Diligently follow all waste disposal regulations when disposing of waste materials.

2.1 Peptide and ON Preparations

1. Peptide stocks: In the below described protocols we have mostly used a peptide designated PepFect 14 (PF14) and its analogues. Weigh the lyophilized peptide powder, which has been brought to room temperature, using the sensitive analytical scales with at least 0.1 mg accuracy (*see* **Note 1**). Dissolve the peptide in appropriate volume of ultrapure water to prepare a stock solution with 1 mM concentration (*see* **Note 2**). Dilute a small amount of the stock solution tenfold with ultrapure

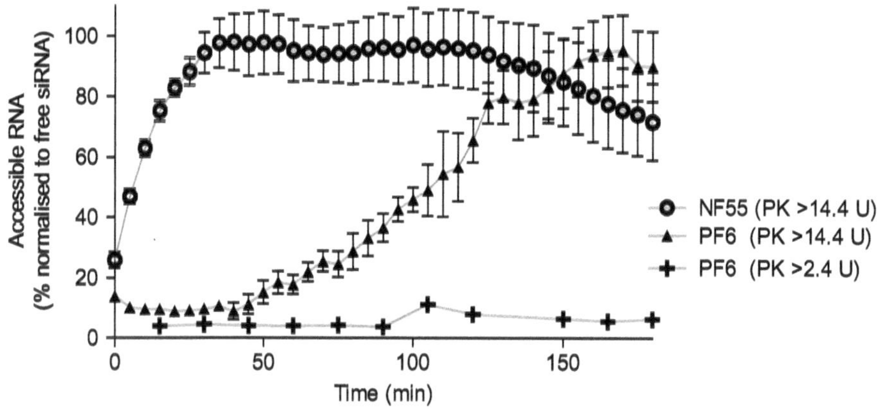

Fig. 3 Protease protection assay of CPP–siRNA nanoparticles. The nanoparticles of CPP–siRNA formed by complexing of PepFect 6 (PF6) and NickFect 55 (NF55) at MR 30 with siRNA in water. For analysis of siRNA accessibility, PicoGreen was added to complexes diluted in MQ water. The emission of fluorescent dye intercalated into accessible siRNA was measured using $\lambda_{ex} = 492$ nm, $\lambda_{em} = 535$ nm for excitation and emission, respectively. The stability of peptide in complexes against degradation was assessed by adding Proteinase K (14.4 U per well for NF55 and PF6, or 2.4 U for PF6 as a comparison) and recording fluorescence signal for 3 h with 15 or 30 min intervals. Results were normalized to free siRNA at the same concentration as used in the complexes (100%) and to siRNA free (0%) wells

water for estimating the concentration. Measure the absorbance of the solution at 278 nm if the peptide contains tryptophan or at 274 nm if tyrosine residue is present (*see* **Note 3**). Calculate the actual concentration of solution considering the ten-fold dilution and molar extinction coefficient 5579 and 1405 cm^{-1}/M for tryptophan and tyrosine, respectively [25]; and adjust the concentration of stock by adding MQ if necessary. Aliquot the solution to 20 or 100 μl stocks and store in freezer at −20 °C or lower. Thaw the stock on the day of experiment and do not freeze it again.

2. Oligonucleotide solutions: Dissolve the lyophilized siRNA and splicing switching ONs in ultrapure water at 20 μM concentrations. Calculate the volume of water based on the ON quantity specified by producer. Make aliquots of 20 or 100 μl, and store in freezer at −20 °C or lower.

2.2 Negative Staining TEM

1. Hexagonal 200-mesh copper grids coated with formvar and carbon layer (*see* **Note 4**).
2. Parafilm M.
3. Uranyl acetate (UA) solution for negative staining of specimens: Dissolve UA in double-distilled water at 2% concentration and filter through 0.22 μm pore sized filter. If sensitive and unstable particles are analyzed, supplement UA stain with 0.1% (w/v) trehalose (*see* **Note 5**).

4. Phosphotungstic acid (PTA) stain: Prepare a 2% aqueous solution of PTA and adjust pH to 7.0 with NaOH, if required. Add trehalose at 0.1% if necessary (*see* **Note 6**).
5. Transmission electron microscope with CCD camera (e.g., Tecnai G2 Spirit BioTWIN with Orius SC1000 camera, FEI Company).

2.3 Measurement of Hydrodynamic Diameter and Zeta Potential of CPP/ON NP

1. 20 μM siRNA stock.
2. 1 mM peptide solutions in MQ water.
3. MQ water.
4. 1.5 ml tubes.
5. UV-transparent disposable cuvettes with lids for hydrodynamic size measurement (*see* **Note 7**).
6. Disposable folded capillary cells with stoppers for zeta potential-measurement (*see* **Note 8**).
7. DLS apparatus (e.g., Zetasizer Nano ZS, Malvern Panalytical).

2.4 Protease Protection Assay/ Fluorescent Dye Intercalation Assay

1. Nucleic acid intercalating dye PicoGreen™ or Ethidium Bromide (for choosing dye *see* **Note 9**).
2. Black 96-well plate suitable for fluorescence measurement.
3. MQ water.
4. Buffers with different pH (e.g., HEPES, MES) (for choosing suitable buffer, *see* **Note 10**).
5. Proteinase K or other suitable enzyme for degrading the peptide component of the nanoparticle (for choosing suitable enzyme, *see* **Note 11**).
6. Spectrofluorometer (e.g., Synergy MX, BioTek Instruments Inc.).

3 Methods

3.1 Preparation of Oligonucleotide Complexes with Peptides

A solution/suspension of particles/complexes is formed in a suitable buffer/media or in distilled water. The protocol for condensing nucleic acid molecules to nanoparticles with CPPs has also been published earlier [11, 13, 15, 16]. As an example, the protocol for assembling 40 μl of PF14–siRNA complexes in water at molar ratio 30 for TEM analysis is presented below.

1. Dilute siRNA to 1 μM and PF14 to 100 μM in MQ water from the respective stock solutions (*see* Subheading 2.1).
2. Pipet into Eppendorf tube 27 μl MQ, add 10 μl of 1 μM siRNA, and mix thoroughly.
3. Add 3 μl of 100 μM PF14 solution upon constant mixing.
4. Incubate for 15–30 min at ambient temperature (*see* **Note 12**).

3.2 Analysis of Morphology of CPP/ON Complexes by Negative Staining TEM

CPP/ON complexes are analyzed on copper grids coated with formvar film and carbon layer.

1. Glow discharge formvar-carbon coated grids before use to increase the hydrophilicity and attachment of complexes to grids (*see* **Note 13**).
2. Pipet 10 μl drops of the sample from Subheading 3.1 and the solutions described in Subheading 2.2 on a piece of Parafilm and place the grids onto the drops with formvar-carbon coated side down. Avoid the migration of the stain to the back side of the grid. If that happens, discard the grid (*see* **Note 14**).
3. Incubate the grid on the sample drop for 2–4 min, remove the grid from the drop, and carefully remove the excess of solution by touching the edge of the grid with a filter paper.
4. Rinse the grid on a drop of UA (or PTA) stain to remove unbound complexes and remove the excess of stain with filter paper as in **step 3** above.
5. Place the grids onto second drop of staining solution for 1–2 min. Remove the excess of stain with filter paper and let the grid dry in air at ambient temperature for at least 30 min (*see* **Note 15**).
6. Examine the specimens under the transmission electron microscope as soon as possible, preferably on the same or next day. Record the images of nanocomplexes at different magnification using CCD camera (*see* **Note 16**).
7. Estimate the size and ellipticity of nanoparticles in recorded images by using ImageJ or other suitable analysis package if necessary (*see* **Note 17**).

3.3 Measurement of Hydrodynamic Diameter and Zeta Potential of ON–CPP NP

Typically the CPP–ON NPs yield in DLS more than one size intensity peaks, indicating the formation of differently sized particles upon manufacturing [24]. The Zetasizer software enables characterization of NPs size-distribution by intensity, volume, or number. In most cases we use the intensity-based characteristics, but if more detailed characterization is needed, the volume or the number distribution can be used (*see* **Note 18**).

1. Prepare CPP–siRNA complexes as described in Subheading 3.1. For measuring the hydrodynamic size, prepare 100 μl of complex solution. For measuring zeta potential prepare 300 μl of complex solution and dilute it with MQ up to 1000 μl (*see* **Note 19**).
2. Pipette gently the siRNA–MQ–CPP mixture into the cuvettes and avoid bubble formation (*see* **Note 20**).
3. Close the cuvettes with the lids or stoppers (*see* **Note 21**).
4. Measure hydrodynamic size or zeta potential at fixed temperature (e.g., 22 °C).

3.4 Protease Protection Assay

1. Add to wells of a black 96-well plate (suitable for fluorescence measurement) 90–110 μl of MQ or buffer depending on the assay. Always include MQ controls (*see* **Note 22**).
2. Prepare PicoGreen solution with appropriate concentration (*see* **Note 23**).
3. Add 20–30 μl of complexes per prepared 96-well plate well (*see* **Note 24**).
4. Mix gently and avoid spillage.
5. Add 20–30 μl of PicoGreen solution to each sample and controls (*see* **Note 25**).
6. Mix gently and incubate in dark at room temperature for 5 min.
7. Measure fluorescence signal of PicoGreen after 10 min, using λ_{ex} 492 nm, λ_{em} 535 nm, for excitation and emission, respectively (*see* **Note 26**).
8. Add 10 μl of proteinase K solution (*see* **Note 27**).
9. Record the changes of fluorescence intensity in time. The interval between the separate time-points should be 5 min or more and in longer measurements 30 min (*see* **Note 28**).
10. Normalize the fluorescence intensities to nucleic acid controls (*see* **Note 29**).

4 Notes

1. Weigh out at least 2 mg of peptide to reduce the relative weighing error.
2. If the peptide contains cysteine residues, degas ultrapure water by vacuum followed by slowly bubbling through helium or argon to avoid oxidation and formation of peptide dimers.
3. If the peptide does not contain aromatic amino acids (Trp, Tyr, Phe, and His) or other similar modifications, the peptide concentration can be estimated based on the absorbance of peptide bond at 205 nm and extinction coefficient 2780 cm^{-1}/M per peptide bond in peptide [25].
4. Hexagonal 200-mesh copper grids with formvar and carbon layer can be purchased from Agar Scientific, EMS and other companies specialized on products for TEM. However, the stability of formvar and carbon coating deteriorates upon storage. Therefore, homemade "fresh" grids are typically more stable and detailed protocol for preparation of formvar and carbon-coated grids is found elsewhere (e.g., www.emsdiasum.com/microscopy/technical/techtips/formvar_film-coated_grids.aspx). We prepare grids with formvar layer of silver color (grey or transparent are too thin and gold too

thick) and 6 nm carbon layer (Leica EM ACE600 high vacuum carbon coater or other).

5. Store the UA stain in the dark at 4 °C and centrifuge before use (4 min, 10,000 × *g*). Stain can be used for 2–3 months.
6. PTA stain yields specimens with lower contrast than UA staining. Still, since UA stain is acidic (pH around 4.5) and might influence the morphology of structures under study; therefore, preferentially stain unstable and sensitive specimens with the neutral PTA solutions in order to avoid artifacts. If the analyzed sample contains phosphates (e.g., PBS) the PTA staining is highly preferable, since UA precipitates in the presence of traces of phosphate.
7. ZEN0118 cuvettes when using Malvern, Zetasizer Nano ZS.
8. DTS1070 cuvettes when using Malvern, Zetasizer Nano ZS.
9. Test the sensitivity of the used dye. For this, dilute nucleic acid cargo in MQ water and in the used solution/buffer. The fluorescent signal should be linear in the range of 0–125% of applied ON concentration used in the nanoparticles. If the signal is too low for detection, increase sensitivity by adding more dye or ON. Start with 0.1–0.5 μg of nucleic acid per 150 μl, and 150-fold dilution of PicoGreen dye.
10. Choose buffer depending on the experiment and required pH. In case when various pH values are required, use the same buffer with different pH-s. Commonly used PBS often leads to aggregation of nanoparticles, therefore 10–20 mM HEPES or MES buffer is more appropriate.
11. Select the protease based on the sequence of used peptides and cleavage sites of enzyme. We prefer Proteinase K since PepFect and NickFect contain multiple aliphatic and aromatic amino acids.
12. Final concentration in the solution is 250 nM for siRNA and 7.5 μM for PF14, and this stock is diluted tenfold with appropriate tissue culture media for cell experiments.
13. The carbon layer deposited on the formvar film has a hydrophobic nature, thus, hydrophilic peptide/ON complexes are repelled from its surface and do not adhere to it upon incubation of the grid on the drop of solution with complexes. In order to make the carbon layer more hydrophilic, the grids are subjected to a brief glow-discharge procedure for 30–60 s (for cleaning, polishing and chemical activation of carbon surface with ionized, plasma-state molecules of air in vacuum), which substantially increases the association of peptide/ON complexes, as well as viruses, exosomes, and other hydrophilic nanoparticles. We use Leica EM ACE600-Carbon Thread Coater equipped with Glow Discharge unit, but any other analogous equipment could be used.

14. Prepare at least two specimens from each sample. Prepare negative control specimen for each series of specimens incubating the grid on the drop of water and staining in parallel with the analyzed samples. Negative control helps to sort out the possible defects in grids and artifacts of stains or staining procedure.

    We also include in series of specimens a positive control, which contains particles formed from PF14 and pDNA in water, and which have a characteristic morphology in electron micro photos.

15. If necessary, wash the specimen on drop of distilled water after drying. This is usually required when the analyzed sample contains buffer or culture media, whose components precipitate upon staining or crystallize during drying. After washing dry the grid again.

16. We use FEI Tecnai G2 Spirit electron microscope (FEI, The Netherlands) at 120 kV accelerating voltage, equipped with Orius SC1000 (Gatan, USA) and Veleta side-mounted CCD camera (Olympus) and record images at 1000 to 50,000-fold magnification depending on the size of observed structures.

17. We typically analyze 600 randomly selected particles from three independent experiments; and estimate the size of particle by measuring the 2D projection area of a particle and calculate the circle equivalent diameter.

18. Switching from intensity to number may vastly over-amplify the small noise in the intensity distribution and lead to erroneous conclusions. Therefore, pay attention to size quality report! On the other hand, the volume contribution of the second peak (e.g., aggregated particles) can be very small, and when transforming from intensity distribution to a volume distribution the second peak disappears. The *Z*-average size can be used if the sample is monomodal/uniform (i.e., only one peak).

19. Zeta-potential cuvettes can also be used for the measurement of hydrodynamic size. In this case dilute the sample up-to 1000 μl with MQ.

20. Air bubbles interfere with the measurement. To remove bubbles, use a pipette.

21. Avoid fingerprints on the cuvette.

22. Calculate the volume of MQ or buffer taking into account the volume of complexes, dye, and proteinase solution. The final volume should not be less than 150 μl per well of 96-well plate.

23. Dilute the stock solution 1:150 to 1:200 shortly before the experiment, and protect from light. Store PicoGreen stocks at −20 °C in freezer and as aliquots for one experiment.

24. Prepare at least 4 parallels from each NP solution, and perform two measurements a minimum. If the number of analyzed samples is low, make 12 parallels and two separate measurements. The optimal amount/concentration of complexes per well should be determined before (*see* **Note 21**), and the amount of dye should be adjusted accordingly.
25. Use a multichannel pipette if the number of samples is high. This is really crucial for the enzyme-adding step.
26. In principle, the time between the addition of PG and measurement should be identical for all samples. However, the signal typically reaches maximum after 5–15 min, that is, before the addition of proteinase.
27. To determine the optimal enzyme concentration in the wells, we suggest to run a pilot experiment with different enzyme concentrations and nanoparticles. Use proteinase K at 1–20 U/ml, as a starting point. If the stability of different analyzed nanocomplexes is low, decrease the enzyme concentration in solution to detect the differences. If the stability of complexes is high, increase the enzyme concentration. However, higher concentration of enzyme will introduce higher scatter since measurement in the last well slightly lags the first, giving the enzyme longer time for cleaving peptide.
28. The interval between the measurement of fluorescence signal and addition of enzyme to each well should be kept constant. The minimal volume of added enzyme solution is 10 μl to reduce the pipetting error. If CPPs in the NPs have similar characteristics, lower the enzyme concentration to discern the differences in stability. If the fluorescence of nucleic acid controls markedly decreases during measurement, decrease the excitation intensity and increase the interval between measurements. (PG dye is considered stable against photobleaching; still its fluorescence might decay upon extended and repeated exposure.)
29. The fluorescence signal of PG from ON released from the nanoparticles may exceed the signal of naked ON control samples, especially, if latter have been measured repeatedly before. After determination of the time-point of the ON release, we suggest to add a new ON control sample for better comparison. Within 6 h, the intensities in ON controls decrease by approximately 10%, leading to possibility of higher signal from ON liberated from NP compared to ON control samples, where PG has been partially bleached.

Acknowledgments

This study was supported by the Estonian Ministry of Education and Research grant 0180019s11, PUT1617P (K.P. and M.P.) and IUT20-26 (L.P. and P.A.) from the Estonian Research Council. The funders had no role in study design, data collection and interpretation, or the decision to submit the work for publication.

References

1. Godfrey C, Desviat LR, Smedsrod B et al (2017) Delivery is key: lessons learnt from developing splice-switching antisense therapies. EMBO Mol Med 9:545–557
2. Aartsma-Rus A (2016) New momentum for the field of oligonucleotide therapeutics. Mol Ther 24:193–194
3. Nikam RR, Gore KR (2018) Journey of siRNA: clinical developments and targeted delivery. Nucleic Acid Ther 28:209–224
4. Kulkarni JA, Cullis PR, van der Meel R (2018) Lipid nanoparticles enabling gene therapies: from concepts to clinical utility. Nucleic Acid Ther 28:146–157
5. Stewart MP, Sharei A, Ding X et al (2016) In vitro and ex vivo strategies for intracellular delivery. Nature 538:183–192
6. Stewart MP, Langer R, Jensen KF (2018) Intracellular delivery by membrane disruption: mechanisms, strategies, and concepts. Chem Rev 118:7409–7531
7. Beierlein JM, McNamee LM, Ledley FD (2017) As technologies for nucleotide therapeutics mature, products emerge. Mol Ther Nucleic Acids 9:379–386
8. Pooga M, Langel Ü (2015) Classes of cell-penetrating peptides. Methods Mol Biol 1324:3–28
9. Lehto T, Ezzat K, Wood MJA et al (2016) Peptides for nucleic acid delivery. Adv Drug Deliv Rev 106:172–182
10. Margus H, Padari K, Pooga M (2012) Cell-penetrating peptides as versatile vehicles for oligonucleotide delivery. Mol Ther 20:525–533
11. Arukuusk P, Pärnaste L, Hällbrink M et al (2015) PepFects and NickFects for the intracellular delivery of nucleic acids. Methods Mol Biol 1324:303–315
12. Veiman KL, Mäger I, Ezzat K et al (2013) PepFect14 peptide vector for efficient gene delivery in cell cultures. Mol Pharm 10:199–210
13. Ezzat K, Helmfors H, Tudoran O et al (2012) Scavenger receptor-mediated uptake of cell-penetrating peptide nanocomplexes with oligonucleotides. FASEB J 26:1172–1180
14. Andaloussi SE, Lehto T, Mäger I et al (2011) Design of a peptide-based vector, PepFect6, for efficient delivery of siRNA in cell culture and systemically in vivo. Nucleic Acids Res 39:3972–3987
15. Urgard E, Lorents A, Klaas M et al (2016) Pre-administration of PepFect6-microRNA-146a nanocomplexes inhibits inflammatory responses in keratinocytes and in a mouse model of irritant contact dermatitis. J Control Release 235:195–204
16. Margus H, Arukuusk P, Langel Ü et al (2016) Characteristics of cell-penetrating peptide/nucleic acid nanoparticles. Mol Pharm 13:172–179
17. Herd H, Daum N, Jones AT et al (2013) Nanoparticle geometry and surface orientation influence mode of cellular uptake. ACS Nano 7:1961–1973
18. Kulkarni JA, Darjuan MM, Mercer JE et al (2018) On the formation and morphology of lipid nanoparticles containing ionizable cationic lipids and siRNA. ACS Nano 12:4787–4795
19. De Carlo S, Harris JR (2011) Negative staining and cryo-negative staining of macromolecules and viruses for TEM. Micron 42:117–131
20. Philo JS (2006) Is any measurement method optimal for all aggregate sizes and types? AAPS J 8:E564–E571
21. Domingues MM, Santiago PS, Castanho MA et al (2008) What can light scattering spectroscopy do for membrane-active peptide studies? J Pept Sci 14:394–400
22. Borm PJ, Robbins D, Haubold S et al (2006) The potential risks of nanomaterials: a review carried out for ECETOC. Part Fibre Toxicol 3:11
23. Pärnaste L, Arukuusk P, Langel K et al (2017) The formation of nanoparticles between small interfering RNA and amphipathic cell-penetrating peptides. Mol Ther Nucleic Acids 7:1–10

24. Freimann K, Arukuusk P, Kurrikoff K et al (2018) Formulation of stable and homogeneous cell-penetrating peptide NF55 nanoparticles for efficient gene delivery in vivo. Mol Ther Nucleic Acids 10:28–35

25. Anthis NJ, Clore GM (2013) Sequence-specific determination of protein and peptide concentrations by absorbance at 205 nm. Protein Sci 22:851–858

Chapter 8

Click-Shielded and Targeted Lipopolyplexes

Philipp Michael Klein and Ernst Wagner

Abstract

Lipopolyplexes present well-established nucleic acid carriers assembled from sequence-defined cationic lipo-oligomers and DNA or RNA. They can be equipped with additional surface functionality, like shielding and targeting, in a stepwise assembly method using click chemistry. Here, we describe the synthesis of the required compounds, an azide-bearing lipo-oligomer structure and dibenzocyclooctyne (DBCO) click agents as well as the assembly of the compounds with siRNA into a surface-functionalized formulation. Both the lipo-oligomer and the DBCO-equipped shielding and targeting agents are produced by solid-phase synthesis (SPS). This enables for precise variation of all functional units, like variation in the amount of DBCO attachment sites or polyethylene glycol (PEG) length. Special cleavage conditions with only 5% trifluoroacetic acid (TFA) must be applied for the synthesis of the shielding and targeting agents due to acid lability of the DBCO unit. The two-step lipopolyplex assembly technique allows for separate optimization of the core and the shell of the formulation.

Key words Click chemistry, Solid phase synthesis, Dibenzocyclooctyne (DBCO), Surface functionalization, Lipopolyplexes, Nanoparticles, Nucleic acid delivery, Gene silencing

1 Introduction

Therapeutic nucleic acids like plasmid DNA (pDNA), microRNA (miRNA), and small interfering RNA (siRNA) offer new opportunities in medical development [1–3]. All these nucleic acids need to enter the cell to show effect. While RNA interference is mediated by cytosolic delivery of miRNA or synthetic siRNA [4, 5], pDNA needs to enter the nucleus. Efficient delivery of nucleic acids, however, still presents a major hurdle for successful clinical application [6, 7]. Negatively charged nucleic acids are larger than conventional drugs and quickly degraded and cleared from the systemic circulation. Therefore, bioresponsive carriers are required, addressing specific extracellular and intracellular barriers in the nucleic acid delivery pathway [8–10].

Cationic lipids or lipo-oligomers present a class of carriers for nucleic acids, which assemble into lipopolyplexes simply upon mixing. The driving force for the assembly is intermolecular

Olof Gissberg et al. (eds.), *Oligonucleotide-Based Therapies: Methods and Protocols*, Methods in Molecular Biology, vol. 2036, https://doi.org/10.1007/978-1-4939-9670-4_8, © Springer Science+Business Media, LLC, part of Springer Nature 2019

hydrophobic and electrostatic interactions. Such cationic amphipathic carriers provide high transfection efficacy and high polyplex stability [11–15].

Precise editing of the chemical structure enables the stepwise optimization of nucleic acid carrier systems [16–19]. Solid phase synthesis (SPS) presents a convenient tool to create monodisperse cationic oligomers by connecting artificial oligoamino acids, natural α-amino acids, and fatty acids sequentially together [20–22]. Thereby, huge libraries with oligomers varying in functional moieties can be set up to systemically evaluate structure activity relations. [16–18, 23–29].

Advanced carrier systems are equipped with shielding domains and ligands to target specific disease tissues, such as cancer cells [30]. There are different ways to integrate those functions into delivery systems. Direct incorporation into a carrier during synthesis of the structure (prefunctionalization) is one option. [18, 20]. In this case, the additional domain of the carrier might influence the formation of polyplexes with nucleic acids. Shielding domains separate units during assembly resulting in smaller or less dense particles with only one nucleic acid incorporated [23, 31–33]. Whereas this effect might be preferable for in vivo application of huge nucleic acids like pDNA, it can also be a disadvantage for systemic circulation of small nucleic acids, like siRNA. A folate targeted mono-siRNA formulation with a hydrodynamic diameter of ~6 nm, for instance, was reported to show efficient gene silencing in vitro and after intratumoral injection, but was rapidly cleared by the kidney a few minutes after systemic injection [23]. The exclusion of the shielding domain and precise integration of hydrophobic domains enables the cationic structures to form multi-siRNA polyplexes, which are quite homogeneous in size (100–200 nm) [27, 34].

For the attachment of the targeting functionality after the core polyplex formation (post-functionalization) an anchor-point is required. Functional groups of cationic oligomers, like thiols or amines, are suitable to attach agents via reactive linkers [35–38]. Thereby, shielding and targeting functions are solely placed on the surface of the formulation. A more advanced linking strategy presents the use of click chemistry, which is orthogonal to all other functional units of a core oligomer [39, 40]. The click anchor, for instance an azide, can precisely be positioned into an established structures, like the sequence-defined T-shaped bis-(cholanic acid amido) oligoaminoamide (ID: ***1106*** [39]) via SPS. Copper-free strain-promoted alkyne-azide cycloaddition (SPAAC) is then used to equip the lipopolyplex surface with a cyclooctine-functionaliced (for example dibenzocyclooctyne (DBCO)) shielding agent optionally with targeting domain, for instance the ligand folate [39]. The orthogonal nature of this click reaction prevents inadvertent effects such as side reactions with amines or thiols of body compounds or the siRNA polyplex.

By using SPS for creating the nanoparticle surface functionalizing agents and the core structures, separate libraries of (1) defined click agents varying in features like polyethylene glycol (PEG) lengths, number of attachment sites (click and double-click agents) and (2) multifunctional cationic core structures can be synthesized with precision (Fig. 1) [39]. Due to acid lability of the DBCO unit, certain cleavage conditions with only 5% trifluoroacetic acid (TFA) are required to ensure functionality.

The click-functionalized polyplexes differ in their physical and biological properties which are strongly influenced by the applied surface-functionalizing agent [39, 40]. Thereby, parameters like size and stability, receptor targeting and gene silencing activity, or the distribution profile in vivo after systemic application (Fig. 2) can be tuned to develop therapeutically active formulations [39].

Here, we describe the SPS of the azide containing core-forming structure ***1106*** and eight DBCO click agents for surface functionalization. We present a method for the assembly of the compounds into siRNA formulations and two basic methods for physical characterization. The current chapter does not describe methods for testing bioactivity of siRNA lipopolyplexes formed with the described reagents. Core lipopolyplexes can be tested for in vitro gene silencing activity analogously to commercial available transfection agents under optimized conditions, such as long-term (48 h) incubations [22]. Note, however, that the advantageous properties of targeted core/shell lipopolyplexes over standard transfection agents will be apparent under special test conditions, such as short term in vitro transfection to highlight receptor targeting or systemic in vivo administration in receptor-positive tumor models as described in [35, 36, 38, 39, 41, 42].

2 Materials

2.1 Solid-Phase Assisted Synthesis (SPS) and Purification of Oligomers and DBCO Agents

Use solvents and reagents of high purity (e.g., peptide grade) for all experiments.

The SPS can be carried out manually or with a semiautomated or an automated peptide synthesizer. Here we describe the method for manual synthesis.

1. Syringe micro reactors with polyethylene filters (Multisyntech GmbH, Witten Germany) (*see* **Note 1**).
2. Overhead shaker (*see* **Note 2**).
3. Solid support: 2-chlorotrityl chloride resin (Iris Biotech, Marktredewitz, Germany).

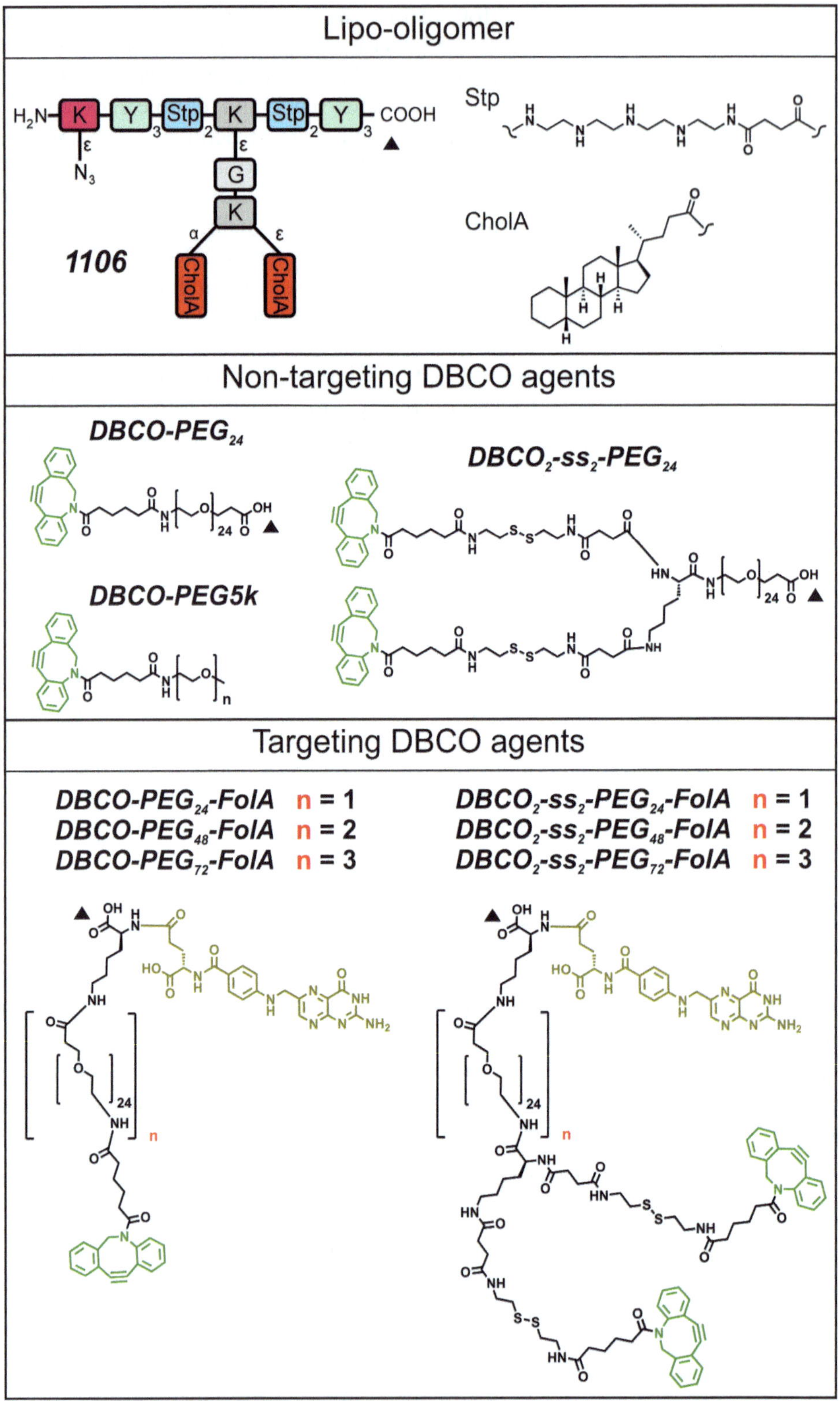

Fig. 1 Overview of chemical compounds. Top: schematic illustration of the sequence-defined oligomer ***1106***. Units of the oligomer: *Y* tyrosine, *K* lysine, *G* glycine, *Stp* succinoyl-tetraethylene-pentamine, *CholA*

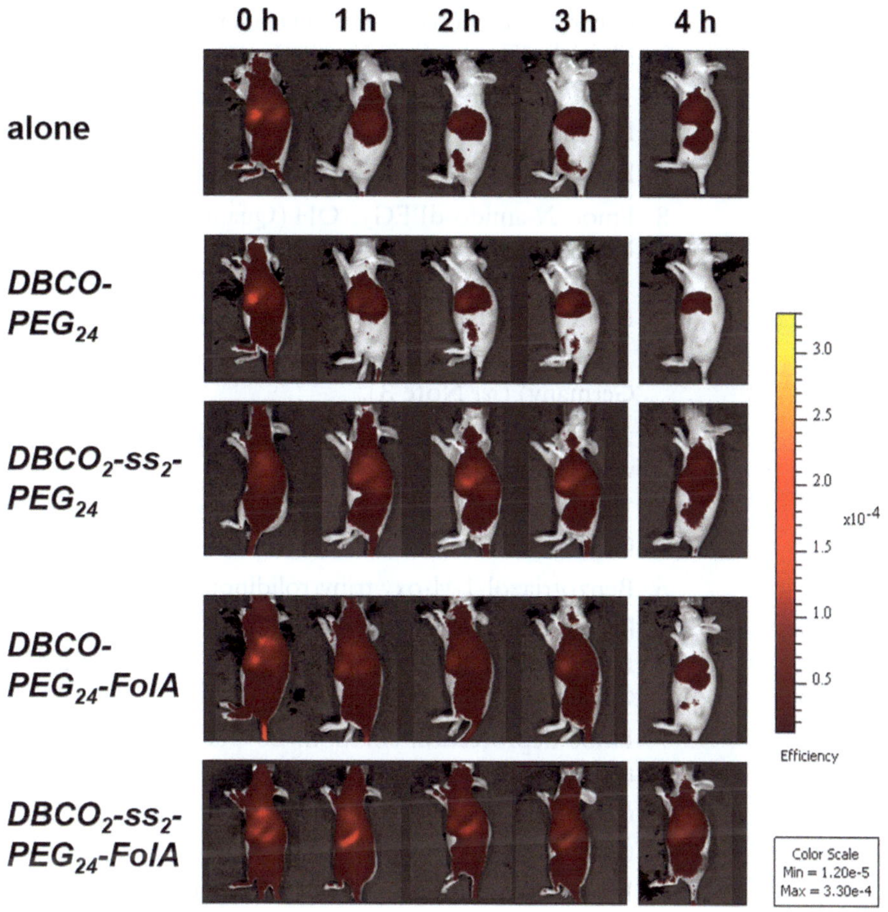

Fig. 2 Biodistribution of ***1106*** siRNA formulations at *N/P* 10 in L1210 tumor-bearing NMRI nude mice after *i. v.* administration. Biodistribution determined by NIR fluorescence bioimaging of 50 μg siRNA (50% Cy7-labeled siRNA) with ***1106*** siRNA polyplexes without shield or surface-modified with 0.5 eq of monovalent and bivalent DBCO agents. Experiments were performed with three animals per group for time points until 1 h, one animal per group for time points 2 h and 3 h and two animals for the 4 h time point. A representative animal of each group is shown. Animals are presented in lateral view. Adapted from (Klein et al., Biomaterials, 2018 [39]) with permission from Elsevier

2.1.1 Amino Acids and Building Blocks

1. Fmoc-Gly-OH, Fmoc-L-Lys(Dde)-OH, Fmoc-L-Lys(Fmoc)-OH, Fmoc-L-Lys(N_3)-OH, and Fmoc-L-Tyr(tBu)-OH (Iris Biotech, Marktredwitz, Germany).
2. Fmoc-Stp(Boc_3)-OH (synthesis described in [43]).
3. Fmoc-succinoylcystamine-OH (synthesis described in [27]).
4. 5β-Cholanic acid (CholA) (Sigma-Aldrich, Munich, Germany).

Fig. 1 (continued) 5β-cholanic acid. The ID ***1106*** is the internal database identification number. Middle: structures of SPS-synthesized, monovalent and bivalent, nontargeted DBCO agents with short PEG_{24}; structure of nontargeted, commercially available ***DBCO-PEG5k*** with a ~5 kDa PEG chain. Bottom: structures of monovalent and bivalent, folate-targeted agents varying in PEG length (PEG_{24}, PEG_{48}, and PEG_{72}). The triangle (▲) indicates the starting point for SPS syntheses. Reproduced from (Klein et al., Biomaterials, 2018 [39]) with permission from Elsevier

5. Dibenzocyclooctyne-acid (DBCO acid) (Sigma-Aldrich, Munich, Germany).
6. N^{10}-(Trifluoroacetyl)pteroic acid (Clauson-Kass A/S, Farum, Denmark).
7. Fmoc-L-Glu-O-2-PhiPr (VWR, Darmstadt, Germany).
8. Fmoc-*N*-amido-dPEG$_{24}$-OH (Quanta Biodesign Powell, OH, USA).

2.1.2 Reagents and Solvents

1. Dichloromethane (DCM) (Bernd Kraft, Duisburg, Germany).
2. *N,N*-Dimethylformamide (DMF) (Iris Biotech, Marktredwitz, Germany) (*see* **Note 3**).
3. *N,N*-Diisopropylethylamine (DIPEA) (Iris Biotech, Marktredwitz, Germany).
4. 1-Hydroxybenzotriazole (HOBt) (Sigma-Aldrich, Munich, Germany).
5. Benzotriazol-1-yl-oxy tripyrrolidinophosphonium hexafluorophosphate (Pybop®) (Multisyntech, Witten, Germany).
6. Di-*tert*-butyl dicarbonate (Boc$_2$O) (Sigma-Aldrich, Munich, Germany).
7. Fmoc-deprotection solution: 20% (v/v) piperidine (Iris Biotech, Marktredwitz, Germany)/DMF.
8. Capping solution: 80:15:5 (v/v/v) DCM–methanol (MeOH)–DIPEA.
9. Kaiser test solution 1: 80% (w/v) phenol in ethanol (EtOH).
10. Kaiser test solution 2: 5% (w/v) ninhydrin in EtOH.
11. Kaiser test solution 3: 20 μM sodium cyanide (KCN) in pyridine (2 mL of 1 mM KCN (aq) in 98 mL of pyridine).
12. Dde-deprotection solution: 2% (v/v) hydrazine monohydrate (Sigma-Aldrich, Munich, Germany) in DMF.
13. TFA deprotection solution: 50:50 (v/v) ammonia solution 25% (Carl Roth, Karlsruhe, Germany)–DMF.
14. DIPEA washing solution: 10% (v/v) DIPEA in DMF.
15. Cleavage cocktail for cationizable oligomers: 95:2.5:2.5 (v/v/v) trifluoroacetic acid (TFA)–triisopropylsilane (TIS)–dH$_2$O.
16. Cleavage cocktail for DBCO agents: 92.5:5:2.5 (v/v/v) DCM–trifluoroacetic acid (TFA)–triisopropylsilane (TIS).
17. Precipitating solution for cationizable oligomers: 50:50 (v/v) methyl *tert*-butyl ether (MTBE)–n-hexane.
18. Precipitating solution for DBCO agents: 25:75 (v/v) methyl *tert*-butyl ether (MTBE)–*n*-hexane.
19. Sodium hydroxide (NaOH) 0.05 M solution.
20. Liquid nitrogen (N$_2$).

2.1.3 Size Exclusion Chromatography of Oligomers

1. Size exclusion column: Tricorn 10/600 column packed with Sephadex G-10 gel filtration resin.
2. Äkta Basic System with fraction collector.
3. Size exclusion running buffer: 70:30 (v/v) 10 mM hydrochloric acid (HCl)–acetonitrile (ACN).

2.1.4 Dialysis of DBCO Agents

1. Spectra/Por 6 Dialysis Membrane, Prewetted RC Tubing MWCO: 1 kDa by Spectrum Labs.
2. Deionized water (dH_2O).

2.2 Analysis of Oligomers and DBCO Agents

2.2.1 Proton ^1H NMR Spectroscopy

1. AVANCE III HD 500 (500 MHz) NMR spectrometer with a 5 mm CPPBBO probe.
2. Deuterium oxide (D_2O).
3. MestreNova (Ver. 9.0 by MestReLab Research).

2.2.2 MALDI Mass Spectrometry

1. Autoflex II MALDI mass spectrometer (Bruker Daltonics, Bremen, Germany).
2. MTP AnchorChip (Bruker Daltonics, Bremen, Germany).
3. sDHB matrix solution: 10 mg/mL sDHB (90:10 (m/m) mixture of 2,5-dihydroxybenzoic acid and 2-hydroxy-5-methoxybenzoic acid) in 70:30:0.1% (v/v/v) dH2O–ACN–TFA.

2.3 Polyplex Formation and Functionalization

2.3.1 Core Polyplex Formation

1. Synthesized oligomer.
2. Ready-to-use siRNA duplex (Axolabs GmbH, Kulmbach, Germany):

   Control siRNA (siCtrl) (sense: 5′-AuGuAuuGGccuGuAuu AGdTsdT-3′; antisense: 5′-CuAAuAcAGGCcAAuAcA UdTsdT-3′) (*see* **Note 4**),

   Small letters: 2′methoxy; s: phosphorothioate.
3. HBG buffer: 5% (w/v) glucose in 20 mM HEPES buffer, pH 7.4.

2.3.2 Functionalization of Polyplex with DBCO Agents

1. Synthesized DBCO agent.
2. HBG buffer (*see* Subheading 2.3.1).

2.4 Biophysical Polyplex Characterization

2.4.1 Agarose Gel Shift Assay for sRNA Polyplexes

1. TBE buffer: 89 mM Tris, 89 mM boric acid, 2 mM ethylenediaminetetraacetic acid disodium salt (EDTA-Na_2) in dH_2O, pH 8.0.
2. Electrophoresis 6× loading buffer: 6 mL of glycerol, 1.2 mL of 0.5 M EDTA-Na_2 solution, pH 8.0, 2.8 mL of dH_2O, 20 mg of bromophenol blue.

3. Agarose NEEO Ultra (Carl Roth GmbH, Karlsruhe, Germany).
4. Gel electrophoresis chamber.
5. GelRed (VWR, Darmstadt, Germany).
6. Dark hood DH-40 with UV transilluminator (Biostep, Burkhardtsdorf, Germany).

2.4.2 Size Measurement Via DLS and Determination of ζ-Potential

1. Zetasizer Nano ZS with backscattering detection and folded capillary cells (Malvern Instruments, Worcestershire, UK).
2. 10 mM sodium chloride (NaCl) solution.

3 Methods

3.1 Solid-Phase Assisted Synthesis (SPS) and Purification of Oligomers and DBCO Agents

SPS is a convenient method for synthesizing defined oligomer structures. A defined chemical structure facilitate the establishment of structure–activity relationships and thereby the rational design and optimization of nucleic acid carriers. The synthesis of the oligomers, as well as the incorporation of the azide function, is carried out by standard Fmoc-SPS following repetitive synthesis cycles (Fig. 3a).

A 2-chlorotrityl chloride resin is used as solid support and loaded with the first amino acid (*see* Subheading 3.1.1). Based on the number of free amines, four equivalents of Fmoc-protected amino acid or another SPS-compatible in combination with also four equivalents of HOBt and PyBOP are used for coupling (unless otherwise stated). DIPEA is added as an auxiliary base with eight equivalents in relation to the free amines. All coupling reagents are dissolved in 50:50 (v/v) DCM–DMF (10 mL/g resin) and mixed for preactivation before adding them to the resin. Couplings are carried out for 90 min at room temperature (RT) using an overhead shaker (*see* **Note 2** for alternative methods). Fmoc deprotection is accomplished by incubating the resin 4 times for 10 min with 20% (v/v) piperidine/DMF (10 mL/g resin).

After each coupling and Fmoc deprotection step, the resin is washed three times with DMF and three times with DCM (10 mL/g of resin). Sufficient coupling and Fmoc deprotection are verified by qualitative detection of free amines by Kaiser test (*see* Subheading 3.1.2) [44]. In case of a positive result of the Kaiser test after coupling, the last coupling step is repeated. In case of a negative result after deprotection, the last deprotection step is redone (Fig. 3a). After the last coupling, the cleavage from the resin is performed. The composition of the cleavage cocktail needs to be adjusted for the respective compound to ensure complete deprotection of side chain protection groups and functionality of the agent (Fig. 3b—*see* Subheadings 3.1.3 and 3.1.4 for details).

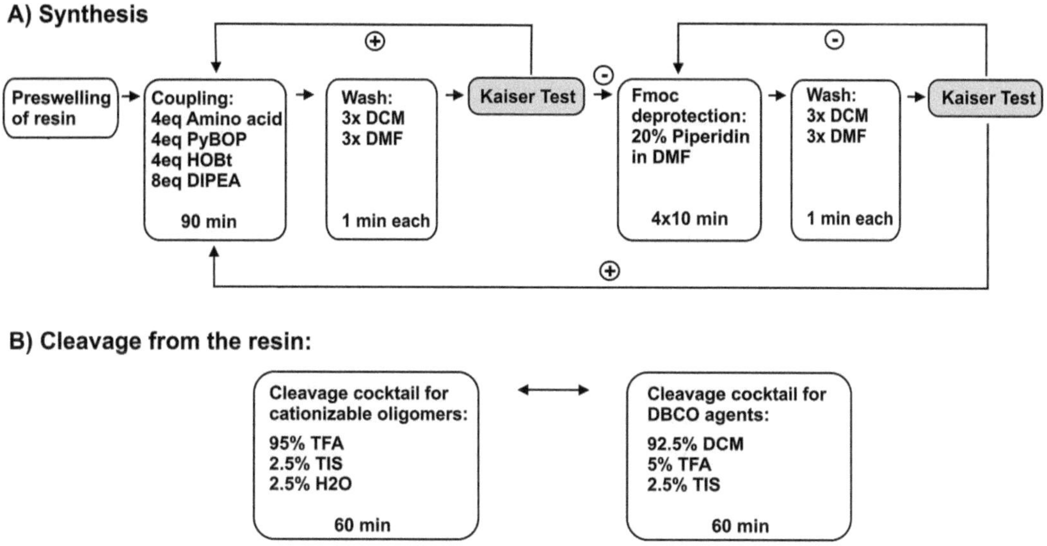

Fig. 3 (**a**) Standard procedure of a solid phase synthesis cycle. (**b**) Different conditions for the cleavage from the resin. Reproduced and modified from (Morys et al., Methods in Molecular Biology, 2016 [21]) with permission from Springer

3.1.1 Resin Loading and Deprotection

1. Place 0.75 g of 2-chlorotrityl chloride resin (1.2 mmol chloride) in a 10 mL syringe reactor (*see* **Note 1**).
2. Swell the resin by shaking for approximately 20 min in 5 mL of water-free DCM (*see* **Note 5**).
3. Discard the DCM.
4. Dissolve 0.35 mmol of the first Fmoc-amino acid, (Fmoc-L-Tyr (tBu)-OH for ***1106***; Fmoc-L-Lys(Dde)-OH or Fmoc-*N*-amido-dPEG$_{24}$-OH for DBCO agents) and 0.7 mmol of DIPEA in 5 mL of dry DCM.
5. Add the amino acid solution from **step 4** to the resin and shake for 60 min.
6. Discard the amino acid solution from **step 5** and add 5 mL of the capping solution for at least 30 min to block remaining active chloride groups on the resin.
7. Discard the capping solution from **step 6** and wash three times with DMF and three times with DCM (5 mL each).
8. Dry the resin under high vacuum and weight triplicate samples (between 5 and 10 mg each) into polystyrene microcentrifuge tubes.
9. Add 1 mL of Fmoc-deprotection solution to the samples and incubate for 90 min at RT in a vortexing unit (*see* **Note 6**).

10. Take 25 μL of the supernatant and dilute it by adding 975 μL DMF.
11. Vortex and calculate the resin loading based on the absorbance at $\lambda = 301$ nm against a blank deprotection solution consisting of 25 μL Fmoc-deprotection solution and 975 μL DMF (*see* **Notes 7** and **8**).
12. Incubate the resin four times for 10 min with 5 mL of Fmoc-deprotection solution.
13. Wash the resin three times with DMF and 3 times with DCM (5 mL each) and perform a Kaiser test.
14. In case of a positive Kaiser test result, dry the resin at high vacuum and store well sealed to exclude air and moisture. In case of a negative Kaiser test result, repeat **step 12** and **13**.

3.1.2 Kaiser Test

1. Transfer a few beads of resin into a polystyrene microcentrifuge tube and add one drop of each Kaiser test solution.
2. Vortex and spin down quickly.
3. Incubate at 100 °C for 4 min. A positive reaction can occur within the first seconds of the incubation time. Blue color indicates free amines.

3.1.3 SPS of Azide-Bearing Oligomer 1106

Here, the synthesis of the azide-bearing, t-shaped lipo-oligomer *1106* is described (*see* **Note 9**).

1. Take the required amount of preloaded L-Tyr(tBu)-OH resin and transfer into the corresponding reactor. A resin amount equivalent to 20 μmol is used for a standard synthesis.
2. Swell the resin for 30 min with 10 mL/g of DCM.
3. Synthesize the linear backbone of the oligomer by sequential coupling (*see* **Note 2** and Fig. 3) and deprotection of two Fmoc-L-Tyr(tBu)-OH amino acids. Continue with two Fmoc-Stp(Boc_3)-OH, one Fmoc-L-Lys(Dde)-OH, two Fmoc-Stp(Boc_3)-OH, three Fmoc-L-Tyr(tBu)-OH and end with a Fmoc-L-Lys(N_3)-OH coupling and deprotection steps.
4. Protect the *N*-terminal amine function of the linear backbone with 10 eq Di-*tert*-butyl dicarbonate (Boc_2O) and 10 eq DIPEA.
5. For Dde deprotection, freshly prepare the Dde-deprotection solution with 2% (v/v) hydrazine hydroxide solution in DMF and apply 5 mL/g of resin and vortex for 2 min. Repeat 15 deprotection cycles and exchange the Dde-deprotection solution after each cycle (*see* **Note 10**).

6. Wash the resin 5 times with DIPEA washing solution, 3 times with DMF and 3 times with DCM (10 mL/g of resin).
7. Continue with the synthesis by coupling and deprotecting Fmoc-Gly-OH and a branching Fmoc-L-Lys(Fmoc)-OH. From this step on, the number of free amines is doubled (*see* **Note 11**).
8. Attach the hydrophobic 5β-Cholanic acid. No Fmoc-deprotection is required after coupling and washing.
9. Dry the resins on high vacuum for approximately 30 min.
10. Prepare the cleavage cocktail for cationizable oligomers and cool the solution to 4 °C (*see* **Note 12**).
11. Apply 10 mL/g of cleavage solution for 1 h at RT while shaking.
12. Precipitate the oligomers by adding the cleavage solution dropwise into 50 mL of ice-cold precipitating solution for cationizable oligomers.
13. Centrifuge for 10 min (4000 × *g*-force (RCF), 4 °C), discard the supernatant and dry the precipitate under nitrogen (N_2) stream.
14. Dissolve the obtained product in 1 mL size exclusion running buffer and purify it by size exclusion chromatography. Collect the first major peak (A214, A280) (*see* **Note 13**).
15. Pool the product containing fractions into a tared 15 mL tube, freeze with liquid nitrogen (N_2) and lyophilize.
16. Determine the product yield by balancing and analyze the samples by ^{1}H-NMR (*see* Subheading 3.2.1 and **Note 14**) and MALDI mass spectrometry (*see* Subheading 3.2.2 and **Note 15**).
17. Store the obtained HCl salts of the oligomers (*see* **Note 16**) dry or as stock solutions tightly sealed under argon at −20 °C (*see* **Notes 17** and **18**).

3.1.4 SPS of DBCO Agents

Due to the acid sensitive nature of DBCO, the complete solid-phase synthesis of DBCO-bearing agents is only possible if a certain concentration of TFA in the cleavage cocktail is not exceeded. For this reason, the cleavage is performed at only 5% of TFA and protecting groups can only be used if they can be deprotected under these mild conditions.

1. Take the required amount of preloaded L-Lys(Dde)-OH or *N*-amido-dPEG$_{24}$-OH resin and transfer into the corresponding reactor. A resin amount equivalent to 10 μmol is used for a standard synthesis.

2. Swell the resin for 30 min with 10 mL/g of DCM.
3. For the control structures, sequentially couple and deprotect the indicated amino acids at the corresponding resin:
   (a) For ***DBCO-PEG$_{24}$*** attach DBCO acid at a *N*-amido-dPEG$_{24}$-OH resin using 3 eq of DBCO acid and coupling agent and 6 eq of DIPEA.
   (b) For ***DBCO$_2$-ss$_2$-PEG$_{24}$*** couple and deprotect Fmoc-L-Lys (Fmoc)-OH at a *N*-amido-dPEG$_{24}$-OH resin. From this step on, the number of free amines is doubled (*see* **Note 11**). Couple and deprotect Fmoc-succinoylcystamine-OH. Do not use 1-hydroxybenzotriazole hydrate for this and the following step. Attach DBCO acid using 3 eq of DBCO acid and coupling agent and 6 eq of DIPEA per amine.
   (c) For ***DBCO-PEG$_x$-FolA*** couple and deprotect Fmoc-Glu-O-2-PhiPr at a L-Lys(Dde)-OH resin. Dissolve N^{10}-(trifluoroacetyl)pteroic acid in DMF and couple it using standard conditions. For Dde deprotection, freshly prepare the Dde-deprotection solution, apply 5 mL/g of resin and vortex for 2 min. Repeat 15 deprotection cycles and exchange the Dde-deprotection solution after each cycle (*see* **Note 10**). Wash the resin five times with DIPEA washing solution, three times with DMF, and three times with DCM (10 mL/g of resin). Repeat the coupling and deprotection of *N*-amido-dPEG$_{24}$-OH according to the number of PEG units in the agent (for PEG$_{24}$ once, for PEG$_{48}$ twice and for PEG$_{72}$ three times). Treat the resin with 25% TFA deprotection solution four times for 30 min. Wash with DMF for 1 min in between each step. Attach DBCO acid using 3 eq of DBCO acid and coupling agent and 6 eq of DIPEA.
   (d) For ***DBCO$_2$-ss$_2$-PEG$_x$-FolA*** couple and deprotect Fmoc-Glu-O-2-PhiPr at a L-Lys(Dde)-OH resin. Dissolve N^{10}-(trifluoroacetyl)pteroic acid in DMF and couple it using standard conditions. For Dde deprotection, freshly prepare the Dde-deprotection solution, apply 5 mL/g of resin and vortex for 2 min. Repeat 15 deprotection cycles and exchange the Dde-deprotection solution after each cycle (*see* **Note 10**). Wash the resin five times with DIPEA washing solution, three times with DMF and three times with DCM (10 mL/g of resin). Repeat the coupling and deprotection of *N*-amido-dPEG$_{24}$-OH according to the number of PEG units in the agent (for PEG$_{24}$ once, for PEG$_{48}$ twice and for PEG$_{72}$ three times). Couple and deprotect Fmoc-L-Lys(Fmoc)-OH. From this step on, the number of free amines is doubled (*see* **Note 11**).

Treat the resin with 25% TFA deprotection solution four times for 30 min. Wash with DMF for 1 min in between each step and three times with DMF and three times with DCM (10 mL/g of resin) after the last treatment. Dissolve Fmoc-succinoylcystamine-OH in DMF and couple and deprotect it. Do not use 1-Hydroxybenzotriazole hydrate for this and the following step. Attach DBCO acid using 3 eq of DBCO acid and coupling agent and 6 eq of DIPEA per amine.

4. Dry the resins on high vacuum for approximately 30 min.
5. Prepare the cleavage cocktail for DBCO agents and cool the solution to 4 °C (*see* **Note 12**).
6. Apply 10 mL/g of cleavage solution for 1 h at RT while shaking.
7. Precipitate the oligomers by adding the cleavage solution dropwise into 50 mL of ice-cold precipitating solution for DBCO agents.
8. Centrifuge for 10 min (4000 × *g*-force (RCF) 4 °C), discard the supernatant and dry the precipitate under nitrogen (N_2) stream.
9. Dissolve the obtained product in 1 mL 0.05 M NaOH solution and adjust the pH to 7.
10. Carefully wash a tubular Spectra/Por 6 Dialysis Membrane MWCO: 1 kDa with deionized water (dH_2O), lock one side with a clamp, fill the tube with the dissolved DBCO agent and lock the other side with a second clamp.
11. Dialyze the sample against 5 L dH_2O for 16 h at 4 ° C.
12. Pipet the dialyzed product out of the tubular membrane into a suitable tube, freeze with liquid N_2 and lyophilize.
13. Determine the product yield by balancing and analyze the samples by MALDI mass spectrometry (*see* Subheading 3.2.2 and **Note 15**).
14. Store the obtained Na^+ salts of the oligomers (*see* **Note 16**) dry or as stock solutions tightly sealed under argon at −20 °C (*see* **Notes 17** and **18**).

3.2 Analytics of Azide-Bearing Cationic Oligomer and DBCO Agents

The identity and the integrity of the compounds are of utmost importance. Nuclear magnetic resonance (NMR) spectroscopy is a well-established method to confirm the identity of chemical structures. Further, mass spectrometry presents a convenient method to confirm the identity of sequence defined structures. Especially for the susceptible DBCO group it is important to show functionality. By mixing azide and DBCO agents, the conjugated product can be detected by mass spectrometry demonstrating the intactness of both compounds (*see* **Note 19**).

3.2.1 Proton ^1H NMR Spectroscopy

1. Dissolve the compound at a concentration of 10 mg/mL in D_2O.
2. Insert at least 6 mL of the solution in a NMR tube.
3. Record the ^1H NMR spectrum at room temperature (300 MHz).
4. Use the residual proton signal of the deuterium oxide (D_2O) solvent as internal standard (D_2O at 4.79).
5. Analyze spectra using MestreNova NMR Software.

3.2.2 MALDI Mass Spectrometry

1. Prepare the sample solution at a concentration of 1 mg/mL in dH_2O. For evaluation of the intactness of azide and DBCO compounds, prepare an equimolar mixture (or slight excess of one compound, to focus on one functional group) at a concentration of ~10 mg/mL in dH_2O and dilute it to 1 mg/mL with dH_2O after 16 h reaction time.
2. One μL of sDHB matrix solution is spotted on the AnchorChip.
3. After the sDHB matrix has crystallized, 1 μL of the sample solution (1 mg/mL in water) is added to the matrix spot.
4. Samples are recorded by mass spectrometry in positive or negative ion mode.

3.3 Polyplex Formation and Functionalization

3.3.1 Core Polyplex Formation

Formation of lipopolyplexes spontaneously occurs due to electrostatic and hydrophobic interactions upon mixing of negatively charged nucleic acids with positively charged lipo-oligomers (Fig. 4). Nucleic acid binding and stability of the resulting lipopolyplexes is highly dependent on the ratio of oligomers to nucleic acid. The N/P value is frequently used to describe the ratio between amines (N) of the oligomer and phosphates (P) of nucleic acid in the formulation (*see* **Note 20**).

1. Prepare a stock solution of 0.5 μg of siRNA per μL HBG.
2. Dilute the calculated amount of oligomer with HBG to a concentration desired to yield the respective N/P (*see* **Note 21**).

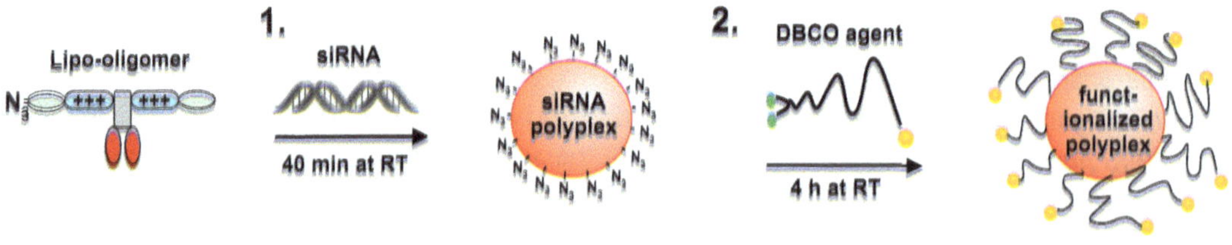

Fig. 4 Formulation of a functionalized polyplex: the azido-bearing lipo-oligomer ***1106*** was mixed with siRNA and incubated for 40 min at room temperature. Then a DBCO agent was added and the solution was incubated for 4 h. Reproduced and modified from (Klein et al., Biomaterials, 2018 [39]) with permission from Elsevier

3. Add the siRNA to the oligomer solution and mix five times by rapid pipetting.
4. Incubate the solution for 40 min at room temperature.

3.3.2 Functionalization of Polyplexes with DBCO Agents

Formation of polyplexes with azide-bearing oligomers results in polyplexes that can further be surface functionalized via strain-promoted azide-alkyne cycloaddition (SPAAC) reaction, for instance by using DBCO agents (Fig. 4).

1. Calculate the required amount of DBCO agent (*see* **Note 16**) according to corresponding equivalents (eq). Equivalents represent the molar ratio of DBCO agents to azide-oligomer.
2. Dilute the calculated amount of DBCO agent with HBG buffer to ¼ of the volume of the previously prepared polyplex solution (*see* Subheading 3.3).
3. Add the DBCO agent solution to the polyplex solution and mix five times by rapid pipetting.
4. Incubate the mixture for 4 h.

3.4 Biophysical Polyplex Characterization

Biophysical properties of polyplexes are important regarding their stability and possible interactions with biological constituents, fluids and membranes, thereby influencing their efficiency and safety. Nucleic acid binding and polyplex stability can be screened by agarose gel retardation assays with or without serum. Negatively charged siRNA migrates in an electric field unless the nucleic acid is complexed by the cationic lipo-oligomers. Upon complexation, the electrophoretic mobility is reduced or even reversed due to loss of negative charge and increased size. The agarose gel shift assay is used to evaluate the ability of the lipo-oligomers to bind siRNA as well as to determine the minimum required *N/P* ratio for complete nucleic acid binding. In case of surface-functionalized polyplexes, the migratory behavior in an agarose gel is sometimes changed. Slight shifts toward the cathode or the anode might be noticed depending on the terminal charge of the surface-functionalizing agent (*see* **Note 22**) [39, 40]. Polyplexes can be exposed to 90% full serum at 37 °C for several hours before electrophoresis, which can be an indicative assay for extracellular stability [39]. Polyplex size, polydispersity and ζ-potential are important biophysical properties and can be assessed by dynamic light scattering (*see* **Note 23**) [39, 40].

3.4.1 Agarose Gel Shift Assay for siRNA Polyplexes

1. Fix a 15 cm × 15 cm UV-transparent gel tray in a gel casting unit.
2. Weigh 1.8 g of agarose powder (1% gel, w/v) into a flask and add 180 mL of TBE buffer.
3. Dissolve agarose by boiling until a clear solution is obtained.

4. Allow the solution to cool down to ~50 °C, then add 180 μL of 1000 × concentrated GelRed™ for nucleic acid staining.
5. Pour the agarose solution into the gel casting unit. Remove bubbles with a pipette tip before fixating a well comb. Allow the gel to solidify (usually within 30 min).
6. Prepare polyplexes containing 0.5 μg of siRNA at different *N/Ps* and/or equivalents of DBCO agent as described under Subheading 3.3 and dilute them to 20 μL with HBG after polyplex incubation is finished. Optionally, instead of HBG, add full serum to a final concentration of 90% (or 87.5% for DBCO functionalized formulations) and incubate at 37 °C for the desired time before performing the gel shift assay.
7. Prepare all relevant controls for the assay. In case of assays with serum, use free siRNA in buffer (0.5 μg of siRNA in 20 μL HBG), buffer in serum (2 μL HBG + 18 μL full serum) and free siRNA in serum (0.5 μg of siRNA in 18 μL full serum +2 μL HBG) as controls. Otherwise, only use free siRNA (0.5 μg of siRNA in 20 μL HBG) as a control.
8. Add 4 μL of 6× loading buffer to all samples and controls.
9. Remove the well comb from the gel and transfer the gel to the electrophoresis unit.
10. Fill the chamber with TBE buffer until the gel is fully covered and all pockets are filled.
11. Load the samples into the sample pockets and apply a voltage of 70 V for 60 min.
12. Observe the gel under UV light exposure.

3.4.2 Size Measurement Via DLS and Determination of ζ-Potential

1. Prepare a polyplex formulation containing 1.5 μg of siRNA as described under Subheading 3.3.
2. Dilute the polyplex solution to a final volume of 60 μL with HBG.
3. Transfer the polyplex solution into a folded capillary cell.
4. For size and polydispersity measurements, set the method of the zetasizer to 3 measurements with 15 sub-runs (*see* **Note 24**).
5. For the determination of the ζ-potential, add 740 μL 10 mM NaCl and measure each sample 3 times with 10 to 15 subruns at 25 °C.

4 Notes

1. Syringe micro reactors with polyethylene filters (Multisyntech GmbH, Witten Germany) are available in different sizes (2–100 mL) and should be chosen according to the resin

amount. The amount of resin depends on the determined resin loading (L) and the scale size (scale size[mmol]/*L*[mmol/g] = resin amount[g]).

2. Any stirring mechanism guaranteeing continuous mixing of the solution can be used, such as overhead shakers, manual stirring fixed in a vacuum manifold, vortex mixers and vortexing units of semiautomated and automated peptide synthesizers. Coupling time can be reduced by performing the reaction at higher temperature. Different manufacturers offer peptide synthesizers equipped with heat block or microwave units with temperature control. For automated synthesis (especially if higher temperature is used), the solvent DCM is usually exchanged by *N*-Methyl-2-pyrrolidon (NMP). The coupling temperature should not exceed 50 °C if 2-chlorotrityl chloride resin is used as solid support. Apparatuses with vortex mixers are usually equipped with vacuum pumps for solvent removal.
3. DMF tends to hydrolyze to formic acid and dimethylamine when exposed to water. This can reduce coupling efficiencies during synthesis and cause false positive results in Kaiser tests. Peptide grade quality DMF should be used and stored well sealed at a dry place at room temperature for maximum 24 months.
4. For therapeutic or biological assays, siRNA against a target mRNAs is required. siRNAs are also available with other chemical modifications and can be customized with linkers, dyes or other compounds attached to the 5′ or 3′-end of a strand.
5. Dry DCM by storage over calcium chloride ($CaCl_2$) to prevent H_2O from reacting with the resin's linker.
6. Make sure that the resin is not sedimenting during the incubation by vortexing with high speed (at least 1000 rpm).
7. Calculate resin load by the following formula

$$\text{Loading}\left[\frac{\text{mmol}}{\text{g}}\right] = \frac{1000 \cdot A_{301}}{D \cdot 7800 \cdot m\,[\text{mg}]}$$

with D as dilution factor (0.025) and 7800 as molar extinction coefficient.

$[L \cdot \text{mol}^{-1} \cdot \text{cm}^{-1}]$ of Fmoc. Calculate the arithmetic mean of the triplicate values as final resin loading.

8. The determined loading should be in a range between 0.2 and 0.4 mmol/g of resin.
9. Sequence (N→C):

1106: H_2N-K(N_3)-Y_3-Stp_2-K-ε[G-K-α,ε(CholA)$_2$]αStp_2-Y_3-OH.

10. The Dde-deprotection is performed with an automated peptide synthesizer. If the Dde-deprotection is performed

manually for example using an overhead shaker, take samples of the Dde-deprotection solution and measure the absorbance against a blank of fresh hydrazine deprotection solution at $\lambda = 290$ nm. Deprotection is finished when the absorbance is well below 0.1 for at least three cycles.

11. After branching with Fmoc-L-Lys(Fmoc)-OH, the molar amounts of coupling reagents (acid, PyBOP, HOBt, and DIPEA) have to be doubled since the number of amines is doubled.
12. Precooling of both cleavage solution and resin neutralizes the heat that emerges during cleavage. In some cases, this is essential to reduce side reactions [45]. TFA is a very aggressive acid, so wear protective clothes and protective goggles.
13. For purification of the lipo-oligomer, the sample is dissolved in 1 mL of size exclusion running solution. A Tricorn 10/600 exclusion column is packed with Sephadex G-10 gel filtration resin and attached to an Äkta Basic System with fraction collector. The system is equilibrated with size exclusion running solution using a flow rate of 2 mL/min at room temperature. The sample is injected and fractions comprising the first major peak (A214, A280) collected.
14. ^{1}H-NMR spectrum of ***1106*** (500 MHz, Deuterium oxide) δ (ppm) = 0.35–2.20 (m, 96 H, βγδH lysine, βγδεH azidolysine, cholanic acid), 2.20–2.60 (m, 20 H, –CO–CH_2–CH_2–CO–Stp, –CO–CH_2– cholanic acid), 2.6–3.05 (m, 16 H, εH lysine and tyrosine), 3.05–3.60 (m, 64 H, –CH_2– Tp), 3.60–4.60 (m, 11 H, αH amino acids), 6.50–7.25 (m, 24 H, –CH– tyrosine).
15. $[M+H]^+$(***1106***): calc: 3234.1 g/mol, found: 3233.0 g/mol; $[M+Na]^+$(***DBCO-PEG$_{24}$***): calc: 1482.8 g/mol, found: 1481.3 g/mol; $[M+Na]^+$(***DBCO$_2$-ss$_2$-PEG$_{24}$***): calc: 2395.1 g/mol, found: 2394.8 g/mol; $[M+Na]^+$(***DBCO-PEG$_{24}$-FolA***): calc: 2033.0 g/mol, found: 2035.5 g/mol; $[M+Na]^+$(***DBCO-PEG$_{48}$-FolA***): calc: 3161.7 g/mol, found: 3158.1 g/mol; $[M+Na]^+$(***DBCO-PEG$_{72}$-FolA***): calc: 4289.4 g/mol, found: 4284.2 g/mol; $[M+H]^+$(***DBCO$_2$-ss$_2$-PEG$_{24}$-FolA***): calc: 2923.4 g/mol, found: 2922.9 g/mol; $[M+Na]^+$(***DBCO$_2$-ss$_2$-PEG$_{48}$-FolA***): calc: 4073.0 g/mol, found: 4073.1 g/mol; $[M+Na]^+$(***DBCO$_2$-ss$_2$-PEG$_{72}$-FolA***): calc: 5200.0 g/mol, found: 5196.2 g/mol;
16. For calculation of the molecular weight the respective salt form of the compound is considered. The HCl salt of the oligomer has a Cl^- counterion at each protonatable amine. 36.5 g/mol is added to the molecular weight for each protonatable amine. The Na^+ salt of the DBCO agents have a Na^+ counterion at each carboxylate function. 23.0 g/mol is added to the molecular weight for each carboxylate function.

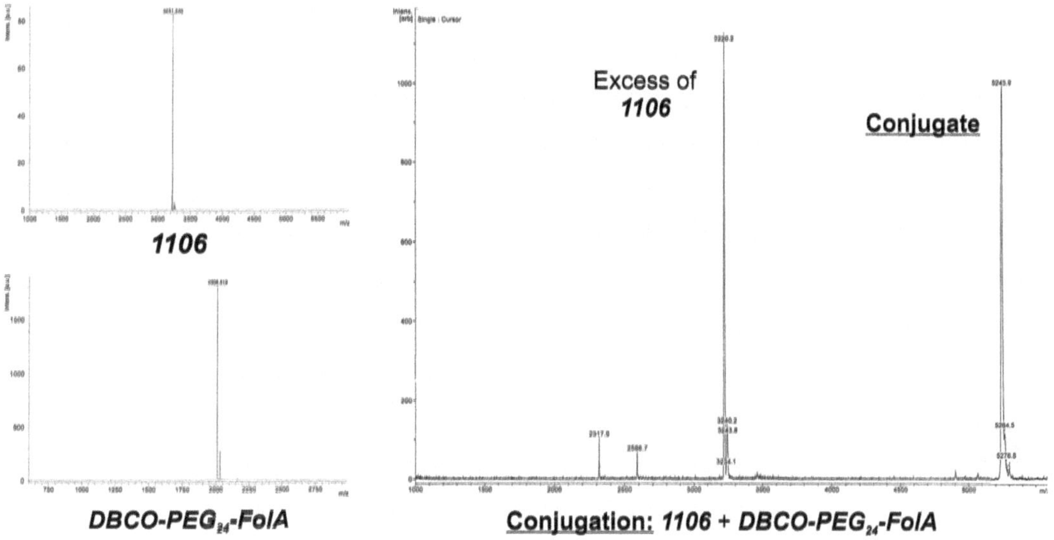

Fig. 5 Reaction of azido-containing oligomer and DBCO-containing agent. Oligomer 1106 and 0.5 eq of DBCO-PEG24-FolA were mixed and incubated for 4 h. MALDI mass spectrometry of the single compounds (left) and the reaction mixture (right) was performed. Calculated mass of the conjugate $[M-H]^-$: 5244.1 Da, found: 5243.9 Da (MALDI negative ion mode). Reproduced from (Klein et al., Biomaterials, 2018 [39]) with permission from Elsevier

17. The generated salts tend to be hygroscopic. Therefore, flush the vials with argon and seal well to preserve the products from air and moisture.
18. Stock solutions should be prepared in H_2O (concentration: 10 mg/mL) and frozen in aliquots.
19. The azide and the DBCO compound, as well as the product resulting from the click reaction of the two compounds can be identified by MALDI mass spectrometry. Thereby, the intactness of both compounds can be confirmed (*see* Fig. 5).
20. The N/P values depict the ratio of protonatable amines (N) of the oligomer to phosphates (P) of the siRNA. As the diaminoethylene motif of Stp is pH-responsive, not all protonatable amines are protonated at neutral pH, which is why the N/P ratio does not present charge ratios during polyplex formation.
21. $n(\text{Phosphate})$

$$= m(\text{siRNA})/\text{Average molecular weight of nucleotide} n(\text{Nitrogen})$$
$$= n(\text{Phosphate}) \times \text{Desired } N/P v(\text{Sample})$$
$$= \frac{n(\text{Nitrogen})}{c(\text{Oligomer}) \times \text{Number of protonatable amines}}$$

Average MW of nucleotides = 311 g/mol. The number of protonatable amines is calculated by all available secondary

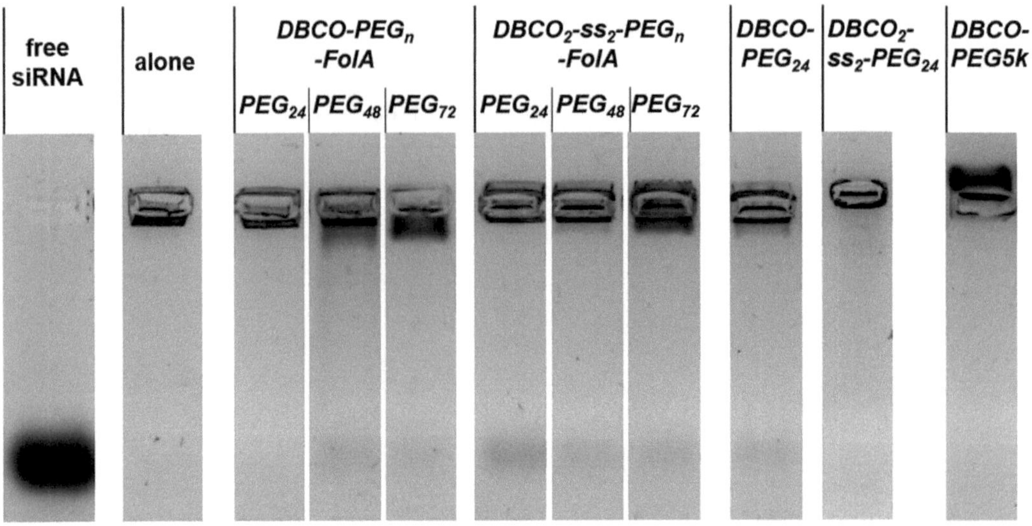

Fig. 6 Electrophoretic mobility of ***1106*** siRNA polyplex formulations analyzed with an agarose gel shift assay. ***1106*** siRNA polyplex without shield and after modification with 0.5 equivalents (eq mol/mol) of the monovalent and bivalent folate targeted DBCO agents with increasing PEG length, monovalent and bivalent DBCO agents and commercial ***DBCO-PEG5k***. The left lane shows the running distance of free siRNA not complexed with a lipo-oligomer. 1% agarose gel, 70 V, 60 min running time. Reproduced from (Klein et al., Biomaterials, 2018 [39]) with permission from Elsevier

(Stp) amines as well as *N*-terminal primary amines. The unit of *c*(oligomer) is mol/L.

22. Full retardation of nucleic acid inside the pockets of the gel indicates complete binding by cationic structures. Further, formulations functionalized with well shielding agents show migratory effects towards the cathode or the anode that cannot be explained by the intrinsic charge of the nucleic acid. The surface charge, largely influenced by the terminal charge of the surface-functionalizing shielding agent, determines the migratory direction and distance (*see* Fig. 6) [39, 40]. Longer PEG chains, for instance, enable a polyplex to migrate towards the cathode. Terminal conjugation of a negatively charged folate ligand inverts the migratory direction towards the anode. For shorter PEG chains with lower shielding efficiency, less or no migration is observed.

23. Surface-functionalizing agents might influence the polyplex size, polydispersity and ζ-potential. Whereas surface-functionalization with a shielding agent, like PEG, strongly influences the ζ-potential toward neutral values, it negligibly changes the polyplex size (*see* Table 1). Terminal conjugation of a hydrophobic, negatively charged ligand, like folate, further influences polyplex size and polydispersity. This might result in

Table 1
Particle size (*z*-average) and zeta potential of *1106* siRNA formulations determined with a DLS zetasizer

1106 siRNA formulation	eq agent	*z*-average (nm)	Mean PDI	Mean ζ-potential (mV)
Nonshielded	–	188.3 ± 1.4	0.26 ± 0.01	34.5 ± 0.8
DBCO-PEG$_{24}$	0.5	367.4 ± 8.0	0.31 ± 0.06	14.6 ± 0.5
DBCO$_2$-ss$_2$-PEG$_{24}$	0.5	251.5 ± 2.9	0.24 ± 0.02	10.5 ± 0.4
DBCO-PEG5k	0.5	165.4 ± 0.9	0.16 ± 0.02	4.1 ± 0.9
DBCO-PEG$_{24}$-FolA	0.5	253.3 ± 2.5	0.24 ± 0.02	23.9 ± 0.4
DBCO-PEG$_{48}$-FolA	0.5	919.6 ± 168.4	0.26 ± 0.01	13.3 ± 0.7
DBCO-PEG$_{72}$-FolA	0.5	923.1 ± 266.3	0.40 ± 0.13	9.2 ± 0.3
DBCO$_2$-ss$_2$-PEG$_{24}$-FolA	0.5	191.8 ± 1.3	0.25 ± 0.01	22.8 ± 0.4
DBCO$_2$-ss$_2$-PEG$_{48}$-FolA	0.5	502.9 ± 97.8	0.30 ± 0.03	12.5 ± 0.6
DBCO$_2$-ss$_2$-PEG$_{72}$-FolA	0.5	854.6 ± 185.8	0.59 ± 0.16	10.2 ± 0.9

The *1106* siRNA polyplexes were prepared at *N/P* 10 and modified with the indicated agents. Reproduced from (Klein et al., Biomaterials, 2018 [39]) with permission from Elsevier

limitations of usability of certain agents and the demand for further optimization.

24. The equilibration time is set to 0 min, the temperature is 25 °C and an automatic attenuator is used. The refractive index of the solvent is 1.330 and the viscosity is 0.8872 mPa s.

Acknowledgments

This work was supported by DFG SFB1032 B4 (P.K. and E.W.), SFB1066 B5 (P.K. and E.W.), and DFG Excellence Cluster Nanosystems Initiative Munich (E.W.).

References

1. Friedmann T, Roblin R (1972) Gene therapy for human genetic disease? Science 175 (4025):949–955
2. Fire A (1999) RNA-triggered gene silencing. Trends Genet 15(9):358–363. https://doi.org/10.1016/S0168-9525(99)01818-1
3. Ginn SL, Amaya AK, Alexander IE, Edelstein M, Abedi MR (2018) Gene therapy clinical trials worldwide to 2017: an update. J Gene Med 20(5). https://doi.org/10.1002/jgm.3015
4. Elbashir SM, Harborth J, Lendeckel W, Yalcin A, Weber K, Tuschl T (2001) Duplexes of 21-nucleotide RNAs mediate RNA interference in cultured mammalian cells. Nature 411 (6836):494–498. https://doi.org/10.1038/35078107
5. Hannon GJ (2002) RNA interference. Nature 418(6894):244–251. https://doi.org/10.1038/418244a
6. Reinhard S, Wagner E (2017) How to tackle the challenge of siRNA delivery with sequence-defined oligoamino amides. Macromol Biosci

17(1). https://doi.org/10.1002/mabi.201600152

7. Wagner E (2012) Functional polymer conjugates for medicinal nucleic acid delivery. Polym Nanomedicine 247:1–29. https://doi.org/10.1007/12_2011_148
8. de Fougerolles A, Vornlocher HP, Maraganore J, Lieberman J (2007) Interfering with disease: a progress report on siRNA-based therapeutics. Nat Rev Drug Discov 6 (6):443–453. https://doi.org/10.1038/nrd2310
9. Wagner E (2007) Programmed drug delivery: nanosystems for tumor targeting. Expert Opin Biol Ther 7(5):587–593. https://doi.org/10.1517/14712598.7.5.587
10. Davis ME, Zuckerman JE, Choi CH, Seligson D, Tolcher A, Alabi CA, Yen Y, Heidel JD, Ribas A (2010) Evidence of RNAi in humans from systemically administered siRNA via targeted nanoparticles. Nature 464 (7291):1067–1070. https://doi.org/10.1038/nature08956
11. Semple SC, Akinc A, Chen JX, Sandhu AP, Mui BL, Cho CK, Sah DWY, Stebbing D, Crosley EJ, Yaworski E, Hafez IM, Dorkin JR, Qin J, Lam K, Rajeev KG, Wong KF, Jeffs LB, Nechev L, Eisenhardt ML, Jayaraman M, Kazem M, Maier MA, Srinivasulu M, Weinstein MJ, Chen QM, Alvarez R, Barros SA, De S, Klimuk SK, Borland T, Kosovrasti V, Cantley WL, Tam YK, Manoharan M, Ciufolini MA, Tracy MA, de Fougerolles A, MacLachlan I, Cullis PR, Madden TD, Hope MJ (2010) Rational design of cationic lipids for siRNA delivery. Nat Biotechnol 28(2):172–U118. https://doi.org/10.1038/nbt.1602
12. Akinc A, Zumbuehl A, Goldberg M, Leshchiner ES, Busini V, Hossain N, Bacallado SA, Nguyen DN, Fuller J, Alvarez R, Borodovsky A, Borland T, Constien R, de Fougerolles A, Dorkin JR, Jayaprakash KN, Jayaraman M, John M, Koteliansky V, Manoharan M, Nechev L, Qin J, Racie T, Raitcheva D, Rajeev KG, Sah DWY, Soutschek J, Toudjarska I, Vornlocher HP, Zimmermann TS, Langer R, Anderson DG (2008) A combinatorial library of lipid-like materials for delivery of RNAi therapeutics. Nat Biotechnol 26(5):561–569. https://doi.org/10.1038/nbt1402
13. Martin B, Sainlos M, Aissaoui A, Oudrhiri N, Hauchecorne M, Vigneron JP, Lehn JM, Lehn P (2005) The design of cationic lipids for gene delivery. Curr Pharm Des 11(3):375–394. https://doi.org/10.2174/1381612053382133
14. Ma JB, Ye KQ, Patel DJ (2004) Structural basis for overhang-specific small interfering RNA recognition by the PAZ domain. Nature 429 (6989):318–322. https://doi.org/10.1038/nature02519
15. Lee ER, Marshall J, Siegel CS, Jiang CW, Yew NS, Nichols MR, Nietupski JB, Ziegler RJ, Lane MB, Wang KX, Wan NC, Scheule RK, Harris DJ, Smith AE, Cheng SH (1996) Detailed analysis of structures and formulations of cationic lipids for efficient gene transfer to the lung. Hum Gene Ther 7(14):1701–1717. https://doi.org/10.1089/hum.1996.7.14-1701
16. Green JJ, Langer R, Anderson DG (2008) A combinatorial polymer library approach yields insight into nonviral gene delivery. Acc Chem Res 41(6):749–759. https://doi.org/10.1021/ar7002336
17. Uchida H, Miyata K, Oba M, Ishii T, Suma T, Itaka K, Nishiyama N, Kataoka K (2011) Odd-even effect of repeating aminoethylene units in the side chain of N-substituted polyaspartamides on gene transfection profiles. J Am Chem Soc 133(39):15524–15532. https://doi.org/10.1021/ja204466y
18. Frohlich T, Edinger D, Klager R, Troiber C, Salcher E, Badgujar N, Martin I, Schaffert D, Cengizeroglu A, Hadwiger P, Vornlocher HP, Wagner E (2012) Structure-activity relationships of siRNA carriers based on sequence-defined oligo (ethane amino) amides. J Control Release 160(3):532–541. https://doi.org/10.1016/j.jconrel.2012.03.018
19. Krzyszton R, Salem B, Lee DJ, Schwake G, Wagner E, Radler JO (2017) Microfluidic self-assembly of folate-targeted monomolecular siRNA-lipid nanoparticles. Nanoscale 9 (22):7442–7453. https://doi.org/10.1039/c7nr01593c
20. Schaffert D, Troiber C, Salcher EE, Frohlich T, Martin I, Badgujar N, Dohmen C, Edinger D, Klager R, Maiwald G, Farkasova K, Seeber S, Jahn-Hofmann K, Hadwiger P, Wagner E (2011) Solid-phase synthesis of sequence-defined T-, i-, and U-shape polymers for pDNA and siRNA delivery. Angew Chem Int Ed 50(38):8986–8989. https://doi.org/10.1002/anie.201102165
21. Morys S, Wagner E, Lachelt U (2016) From artificial amino acids to sequence-defined targeted oligoaminoamides. Methods Mol Biol 1445:235–258. https://doi.org/10.1007/978-1-4939-3718-9_15
22. Lee DJ, Wagner E, Lehto T (2015) Sequence-defined oligoaminoamides for the delivery of siRNAs. Methods Mol Biol 1206:15–27.

https://doi.org/10.1007/978-1-4939-1369-5_2

23. Dohmen C, Edinger D, Frohlich T, Schreiner L, Lachelt U, Troiber C, Radler J, Hadwiger P, Vornlocher HP, Wagner E (2012) Nanosized multifunctional polyplexes for receptor-mediated siRNA delivery. ACS Nano 6(6):5198–5208. https://doi.org/10.1021/nn300960m
24. Gilleron J, Querbes W, Zeigerer A, Borodovsky A, Marsico G, Schubert U, Manygoats K, Seifert S, Andree C, Stoter M, Epstein-Barash H, Zhang L, Koteliansky V, Fitzgerald K, Fava E, Bickle M, Kalaidzidis Y, Akinc A, Maier M, Zerial M (2013) Image-based analysis of lipid nanoparticle-mediated siRNA delivery, intracellular trafficking and endosomal escape. Nat Biotechnol 31 (7):638–646. https://doi.org/10.1038/nbt.2612
25. Sahay G, Querbes W, Alabi C, Eltoukhy A, Sarkar S, Zurenko C, Karagiannis E, Love K, Chen D, Zoncu R, Buganim Y, Schroeder A, Langer R, Anderson DG (2013) Efficiency of siRNA delivery by lipid nanoparticles is limited by endocytic recycling. Nat Biotechnol 31 (7):653–658. https://doi.org/10.1038/nbt.2614
26. Wittrup A, Lieberman J (2015) Knocking down disease: a progress report on siRNA therapeutics. Nat Rev Genet 16(9):543–552. https://doi.org/10.1038/nrg3978
27. Klein PM, Reinhard S, Lee DJ, Muller K, Ponader D, Hartmann L, Wagner E (2016) Precise redox-sensitive cleavage sites for improved bioactivity of siRNA lipopolyplexes. Nanoscale 8(42):18098–18104. https://doi.org/10.1039/c6nr05767e
28. Meyer M, Philipp A, Oskuee R, Schmidt C, Wagner E (2008) Breathing life into polycations: functionalization with pH-responsive endosomolytic peptides and polyethylene glycol enables siRNA delivery. J Am Chem Soc 130(11):3272–3273. https://doi.org/10.1021/ja710344v
29. Leng Q, Chou ST, Scaria PV, Woodle MC, Mixson AJ (2014) Increased tumor distribution and expression of histidine-rich plasmid polyplexes. J Gene Med 16(9-10):317–328. https://doi.org/10.1002/jgm.2807
30. Hughes JA, Rao GA (2005) Targeted polymers for gene delivery. Expert Opin Drug Deliv 2 (1):145–157. https://doi.org/10.1517/17425247.2.1.145
31. Kos P, Lachelt U, Herrmann A, Mickler FM, Doblinger M, He DS, Levacic AK, Morys S, Brauchle C, Wagner E (2015) Histidine-rich stabilized polyplexes for cMet-directed tumor-targeted gene transfer. Nanoscale 7 (12):5350–5362. https://doi.org/10.1039/c4nr06556e
32. Morys S, Levacic AK, Urnauer S, Kempter S, Kern S, Radler JO, Spitzweg C, Lachelt U, Wagner E (2017) Influence of defined hydrophilic blocks within oligoaminoamide copolymers: compaction versus shielding of pDNA nanoparticles. Polymers 9(4). https://doi.org/10.3390/polym9040142
33. Tockary TA, Osada K, Motoda Y, Hiki S, Chen QX, Takeda KM, Dirisala A, Osawa S, Kataoka K (2016) Rod-to-globule transition of pDNA/PEG-poly(L-lysine) polyplex micelles induced by a collapsed balance between DNA rigidity and PEG crowdedness. Small 12 (9):1193–1200. https://doi.org/10.1002/smll.201501815
34. Troiber C, Edinger D, Kos P, Schreiner L, Klager R, Herrmann A, Wagner E (2013) Stabilizing effect of tyrosine trimers on pDNA and siRNA polyplexes. Biomaterials 34 (5):1624–1633. https://doi.org/10.1016/j.biomaterials.2012.11.021
35. Muller K, Kessel E, Klein PM, Hohn M, Wagner E (2016) Post-PEGylation of siRNA lipo-oligoamino amide polyplexes using tetra-glutamylated folic acid as ligand for receptor-targeted delivery. Mol Pharm 13 (7):2332–2345. https://doi.org/10.1021/acs.molpharmaceut.6b00102
36. Muller K, Klein PM, Heissig P, Roidl A, Wagner E (2016) EGF receptor targeted lipo-oligocation polyplexes for antitumoral siRNA and miRNA delivery. Nanotechnology 27 (46):464001. https://doi.org/10.1088/0957-4484/27/46/464001
37. Morys S, Urnauer S, Spitzweg C, Wagner E (2018) EGFR targeting and shielding of pDNA lipopolyplexes via bivalent attachment of a sequence-defined PEG agent. Macromol Biosci 18(1). https://doi.org/10.1002/mabi.201700203
38. Zhang W, Muller K, Kessel E, Reinhard S, He D, Klein PM, Hohn M, Rodl W, Kempter S, Wagner E (2016) Targeted siRNA delivery using a lipo-oligoaminoamide nanocore with an influenza peptide and transferrin shell. Adv Healthc Mater 5(12):1493–1504. https://doi.org/10.1002/adhm.201600057
39. Klein PM, Kern S, Lee DJ, Schmaus J, Hohn M, Gorges J, Kazmaier U, Wagner E (2018) Folate receptor-directed orthogonal click-functionalization of siRNA lipopolyplexes for tumor cell killing in vivo. Biomaterials 178:630–642. https://doi.org/10.1016/j.biomaterials.2018.03.031

40. Klein PM, Klinker K, Zhang W, Kern S, Kessel E, Wagner E, Barz M (2018) Efficient shielding of polyplexes using heterotelechelic polysarcosines. Polymers 10(6). https://doi.org/10.3390/polym10060689
41. Lee DJ, Kessel E, Edinger D, He D, Klein PM, Voith von Voithenberg L, Lamb DC, Lachelt U, Lehto T, Wagner E (2016) Dual antitumoral potency of EG5 siRNA nanoplexes armed with cytotoxic bifunctional glutamyl-methotrexate targeting ligand. Biomaterials 77:98–110. https://doi.org/10.1016/j.biomaterials.2015.11.004
42. Lee DJ, Kessel E, Lehto T, Liu X, Yoshinaga N, Padari K, Chen YC, Kempter S, Uchida S, Radler JO, Pooga M, Sheu MT, Kataoka K, Wagner E (2017) Systemic delivery of folate-PEG siRNA lipopolyplexes with enhanced intracellular stability for in vivo gene silencing in leukemia. Bioconjug Chem 28(9):2393–2409. https://doi.org/10.1021/acs.bioconjchem.7b00383
43. Schaffert D, Badgujar N, Wagner E (2011) Novel Fmoc-polyamino acids for solid-phase synthesis of defined polyamidoamines. Org Lett 13(7):1586–1589. https://doi.org/10.1021/ol200381z
44. Kaiser E, Colescott RL, Bossinger CD, Cook PI (1970) Color test for detection of free terminal amino groups in the solid-phase synthesis of peptides. Anal Biochem 34(2):595–598
45. Reinhard S, Zhang W, Wagner E (2017) Optimized solid-phase-assisted synthesis of oleic acid containing siRNA nanocarriers. ChemMedChem 12(17):1464–1470. https://doi.org/10.1002/cmdc.201700350

Chapter 9

Attachment of Peptides to Oligonucleotides on Solid Support Using Copper(I)-Catalyzed Huisgen 1,3-Dipolar Cycloaddition

Malgorzata Honcharenko, Dmytro Honcharenko, and Roger Strömberg

Abstract

In vivo bioavailability and delivery of nucleic acids to the site of action is a severe limitation in oligonucleotide (ON) therapeutics. Equipping the ONs with cell penetrating, homing or endosomal escape peptides can enhance specificity and/or uptake efficiencies. We describe here a general procedure for the preparation of peptide–oligonucleotide conjugates (POCs) on solid support utilizing a novel activated alkyne containing linker which enhances the Cu(I) catalyzed Huisgen 1,3-dipolar cycloaddition. Conjugation reaction is efficient in millimolar concentration and submicromolar amounts at ambient temperature. The route for POC preparation involves two subsequent conjugation steps: to solid-supported ONs containing a 5′-amino modifier (1) the triple bond donor (*p*-(*N*-propynoylamino)toluic acid (PATA), *p*-([2-(propynyloxy)acetamido]methyl)benzoic acid (PAMBA) or 2-(propynyloxy)acetic acid (PAA)) is first coupled and then (2) an azido-functionalized peptide is attached via a triazole linkage by copper(I) catalyzed Huisgen 1,3-dipolar cycloaddition. The fragment-conjugated POC is released from the solid support by concentrated ammonia. The method gives high conversion of ON to the POC and only involves a single purification step after complete assembly and release from the solid support. The synthesis is flexible and designed to utilize commercially available oligonucleotide and peptide derivatives without the need for specific automated synthesizers.

Key words Peptide–oligonucleotide conjugates, Huisgen 1,3-dipolar cycloaddition, Click chemistry, Solid-phase synthesis, Conjugation, Activated triple bond donor, Azido-containing peptides

1 Introduction

Delivery is a seriously limiting factor for antisense, siRNA and gene therapy in vivo [1–3]. One approach to enhance nucleic acid uptake into cells is to utilize cell penetrating peptides (CPPs), either in the form of complexes or in the form of covalent conjugates, which also protects from digestion by intracellular enzymes [4, 5]. A recent successful example involves a CPP conjugate of a morpholino phosphorodiamidate oligomer that when given in low doses leads to highly efficient splice-switching and production of therapeutically

Olof Gissberg et al. (eds.), *Oligonucleotide-Based Therapies: Methods and Protocols*, Methods in Molecular Biology, vol. 2036,
https://doi.org/10.1007/978-1-4939-9670-4_9,

useful levels of dystrophin in skeletal and heart muscles [6, 7]. This provides a promising approach for the treatment of, for example, Duchenne muscular dystrophy (DMD) [6, 7]. One of the main strategies for the synthesis of peptide–oligonucleotide conjugates (POCs) is the fragment conjugation. For this purpose, a reaction that would seem ideal, due to the compatibility with many other functional groups, is the copper(I) catalyzed Huisgen 1,3-dipolar cycloaddition between an azide and an alkyne, commonly referred to as click chemistry [8, 9]. Conjugation in solution of highly cationic peptides can be problematic due to the tendency to form complexes with anionic oligonucleotide (ON) phosphate backbones. The reaction mixture can even become highly heterogeneous due to precipitation and results in considerably reduced conjugation yields. One way to avoid this problem, and at the same time gain simplicity and reduce number of purification steps, is to perform the fragment conjugation of ONs and peptides with one of the oligomers still protected and attached to the solid support.

We describe here a method for solid-phase fragment conjugation (SPFC) in preparation of 5′-POCs by copper(I) catalyzed Huisgen 1,3-dipolar cycloaddition that is possible to carry out without the need for specific synthesizers, through limited manipulation of commercially available ONs and peptide derivatives [10–14]. The method is a general approach (*see* Fig. 1) and is also suitable for the conjugation of other biomolecules to ONs under mild conditions. ONs which are still attached to the solid support and 5′-modified with amino linkers can be purchased from most companies marketing oligonucleotides. The azido-containing peptides can also be acquired, for example, by adding an azido-lysine to the amino acid sequence. Furthermore, the described method is enabled by use of a new activated triple bond donor and allows for near quantitative conjugation in submicromolar scale at a low concentration under mild conditions and at ambient temperature

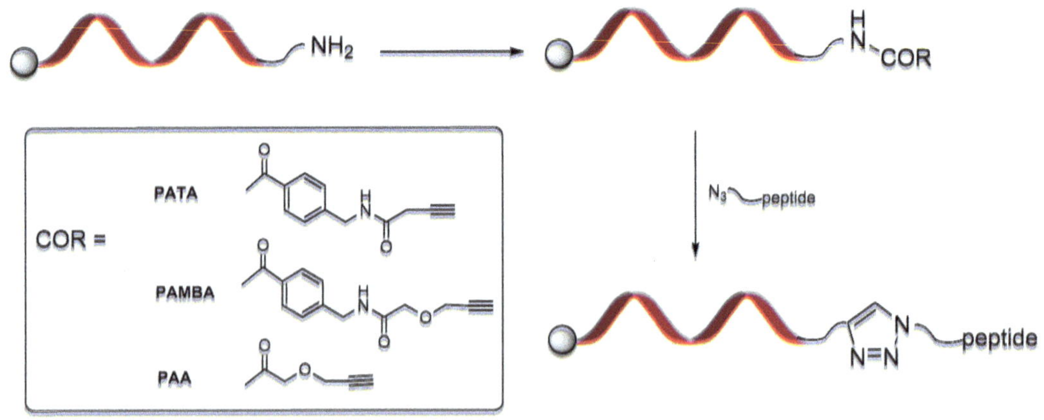

Fig. 1 Schematic representation of the conjugation steps for the POC preparation

(*see* **Note 1**). Linkers used for conjugations: PATA, PAMBA and PAA, are equipped with electron-withdrawing substituent on the dipolarophile that accelerate Huisgen 1,3-dipolar cycloaddition as compared to other not activated triple bond donors (e.g., 4-pentynoic acid). However, this also makes the triple bond donor PATA, but not PAMBA or PAA, to be prone to the side reactions when good nucleophiles are present, probably due to Michael-type addition to the triple bond.

2 Materials

2.1 Conjugation on Solid Support

1. 0.5 mL microcentrifuge tubes equipped with a screw cap and a seal.
2. 1.5 mL microcentrifuge tubes.
3. 1 mL syringes.
4. Needles.
5. Copper(I) in DMSO: stock solution of 1.52 mg of CuI in 1 mL of DMSO.
6. *N,N*-Diisopropylethylamine (DIPEA).
7. *Tert*-Butanol: *tert*-BuOH)–water, (1:1 v/v).
8. Dimethyl sulfoxide (DMSO).
9. Acetonitrile (MeCN).
10. PATA linker.
11. *N,N,N′,N′*-tetramethyl-*O*-(1*H*-benzotriazol-1-yl)uronium hexafluorophosphate (HBTU).
12. *N*-methylmorpholine (NMM).
13. *N,N*-dimethylformamide (DMF).
14. Azido-containing peptide.
15. 10 mM solution (aq.) of ethylenediaminetetraacetic acid (EDTA).

2.2 Deprotection of Protecting Groups and Cleavage from Solid Support

1. 28% NH_3 (aq.)
2. Vortex.
3. 10 mL glass flask for evaporation.
4. Rotary evaporator with a pump and water bath adjusted to 35 °C.
5. Milli-Q Water.

2.3 HPLC Purification

1. HPLC system equipped with an analytical RP-C18 column (e.g., Discovery BIO Wide Pore C18, 5 μm (250 × 4.6 mm).
2. Milli-Q Water.

3. Acetonitrile (MeCN) (HPLC grade).
4. Triethylamine (freshly distilled).
5. Acetic acid.
6. pH Meter,
7. Buffer A: 50 mM TEAA (triethylammonium acetate, pH 6.5) (*see* **Note 2**).
8. Buffer B: 50 mM TEAA (triethylammonium acetate pH 6.5 in 50% MeCN) (*see* **Note 2**).
9. Rotary evaporator with a pump and water bath adjusted to 35 °C.
10. Round bottom glass flasks.
11. Freeze-drier.

3 Methods

3.1 Conjugation on Solid Support

1. Place 0.1 μmol of commercially available solid-supported 5′-amino-modified oligonucleotide in a 0.5 mL microcentrifuge tube with a screw cap (3–6 mg support, depending on the loading) (*see* **Note 3**).
2. In separate 1.5 mL microcentrifuge tube, place HBTU (48 μmol) and active linker PATA (50 μmol) followed by 560 μL of dry DMF and 55 μL of NMM (495 μmol).
3. Close the microcentrifuge tube and place on a vortex and agitate for 0.5 h. Remove the solution with a syringe equipped with a needle and add to the solid supported ON in a 0.5 mL microcentrifuge tube with a screw cap.
4. Seal the 0.5 mL microcentrifuge tube with the reaction mixture and the solid supported ON and place it horizontally on a vortex for agitation over 2 h.
5. Place the 0.5 mL microcentrifuge tube in the centrifuge and separate the solid supported ON from solution by centrifugation (75 s at 13.3 rpm).
6. Remove the solution carefully from the solid support with a syringe and add 200 μL of DMF to the tube.
7. Wash the solid supported ON with the DMF by placing the microcentrifuge tube on a vortex for 0.5 min and repeat the centrifugation as in **step 5**.
8. Repeat the washing in **steps 5–7** with new portions of DMF (200 μL) to have in total 10 washing steps with DMF.
9. Finally repeat the washing **step 2** times with *tert*-BuOH–H_2O (1:1 v/v).

10. Dissolve the azido group containing peptide (4 eq., 0.4 mmol) in 35 μL of *tert*-BuOH–H_2O (1:1 v/v) and add to the solid supported ON (*see* **Note 4**).
11. Add a solution of DIPEA (2 eq., 0.2 μmol) in 25 μL of *tert*-BuOH–H_2O (1:1 v/v) (from a stock solution of 2 μL DIPEA in 1 mL of *tert*-BuOH–H_2O (1:1 v/v)), and 1 eq. (0.1 μmol of CuI dissolved in 25 μL of DMSO (*see* **Note 5**).
12. Seal the microcentrifuge tube and place on a vortex for 24 h. Remove the conjugation solution by centrifugation of the solid support.
13. Repeat **steps 6** and 7 with DMSO (3 × 0.5 mL).
14. Repeat **steps 6** and 7 with 10 mM EDTA (aq.).
15. Repeat **steps 6** and 7 with MeCN (2 × 0.5 mL).

3.2 Deprotection of Protecting Groups and Cleavage from Solid Support

1. Add 300 μL of 28% NH_3 (aq.) solution to dry solid supported ON conjugate in a 0.5 mL microcentrifuge tube.
2. Seal the microcentrifuge tube and place it on the vortex overnight at room temperature.
3. Place the 0.5 mL microcentrifuge tube in the centrifuge and separate the solid support from solution by centrifugation.
4. Remove the solution carefully from the solid support with a syringe equipped with a needle and place it in a round bottom glass flask suitable for evaporation under reduced pressure.
5. Wash the support with another portion of ammonia solution, by repeating 1, 3 and 4.
6. Evaporate the combined solutions under reduced pressure with the temperature of the water bath not higher than 35 °C.
7. Redissolve the crude product by adding 1 mL of milli-Q water.

3.3 HPLC Purification

1. Transfer 50 μL of the solution from Subheading 3.2, **step** 7 to a 1 mL microcentrifuge tube, add 50 μL of 10 mM EDTA solution and inject the resulting solution to the RP-HPLC system.
2. Elute using a linear gradient of buffer B in buffer A from 0% to 100% in 30 min at 50 °C (UV detection at 260 nm) (*see* **Notes 2** and **6**).
3. Confirm presence and authenticity of the ON conjugate in the fraction using ESI-MS in negative mode.
4. Collect fractions containing ON conjugate, and evaporate solution under reduced pressure with the temperature of the water bath not higher than 35 °C.

5. Add 10 mL of milli-Q water to the collected fraction, freeze using liquid nitrogen and assembly for freeze-drying on the lyophilizer.
6. Repeat the procedure in **step 4**.
7. Repeat the procedure in **step 4** using 1 mL of water and transfer the liquid to the microcentrifuge tube.
8. Wash the remaining flask with 0.5 mL of water and combine the liquids in a microcentrifuge tube.
9. Freeze the resulted solution in the microcentrifuge tube using liquid nitrogen and assembly for freeze-drying on the lyophilizer.

4 Notes

1. The activated triple bond donor linkers PATA, PAMBA and PAA (*see* Fig. 1) can be synthesized using established procedures [10, 12] and stored at −20 °C for at least several months. The PAA linker is also commercially available.
2. Buffer A: 50 mM TEAA (triethylammonium acetate, pH 6.5) prepared by adding 14 mL triethylamine to 2 L of milli-Q water followed by 5.6 mL of acetic acid. Adjust pH to 6.5 using pH meter. Buffer B: 50 mM TEAA (triethylammonium acetate pH 6.5) prepared by adding 14 mL triethylamine to 2 L of 50% milli-Q water/MeCN followed by 5.6 mL of acetic acid. Adjust pH to 6.5 using pH meter.
3. It is recommended to purchase solid supported ON with 5′-amino modifier that still possesses the amino protecting group, e.g., 4,4′-dimethoxytrityl (DMTr) and to deprotect this group manually just before conjugation with the triple bond donor. Deprotection can be done using 5% dichloroacetic acid (DCA) in dichloromethate (DCM). Add 0.5 mL of the DCA solution to the microcentrifuge tube containing solid supported ON and mix on the vortex. After 1 min, centrifuge and remove the liquid with a syringe equipped with a needle and then repeat the procedure once. Wash the solid support with DCM (3 × 0.5 mL), centrifuge and remove the solution above the solid support each time.
4. For peptides that are not soluble in *tert*-BuOH–H_2O (1:1 v/v) use a DMSO–water (4:1 v/v) mixture.
5. Dissolving CuI in DMSO may take time. Use an ultrasonic bath if necessary. Always use freshly dissolved CuI for the conjugation reaction.

6. It is recommended to use 10 mM EDTA as an addition to every fraction that is HPLC purified to remove the last traces of copper from the ON conjugates.

References

1. Akhtar S, Hughes MD, Khan A et al (2000) The delivery of antisense therapeutics. Adv Drug Deliv Rev 44:3–21
2. Lundin P, Johansson H, Guterstam P et al (2008) Distinct uptake routes of cell-penetrating peptide conjugates. Bioconjug Chem 19:2535–2542
3. Lebleu B, Moulton HM, Abes R et al (2008) Cell penetrating peptide conjugates of steric block oligonucleotides. Adv Drug Deliv Rev 60:517–529
4. Heitz F, Morris MC, Divita G (2009) Twenty years of cell-penetrating peptides: from molecular mechanisms to therapeutics. Br J Pharmacol 157:195–206
5. Borrelli A, Tornesello AL, Tornesello ML et al (2018) Cell penetrating peptides as molecular carriers for anti-cancer agents. Molecules 23:295
6. Jirka SMG, 'tHoen PAC, Diaz Parillas V et al (2018) Cyclic peptides to improve delivery and exon skipping of antisense oligonucleotides in a mouse model for Duchenne muscular dystrophy. Mol Ther 26:132–147
7. Jirka SMG, Heemskerk H, Tanganyika-de Winter CL et al (2014) Peptide conjugation of 2'-O-methyl phosphorothioate antisense oligonucleotides enhances cardiac uptake and exon skipping in mdx mice. Nucleic Acid Ther 24:25–36
8. Astakhova K, Ray R, Taskova M et al (2018) "Clicking" gene therapeutics: a successful union of chemistry and biomedicine for new solutions. Mol Pharm 15:2892–2899
9. El-Sagheer AH, Brown T (2012) Click chemistry - a versatile method for nucleic acid labelling, cyclisation and ligation. In: Fox KR, Brown T (eds) DNA conjugates and sensors. RSC Biomolecular Sciences
10. Jezowska-Herrera M, Honcharenko D, Ghidini A et al (2016) Enabling multiple conjugation to oligonucleotides using "click cycles". Bioconjug Chem 27:2620–2628
11. Honcharenko M, Bestas B, Jezowska M et al (2016) Synthetic m3G-CAP attachment necessitates a minimum trinucleotide constituent to be recognised as a nuclear import signal. RSC Adv 6:51367–51373
12. Wenska M, Alvira M, Steunenberg P et al (2011) An activated triple bond linker enables "click" attachment of peptides to oligonucleotides on solid support. Nucleic Acids Res 39:9047–9059
13. Honcharenko M, Romanowska J, Alvira M et al (2012) Capping of oligonucleotides with "clickable" m3G-CAPs. RSC Adv 2:12949–12962
14. Jezowska M, Romanowska J, Bestas B et al (2012) Synthesis of biotin linkers with the activated triple bond donor [p-(N-propynoylamino)toluic acid] (PATA) for efficient biotinylation of peptides and oligonucleotides. Molecules 17:14174–14185

Chapter 10

Characterizing Oligonucleotide Uptake in Cultured Cells: A Case Study Using AS1411 Aptamer

Elsa M. Reyes-Reyes and Paula J. Bates

Abstract

Oligonucleotides can be designed or evolved to bind to specific DNA, RNA, protein, or small molecule targets and thereby alter the biological function of the target. The therapeutic potential of oligonucleotides targeted to intracellular molecules will depend largely on their ability to be taken up by the cells of interest, as well as their subsequent subcellular distribution. Here we describe methods to characterize the extent and mechanism of cellular uptake of AS1411, an aptamer oligonucleotide that has progressed to human clinical trials and which is also widely used by researchers as a cancer-targeting ligand.

Key words Oligonucleotide, AS1411, Aptamer, G-quadruplex, Nucleolin, Endocytosis, Macropinocytosis, Cancer, Flow cytometry, Confocal microscopy

1 Introduction

Oligonucleotides consisting of synthesized DNA or RNA strands, or chemically modified versions thereof, are a promising class of therapeutic agents with the potential to regulate molecular targets that are conventionally "undruggable" [1–3]. Oligonucleotides can specifically recognize nucleic acid, protein, or small molecule targets by either sequence-dependent base pairing or structure-dependent shape complementarity. The intended targets of many therapeutic oligonucleotides are located inside the cell, in the nucleus or cytoplasm. Therefore, the biological activities of such oligonucleotides will depend on their ability to be internalized by the cells of interest and also by their subsequent localization within those cells. The cellular uptake and trafficking of oligonucleotides can depend on their concentration, sequence, and chemical modifications, and can vary by cell type [4]. Determining the extent and mechanism of oligonucleotide uptake in cells, as well as their subcellular distribution, is essential for evaluating their therapeutic potential and mechanism of action. More generally, a better understanding of how oligonucleotides are internalized and trafficked by

Olof Gissberg et al. (eds.), *Oligonucleotide-Based Therapies: Methods and Protocols*, Methods in Molecular Biology, vol. 2036, https://doi.org/10.1007/978-1-4939-9670-4_10, © Springer Science+Business Media, LLC, part of Springer Nature 2019

cells should enable much-needed strategies to increase oligonucleotide internalization efficiency and endosomal escape [1, 2].

Molecules can enter cells by passive diffusion (for some small, non-charged molecules), via specific transporters (for some ions and metabolites), or by endocytosis (for large, charged, or highly polar molecules) [5]. Molecule uptake by passive diffusion is rapid and does not require energy. Endocytosis is an energy-dependent process by which cells engulf and internalize extracellular materials and cell surface proteins via invagination or deformation of their plasma membrane to form membrane-bound endocytic vesicles. Once internalized, these vesicles are trafficked via the endolysosomal system and their contents can end up being recycled to the cell surface, degraded in lysosomes, or (rarely) released into the cytosol [1, 2, 6–10]. Most cells have several distinct known pathways of endocytosis such as clathrin-mediated, caveolar, macropinocytosis, and the clathrin-independent carriers/glycosylphosphatidylinositol- anchored protein enriched compartments (CLIC/GEEC) pathways (Fig. 1). These pathways may overlap in their characteristic dependencies (e.g., on actin or dynamin) but can be distinguished by their unique characteristics (Fig. 1). Pharmacological and genetic approaches have both been used to elucidate endocytosis mechanisms, including several chemical inhibitors that preferentially target different forms of endocytosis [8–10]. The endocytic mechanism can be further characterized based on the size of

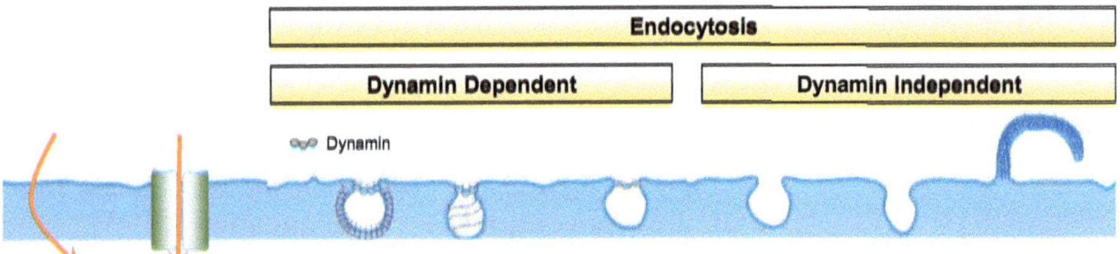

	Passive Diffusion	Transporter	Clathrin	Caveolar	RhoA	CLIC/GEEC	Flotillin	Macro-pinocytosis
Temperature-dependent?	No	Sometimes	Yes	Yes	Yes	Yes	Yes	Yes
Inhibited by cytochalasin?	No	No	Yes	Yes	Yes	Yes	Yes	Yes
Inhibited by Dynasore?	No	No	Yes	Yes	Yes	No	No	No
Inhibited by amiloride?	No	No	No	No	No	No	Maybe	Yes
Marker			Transferrin					Dextran
Endocytic vesicle size	None	None	~ 0.1 μm	~ 0.1 μm	~ 0.1 μm	~ 0.1 μm	~ 0.1 μm	~ 1.0 μm

Fig. 1 Illustration of some major pathways for cellular uptake. Oligonucleotides are too large to enter cells by passive diffusion and no specific transporter has been identified, so uptake occurs predominantly via endocytosis. The various forms of endocytosis can be distinguished based on their sensitivities to pharmacological inhibitors of actin (cytochalasin), dynamin (Dynasore), and Na^+/H^+ exchange (amiloride). Dynamin-dependent mechanisms can be further distinguished if necessary, by their sensitivities to methyl-β-cyclodextrin (inhibits caveolar) and chlorpromazine (inhibits clathrin-dependent). Observation of specific markers and endocytic vesicles can provide additional information to confirm mechanisms. Phagocytosis is another form of endocytosis (for engulfing large solid particles or cells), but only occurs in specialized immune cells and is not listed here

endocytic vesicles formed, intracellular distribution, and colocalization with specific markers. The role of specific proteins, including transporters or receptors, can be determined through pharmacological means (if inhibitors are available) or by genetic approaches such as depletion (mediated by RNA interference or gene editing) or overexpression (of wild-type or mutant proteins).

In this chapter we describe the protocols that were used to investigate the mechanism of cellular uptake for a G-rich DNA oligonucleotide named AS1411 in two human cell lines that are sensitive (DU145 prostate cancer cells) or resistant (Hs27 nonmalignant skin fibroblasts) to its antiproliferative effects [4]. We have previously shown that AS1411 can form G-quadruplex structures that bind as aptamers to nucleolin, a protein that is present in the nucleus of proliferating cells (both normal and malignant) but is also found on the cell surface and in the cytoplasm in the case of cancer cells [11, 12]. AS1411 can induce proliferation arrest and cell death in a wide range of cancer cells but has little effect on normal cells, and human clinical trials have indicated that some patients with advanced cancers have durable clinical responses to AS1411 [12, 13]. Unusually for unmodified oligonucleotides in general, but consistent with other G-rich, quadruplex-forming oligonucleotides [3, 14], AS1411 is resistant to nucleases and can efficiently enter cells without the need for a transfection agent [3, 4, 15]. Furthermore, many researchers have reported using AS1411 as a cancer-targeting ligand to direct various cargoes specifically to cancer cells [12]. Yet, despite the extraordinary characteristics and therapeutic potential of AS1411, the mechanism of action by which this oligonucleotide exerts its selective effects on cancer cells is not fully understood and this prompted us to compare its uptake in cancerous and nonmalignant cultured cells. In particular, we wanted to test the hypothesis that nucleolin mediates receptor-mediated uptake (i.e., clathrin-dependent endocytosis) of AS1411 in cancer cells. Our studies [4] ultimately revealed this hypothesis to be incorrect and led instead to several unexpected but significant findings about AS1411 uptake. We found that AS1411 was taken up by endocytosis to a similar degree in both the cancer and normal cells but was taken up specifically by macropinocytosis in cancer cells while normal cells displayed a different endocytosis mechanism [4]. We noted that the cancer cells displayed much higher levels of macropinocytosis than normal cells [4], a finding that was subsequently confirmed and explained by others [16]. Our results suggested that nucleolin is not responsible for initial receptor-mediated uptake of AS1411 but plays a role in induction of additional macropinocytosis and subsequent uptake of AS1411 [4]. Notably, we found no evidence that AS1411 escapes from endosomes into the cytoplasm or nucleus, suggesting its target (s) may be on the cell surface or endosomal. Our uptake studies eventually led to a new model to explain AS1411's cancer-selective activities [4, 17], though the detailed molecular mechanisms remain to be elucidated [12]. This chapter describes the protocols we used to evaluate the mechanism of uptake of AS1411 in cultured cell lines; these methods are applicable for assessing the cellular uptake of any type of potentially therapeutic oligonucleotides or other molecules of interest.

2 Materials

We have listed the specific suppliers and catalog numbers for some reagents and equipment that are used in our studies. However, it is likely that reagents or equipment from any reputable supplier would be equivalent.

2.1 Oligodeoxynucleotides

1. High-performance liquid chromatography (HPLC)-purified oligonucleotides with an unmodified DNA backbone and labeled at the 5′-terminus with fluorophore, are purchased from Thermo Fisher or Integrated DNA Technologies (IDT) company. The oligonucleotides consist of the AS1411 or control (CRO) 26-nucleotide sequence with three additional thymidine bases at the 5′-end (to avoid quenching of the fluorophore), that is, FL-AS1411 is 5′-FL-TTTGGTGGT GGTGGTTGTGGTGGTGGTGG-3′ and FL-CRO is 5′-FL--TTTCCTCCTCCTCCTTCTCCTCCTCCTCC-3′, where FL is Alexa Fluor 488 (*see* **Notes 1** and **2**).
2. Ultrapure distilled water: DNase/RNase-free sterile distilled water.
3. A UV-visible spectrophotometer capable of recording absorbance at 260 nm to determine FL-AS1411 and FL-CRO concentration according to Beer's law.

2.2 Cell Culture

1. Hs27 (nonmalignant human foreskin fibroblast) and DU145 (hormone refractory prostate cancer) cell lines are obtained from ATCC (*see* **Note 3**).
2. DMEM cell culture medium: supplemented with 10% heat-inactivated fetal bovine serum (FBS), inactivated for 15 min at 65 °C, and 1% penicillin–streptomycin (10,000 U each per 1 mL).
3. 1× trypsin–ethylenediamine tetraacetic acid (EDTA 4 Na) (Thermo Fisher Scientific # 25300054).
4. 1× Dulbecco's phosphate buffered saline (DPBS) (Thermo Fisher Scientific # 14190250)
5. 0.4% trypan blue solution (Thermo Fisher Scientific # 15250061).

2.3 AS1411 Uptake Mechanism Analysis

1. 10 mM cytochalasin D (Millipore Sigma #250255) in DMSO.
2. 10 mM Dynasore (Millipore Sigma # 324410) in DMSO.
3. 3 mM Amiloride (Millipore Sigma # 129876) in serum-free cell media solution filtered using a 0.2 μm membrane filter.
4. 5 mg "Dextran-10 K": Macropinocytosis marker Dextran (10,000 Da molecular weight) anionic fixable labeled with Alexa Fluor 594 (Thermo Fisher Scientific # D22910) reconstituted in DPBS to obtain a 10 mg/mL (*see* **Note 4**).
5. 5 mg Transferrin conjugated with Alexa Fluor 488 (Thermo Fisher Scientific # T13342) reconstituted in deionized water to obtain a 5 mg/mL.

2.4 Assessing the Role of Nucleolin in AS1411 Uptake

1. Small interfering RNA (siRNA) duplex sequences that are targeted specifically to the protein of interest or that can serve as negative control siRNAs. siRNAs are purchased from Thermo Fisher Scientific (Ambion, Silencer®) including negative control siRNAs (AM4611 and AM4613) and three different siRNAs targeted to nucleolin (NCL) with sequences 5′-GGUCGUCAUACCUCAGAAGtt (NCL1, ID #144014), 5′-GGCAAAGCAUUGGUAGCAAtt (NCL2, ID #144015), and 5′-CGGUGAAAUUGAUGGAAAUtt (NCL3, ID #144016).
2. Lipofectamine™ RNAiMAX Transfection Reagent (Thermo Fisher Scientific, #13778030).
3. Opti-MEM medium (Thermo Fisher Scientific, #31985088).
4. Equipment and reagents for SDS-PAGE electrophoresis and western blot (*see* **Note 7**).
5. Monoclonal anti-nucleolin and goat anti-mouse IgG HRP antibody; Santa Cruz # sc-8031 and sc-2005 respectively.

2.5 Analysis Using Flow Cytometry

1. Flow cytometry tubes: 5 mL polystyrene tubes 12 × 75 mm.
2. 1 mg/mL propidium iodide (PI) (Thermo Fisher Scientific # P3566).
3. 1% Paraformaldehyde, methanol-free (Electron Microscopy Science #15700) in DPBS.
4. Flow cytometer (e.g., FACScalibur cytometer, BD Biosciences, Mountain View, CA).

2.6 Analysis Using Confocal Microscopy

1. Sterile round cover glasses, 18 mm, 0.17 mm thickness (Warner Instrument, #64-0714).
2. 4% paraformaldehyde, methanol-free (Electron Microscopy Science #15700) in DPBS.
3. ProLong™ Gold Antifade with DAPI (Thermo Fisher, #P36941).

4. Confocal microscope (e.g., LSM 510 inverted confocal laser-scanning microscope, Carl Zeiss, Oberkochen, Germany, equipped with an Omnichrome argon-krypton laser.
5. Oil immersion objective 1.4 NA, Zeiss Plan-Apo 63×.

3 Methods

3.1 Resuspension of Oligonucleotides

Oligonucleotides are resuspended in an amount of sterile ultrapure distilled water to give a stock solution concentration of 500 μM–1 mM. The oligonucleotides are dissolved by vortexing. The accurate concentration of the stock solution is determined by measuring absorbance at 260 nm and stock solutions of oligonucleotides are stored in aliquots at −20 °C.

3.2 Cells

1. Adhered cells are harvested by trypsinization, assessed for cell viability, and adjusted to the desired cell concentration. The cell suspensions used had >90% viability as determined using trypan blue exclusion or any conventional cell viability assay.
2. *For flow cytometry:* 2×10^5 cells are plated in 2 mL of DMEM medium supplemented with FBS on six-well plates.

   For confocal microscopy: 1×10^5 cells are plated in 1 mL of DMEM medium supplemented with FBS on sterile 18-mm diameter glass coverslips inside 12-well plates.

   Transfection: 1×10^5 cells are plated in 2 mL of DMEM medium supplemented with FBS on six-well plates.
3. Cells are incubated for 18 h to allow adherence.

3.3 Characterizing the AS1411 Uptake Mechanism

Cells are treated as follows to determine the following:

3.3.1 Time Course of Oligonucleotide Uptake

1. The culture medium is changed for DMEM medium supplemented with FBS. FL-AS1411 or FL-CRO stock solution is added directly to medium to give a final concentration of 10 μM, or an equivalent volume of vehicle (sterile water) is added for "no DNA" cells.
2. Cells are incubated for different periods of time (5 min to 8 h) in a humidified incubator at 37 °C with 5% CO_2.
3. Cells are processed to be analyzed by flow cytometry (Subheading 3.5 and *see* **Note 5**) or confocal microscopy (Subheading 3.6).

3.3.2 Temperature Dependence of Uptake Process

1. The cell culture medium is changed for ice-cold cell culture medium supplemented with FBS containing 10 μM FL-AS1411, 10 μM FL-CRO, or no DNA.

2. Cells are incubated at 37 °C or 4 °C for 2 h.
3. Cell are processed to be analyzed by flow cytometry (Subheading 3.5 and *see* **Note 5**) or confocal microscopy (Subheading 3.6).

3.3.3 Endocytosis Mechanism Using Inhibitors (See Note 6)

1. Cell culture medium is changed for serum-free medium containing 5 μM cytochalasin D, or 80 μM Dynasore, or 3 mM amiloride, or vehicle (DMSO or cell media).
2. FL-AS1411 or FL-CRO stock solution is added directly to the medium to give a final concentration of 10 μM, or an equivalent volume of vehicle (sterile water) is added for "no DNA" cells.
3. Cells are incubated at 37 °C for 2 h.
4. Cells are analyzed by flow cytometry (Subheading 3.5 and *see* **Note 5**) and confocal microscopy (Subheading 3.6).

3.3.4 Characterizing Endocytic Vesicles

1. The cell culture medium is changed to serum-free medium.
2. FL-AS1411 or FL-CRO stock solution is added directly to the medium to give a final concentration of 10 μM, or an equivalent volume of vehicle (sterile water) is added for "no DNA" cells.
3. Alexa Fluor 594-labeled dextran-10 K (macropinocytic marker) is added to give a final 0.2 mg/mL concentration, or Alexa Fluor 594-labeled transferrin (clathrin-mediated endocytosis marker) is added to give a final concentration of 5 μg/mL.
4. The colocalization of FL-oligonucleotides and endocytic markers is examined by using confocal microscopy (Subheading 3.6).

3.4 Assessing the Role of Nucleolin in AS1411 Uptake

1. The cell culture medium is changed for Opti-MEM I medium.
2. Cells are transfected with nucleolin-targeted or negative control (scramble) siRNAs using Lipofectamine™ RNAiMAX Transfection Reagent (*see* **Note 7**).
3. siRNA/transfection agent complexes are prepared in sterile polystyrene tubes and distributed into culture plates.
   (a) The transfection agent is diluted in Opti-MEM I medium.
   (b) The siRNAs are diluted in Opti-MEM I medium.
   (c) The siRNA and transfection agent are mixed and incubated at room temperature for 10 min to form siRNA/transfection agent complex.
   (d) The siRNA/transfection agent complex are dispensed into the plated cells.
4. Cell medium is replaced for fresh medium supplemented with FBS at 8 h and again at 24 h posttransfection.

5. Cell medium is changed at 48 h posttransfection with FBS-supplemented medium containing 10 μM FL-AS1411 or 10 μM FL-CRO or no DNA.
6. Cells are incubated at 37 °C for 2 h.
7. Cells are analyzed by flow cytometry and/or confocal microscopy (Subheadings 3.5 and 3.6).

3.5 Analysis Using Flow Cytometry

1. The cells are washed once with ice-cold PBS.
2. A solution of 2 mL of ice-cold DPBS containing 1 μg/mL PI is added and plates are incubated for 3 min on ice. This allowed the exclusion of nonviable cells (*see* **Note 8**).
3. Cells are washed twice with ice-cold DPBS.
4. Cells are harvested by adding 1× trypsin–EDTA (300 μL) and incubating until cells are detached (approximately 1–3 min), then 4 mL of ice-cold FBS-supplemented culture medium is added (*see* **Note 9**).
5. The cell suspension is transferred into flow cytometry tubes and centrifuged at 400 × *g* at 4 °C for 5 min.
6. The cell pellet is gently resuspended in 0.5 mL of 1% paraformaldehyde and incubated for 10 min.
7. Cell are centrifuged at 400 × *g* at 4 °C for 5 min and the cell pellet is resuspended in 0.5 mL of DPBS.
8. The fluorescence is measured using a FACScalibur cytometer. Cells are gated to exclude cell debris and PI labeled (nonviable cells) (Fig. 2). Relative uptake is determined by comparing histograms and mean fluorescence intensities (Fig. 3).

3.6 Confocal Microscopy

1. Cells are washed three times with ice-cold DPBS.
2. Cells are fixed by adding 4% paraformaldehyde in PBS and incubating for 15 min at room temperature.
3. Cells are washed three times with DPBS.
4. The coverslips are mounted on glass slides with ProLong Antifade containing DAPI (Molecular Probes) according to the manufacturer's directions.
5. Fluorescence is observed with an inverted confocal laser-scanning microscope. Images are documented using an oil immersion 63× objective. Localization of FL-oligonucleotide and vesicle marker are compared (Fig. 4) (*see* **Notes 10** and **11**).

4 Notes

1. Check that addition of the fluorophore does not affect the biological activities of the oligonucleotide in question by comparing unlabeled and fluorophore-labeled sequences in a relevant assay (antiproliferative activity for AS1411 [4]).

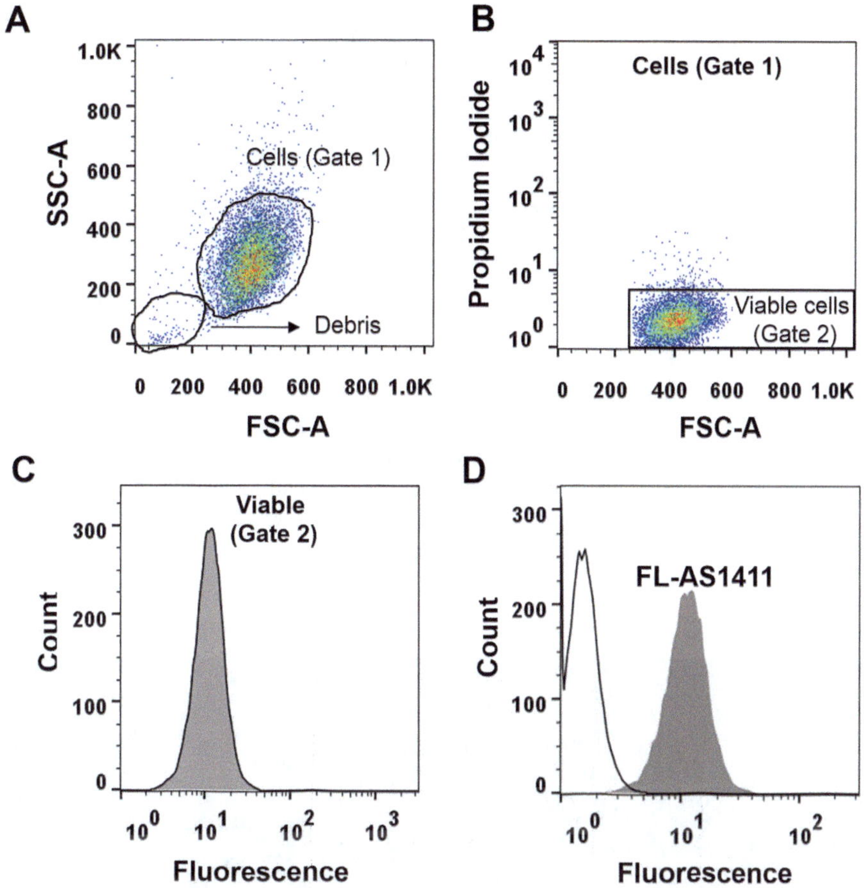

Fig. 2 Uptake analysis using flow cytometry. DU145 cells were left untreated or were incubated with fluorescently labeled AS1411 (FL-AS1411) for 2 h at 37 °C. After incubation, cells were processed for flow cytometry analysis and stained with a viability dye, such as propidium iodide or 7-AAD, which selectively stains dead cells. Unstained (viable) cells are used to set flow cytometer parameters. (**a**) Forward (FSC) versus side scatter (SSC) gating is used to exclude cell debris. (**b**) Propidium iodide (FL-3 channel) vs. FSC to exclude dead cells. Parameters are setting using unstained cells. (**c**) Single parameter (FL-1 channel) histogram of viable gated cells to determine uptake of FL-AS1411. (**d**) Histogram shows untreated cells (black line) and FL-AS1411 treated cells (solid gray)

2. A variety of fluorophore labels are available to be attached to oligonucleotides. We have also used fluorescein (6-FAM, Integrated DNA Technologies) for flow cytometry studies, but prefer Alex Fluor 488 for confocal microscopy because of reduced photobleaching.
3. If cell lines are not obtained directly from a reliable supplier, we recommend cell line authentication and testing for mycoplasma infection. Cross contamination or misidentification of cell lines is common [18] and mycoplasma infection has been reported to influence oligonucleotide uptake [19, 20].

	Mean Fluorescence	
Amiloride (mM)	**0**	**3**
No oligonucleotide	2.71	3.27
FL-CRO	7.65	3.21
FL-AS1411	21.2	11.1

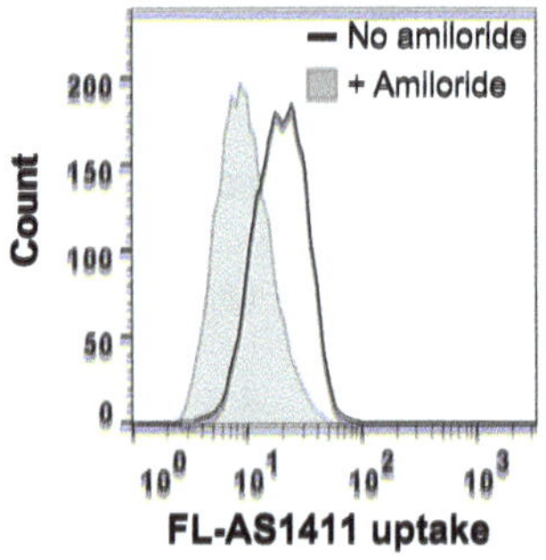

Fig. 3 Uptake analysis to determine the effect of an endocytic inhibitor. DU145 cells were pretreated for 1 h with 3 mM amiloride (macropinocytosis inhibitor) or with vehicle as control. After 1 h, oligonucleotide (10 μM FL-AS1411, 10 μM FL-CRO) or vehicle was added, and cells were incubated at 37 °C for a further 2 h. (**a**) Table shows mean fluorescence intensities of viable gated cells. (**b**) Histogram shows cells treated with FL-AS1411 in the absence (black line) or presence (solid gray) of amiloride

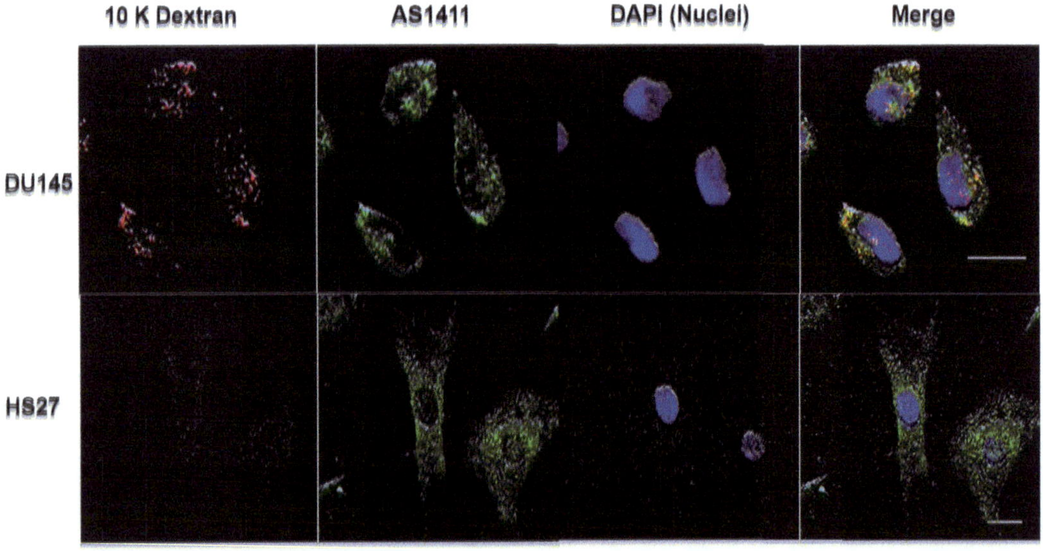

Fig. 4 AS1411 colocalizes with the macropinocytic marker in cancer cells. DU145 cancer cells or Hs27 nonmalignant cells were incubated with 10 μM AS1411 labeled with Alexa Fluor 488 (green) and 0.2 mg/mL dextran-10 K (macropinocytosis marker) labeled with Alexa Fluor 594 (red) for 2 h at 37 °C. Then cells were washed and fixed, then nuclei were stained with 4′,6-diamidino-2- phenylindole (DAPI; blue) and visualized by confocal microscopy. Scale bar, 10 μm

4. A variety of other fluorescently labeled markers for different endocytic mechanisms can be obtained from Thermo Fisher Scientific (Molecular Probes Handbook, Chapter 16). It has been reported recently that 70 kDa dextran may be a better marker for macropinocytosis than 10 kDa dextran [21], though in our studies the 10 kDa dextran appears to accurately mark macropinosomes judging by the size of vesicles detected.

5. Although harvesting cells by using trypsin–EDTA is usually enough to remove any extracellular oligonucleotide, it is important to document that the fluorescence observed is due to internalized rather than surface-bound oligonucleotide. This can be achieved by demonstrating that incubation of cells with trypan blue, which quenches any extracellular Alexa Fluor 488 fluorescence, has no effect on the fluorescence signal. After incubation with PI, cells can be incubated at 0.25 mg/mL trypan blue in serum-free media (or vehicle as control) for 1 min on ice before being assessed by flow cytometry.
6. Pharmacological inhibitors of different endocytic mechanisms can be used as an initial tool to evaluate the mechanism of oligonucleotide cellular uptake [4, 8, 9]. Genetic approaches can confirm the endocytic mechanism by altering the expression of specific proteins that control particular endocytic process. However, it is critical to ascertain that pharmacological inhibitors are used at a dose at which they are both nontoxic to cells and have their desired activity. Nontoxic concentrations for the cell line of interest can be determined by generating a dose response curve using any standard cytotoxicity assay. Pharmacological activity can be confirmed by assessing uptake of an appropriate fluorescently labeled marker (e.g., 10 kDa dextran for macropinocytosis or transferrin for dynamin-dependent endocytosis) in the absence or presence of the inhibitor at the selected nontoxic dose.
7. See the manufacturer's protocol instructions for a detailed RNAiMAX transfection procedure. To validate siRNAs, confirm knockdown of the target protein at various time points after transfection using standard immunoblotting assays. When performing experiments to assess the effects of siRNAs on uptake, retain an aliquot of cells to verify knockdown of the protein of interest under the conditions used. Lyse the cells using SDS-PAGE electrophoresis buffer, electrotransfer onto polyvinylidene fluoride membranes, and blot using any conventional immunoblotting assay. Immunoblotting/western blotting is a basic methodology that is well established in many laboratories. This technique requires equipment for electrotransfer onto polyvinylidene fluoride membranes and immunoblotting, such as: glass plates, spacers, comb, stand, power supply, primary and secondary antibodies, autoradiographic film (Biomax MR or X-Omat, Kodak), film cassettes with intensifying screen (Kodak) and developer.
8. Excluding nonviable cells is a critical step when assessing oligonucleotide uptake. Nonviable cells will take up high levels of fluorophore-labeled oligonucleotides by a nonendocytic, energy-independent process and this will confound the results.

9. This is a critical step. Cells should be observed to determine optimal timing as overtrypsinizing the cells is cytotoxic.
10. Observing the subcellular distribution of fluorophore-labeled oligonucleotides can indicate whether oligonucleotides remain trapped in endosomes (punctate staining in the cytoplasm) or whether they escape endosomes to assess targets in the cytosol or nucleus (diffuse cytoplasmic or nuclear staining). This is important because some mechanisms, including antisense and RNA interference, should require oligonucleotides to be cytosolic or nuclear in order to reach their targets and have the expected activity. However, even if the observed fluorescence is predominantly endosomal, it is theoretically possible that an undetectable amount of oligonucleotide could escape from the endosome.
11. To avoid artifacts using this technique, it is essential that cells are viable (to avoid nonspecific uptake) and that cells are not permeabilized during the fixation process (this would disrupt cell membranes and allows oligonucleotides to move between cellular compartments). In our experience with AS1411, strong nuclear staining is only seen in nonviable or permeabilized cells. To rule out such artifacts, care should be taken to ensure that treatments are nontoxic to cells under the conditions being studied (e.g., by coincubation with a viability dye) and results can be confirmed by studying uptake in live cells. Another limitation of this technique is that it cannot determine if the observed intracellular fluorescence is associated with intact or degraded oligonucleotide. There are a number of ways to assess whether oligonucleotides remain intact in the cell culture medium [15, 22] and an additional control is to compare uptake of FL-oligonucleotide with that of the free fluorophore, but determining oligonucleotide intactness inside cells requires additional methods such as FRET analysis [23]. In the case of AS1411, it is clear that this sequence has unusual cellular uptake properties that can be exploited for delivery of various molecules into cells, but it remains to be seen exactly how it achieves this and how this property is related to its cancer-selective antiproliferative activities [12].

Acknowledgments

The work described was funded by NIH grant R01CA122383 (Bates). The authors are named coinventors on issued patents or patent applications pertaining to AS1411

References

1. Crooke ST, Wang S, Vickers TA, Shen W, Liang XH (2017) Cellular uptake and trafficking of antisense oligonucleotides. Nat Biotechnol 35(3):230–237. https://doi.org/10.1038/nbt.3779
2. Juliano RL (2016) The delivery of therapeutic oligonucleotides. Nucleic Acids Res 44(14):6518–6548. https://doi.org/10.1093/nar/gkw236
3. Bates PJ, Laber DA, Miller DM, Thomas SD, Trent JO (2009) Discovery and development of the G-rich oligonucleotide AS1411 as a novel treatment for cancer. Exp Mol Pathol 86(3):151–164. https://doi.org/10.1016/j.yexmp.2009.01.004
4. Reyes-Reyes EM, Teng Y, Bates PJ (2010) A new paradigm for aptamer therapeutic AS1411 action: uptake by macropinocytosis and its stimulation by a nucleolin-dependent mechanism. Cancer Res 70(21):8617–8629. https://doi.org/10.1158/0008-5472.CAN-10-0920
5. Yang NJ, Hinner MJ (2015) Getting across the cell membrane: an overview for small molecules, peptides, and proteins. Methods Mol Biol 1266:29–53. https://doi.org/10.1007/978-1-4939-2272-7_3
6. Doherty GJ, McMahon HT (2009) Mechanisms of endocytosis. Annu Rev Biochem 78:857–902. https://doi.org/10.1146/annurev.biochem.78.081307.110540
7. Mayor S, Parton RG, Donaldson JG (2014) Clathrin-independent pathways of endocytosis. Cold Spring Harb Perspect Biol 6(6). https://doi.org/10.1101/cshperspect.a016758
8. Ivanov AI (2014) Pharmacological inhibitors of exocytosis and endocytosis: novel bullets for old targets. Methods Mol Biol 1174:3–18. https://doi.org/10.1007/978-1-4939-0944-5_1
9. Ivanov AI (2008) Pharmacological inhibition of endocytic pathways: is it specific enough to be useful? Methods Mol Biol 440:15–33. https://doi.org/10.1007/978-1-59745-178-9_2
10. Vassilieva EV, Nusrat A (2008) Vesicular trafficking: molecular tools and targets. Methods Mol Biol 440:3–14. https://doi.org/10.1007/978-1-59745-178-9_1
11. Bates PJ, Kahlon JB, Thomas SD, Trent JO, Miller DM (1999) Antiproliferative activity of G-rich oligonucleotides correlates with protein binding. J Biol Chem 274(37):26369–26377
12. Bates PJ, Reyes-Reyes EM, Malik MT, Murphy EM, O'Toole MG, Trent JO (2017) G-quadruplex oligonucleotide AS1411 as a cancer-targeting agent: uses and mechanisms. Biochim Biophys Acta Gen Subj 1861(5 Pt B):1414–1428. https://doi.org/10.1016/j.bbagen.2016.12.015
13. Rosenberg JE, Bambury RM, Van Allen EM, Drabkin HA, Lara PN Jr, Harzstark AL, Wagle N, Figlin RA, Smith GW, Garraway LA, Choueiri T, Erlandsson F, Laber DA (2014) A phase II trial of AS1411 (a novel nucleolin-targeted DNA aptamer) in metastatic renal cell carcinoma. Investig New Drugs 32(1):178–187. https://doi.org/10.1007/s10637-013-0045-6
14. Choi EW, Nayak LV, Bates PJ (2010) Cancer-selective antiproliferative activity is a general property of some G-rich oligodeoxynucleotides. Nucleic Acids Res 38(5):1623–1635. https://doi.org/10.1093/nar/gkp1088
15. Dapić V, Bates PJ, Trent JO, Rodger A, Thomas SD, Miller DM (2002) Antiproliferative activity of G-quartet-forming oligonucleotides with backbone and sugar modifications. Biochemistry 41(11):3676–3685. https://doi.org/10.1021/bi0119520
16. Commisso C, Davidson SM, Soydaner-Azeloglu RG, Parker SJ, Kamphorst JJ, Hackett S, Grabocka E, Nofal M, Drebin JA, Thompson CB, Rabinowitz JD, Metallo CM, Vander Heiden MG, Bar-Sagi D (2013) Macropinocytosis of protein is an amino acid supply route in Ras-transformed cells. Nature 497(7451):633–637. https://doi.org/10.1038/nature12138
17. Reyes-Reyes E, Salipur FR, Shams M, Forsthoefel MK, Bates PJ (2015) Mechanistic studies of anticancer aptamer AS1411 reveal a novel role for nucleolin in regulating Rac1 activation. Mol Oncol 9(7):1392–1405. https://doi.org/10.1016/j.molonc.2015.03.012
18. Horbach SP, Halffman W (2017) The ghosts of HeLa: how cell line misidentification contaminates the scientific literature. PLoS One 12(10):e0186281. https://doi.org/10.1371/journal.pone.0186281
19. de Diesbach P, N'kuli F, Delmée M, Courtoy PJ (2003) Infection by mycoplasma hyorhinis strongly enhances uptake of antisense oligonucleotides: a reassessment of receptor-mediated endocytosis in the HepG2 cell line. Nucleic Acids Res 31(3):886–892. https://doi.org/10.1093/nar/gkg181
20. Rosenblatt MN, Burns JR, Duncan VE, Hughes JA (2000) Infection of the macrophage cell line NR8383 with Mycobacterium tuberculosis (H37Ra) leads to an increase in oligodeoxynucleotide accumulation. Antisense

Nucleic Acid Drug Dev 10(1):1–9. https://doi.org/10.1089/oli.1.2000.10.1

21. Li L, Wan T, Wan M, Liu B, Cheng R, Zhang R (2015) The effect of the size of fluorescent dextran on its endocytic pathway. Cell Biol Int 39(5):531–539. https://doi.org/10.1002/cbin.10424
22. Bates PJ, Choi EW, Nayak LV (2009) G-rich oligonucleotides for cancer treatment. Methods Mol Biol 542:379–392. https://doi.org/10.1007/978-1-59745-561-9_21
23. Remaut K, Lucas B, Braeckmans K, Sanders NN, De Smedt SC, Demeester J (2005) FRET-FCS as a tool to evaluate the stability of oligonucleotide drugs after intracellular delivery. J Control Release 103(1):259–271. https://doi.org/10.1016/j.jconrel.2004.11.019

Chapter 11

Measuring the Action of Oligonucleotide Therapeutics in the Lung at the Cell Type-Specific Level by Tissue Disruption and Cell Sorting (TDCS)

Helen Graves, Steven Evans, Michael Fauler, Manfred Frick, and Sterghios A. Moschos

Abstract

The clinical potential of DNA and RNA-targeting therapeutics for airways disease has been hampered by the poor translation of promising drug candidates from cell culture to in vivo models and the clinic. For example, classical preclinical approaches routinely report 20–60% target knockdown effects in the lung, where 1 or 2 log effects are observed in isolated cell cultures in vitro. Preparation of monocellular suspensions of tissues by mechanoenzymatic disruption followed by cell sorting (TDCS) after in vivo drug dosing, however, can offer pharmacokinetic and pharmacodynamic insights on the effects of drugs to precise cell subpopulations. Moreover, this can be reliably achieved with up to 66% fewer animals than standard in vivo pharmacology approaches due to lower data variance afforded through analytics on defined, viable cell numbers. Here we describe the TDCS methodology for the isolation of total lung epithelia, lung macrophages, and epithelium/macrophage-depleted cell fractions from mouse lungs using a two-stage sorting process of immunomagnetic bead separation followed by flow cytometric sorting using fluorescent antibodies against well-established surface markers such as F4/80, CD11b, and CD326. Validated antibodies for additional cell types and markers are also provided.

Key words Lung, Cell type-specific in vivo pharmacology, Oligonucleotides, Fluorescence activated cell sorting, Magnetic cell sorting, RNAi, siRNA, Antisense, MicroRNA

1 Introduction

Pharmacokinetic and pharmacodynamic assessment of oligonucleotide and other DNA or RNA-targeting therapeutics in vivo typically involves bioanalytical procedures carried out at tissue level. After following standardized procedures on animal models of disease, animals are terminally anaesthetized at set time points, tissues are excised, and homogenized, to extract and purify protein, DNA or RNA [1]. Analytes are then processed for the measurement of specific gene/protein expression or, more recently, full proteomic and transcriptomic analysis. Where possible, drug loading can also

Olof Gissberg et al. (eds.), *Oligonucleotide-Based Therapies: Methods and Protocols*, Methods in Molecular Biology, vol. 2036, https://doi.org/10.1007/978-1-4939-9670-4_11,

be assessed (e.g., using mass spectrometry [2], hybridization-based nucleic acid capture assays, or amplification methods such as PCR), provided oligonucleotide drug chemistry is compatible with DNA polymerases. Unfortunately, the 1–2 log knockdown effects of antisense and short interfering RNA (siRNA) therapeutics typically measured in cell culture only translates to 40–60% target RNA reduction at the whole lung tissue level in animals; clinical data can be even more disappointing [3].

The reasons for these discrepancies have been the subject of intense debate, speculation, and assumptions, as extensively discussed elsewhere [3, 4]. From a mathematical perspective, analysing target RNA levels in homogenized lung tissues can only yield lower levels of drug effect as compared to cell line experiments, due to poor signal-to-noise ratios. The problem occurs because the levels of an RNA target measured in an extract from a whole lung lobe reflect the average level of that RNA molecular species across the pool of different cell types that constitute the lung tissue. Furthermore, the relative numbers of each cell type are not fixed and can vary on account of disease, especially when inflammation is involved. At the same time, the extent to which target RNA levels may change on account of oligonucleotide treatment in a given cell is, as a minimum, a function of oligonucleotide transfection efficiency: this efficiency also varies between cell types. Furthermore, it is still unknown if downregulation of a target gene in some cells leads to compensatory gene expression changes in untransfected bystander cells.

In an ideal scenario, therefore, the effect of an oligonucleotide drug on a tissue as complex as the lung should be measured by cell type, and in relation to its degree of transfection. This can be achieved by applying mechanoenzymatic Tissue Disruption and Cell Sorting (TDCS) on in vivo pharmacology experiments. Indeed, industry evidence on what makes for successful drug discovery [5] points to TDCS as a tool that would offer added value to project decision making. By sorting tissue cells by type, measuring drug loading, and on-target effect, one can obtain evidence of target engagement, and an on-target mechanism of action [6] in cells relevant to disease, in vivo, and potentially even in patients. Obtaining such pharmacological evidence is now considered pivotal to drug development efforts [7].

Many of the tools and materials necessary to implement TDCS are well-established from basic research studies involving primary tissue cell isolation. Over the past decade, increasingly complicated cell separation approaches have been used to study cell type specific biology in primary human tissue, tumor biopsies, as well as animal models of disease. Two important methods are fluorescence-activated cell sorting (FACS), and magnetic cell sorting (MACS). The FACS method is good for high cell purity and high cell recovery, low cell surface marker expression, detection of intracellular markers, as well as sorting cells by cell surface marker expression levels. In contrast, MACS, being suitable only for surface markers, is good for bulk cell depletion/enrichment for a single surface marker (e.g., in the preparation for FACS) or situations where the optical properties of the cell interfere with marker sensitivity such as autofluorescence, either in large-scale instruments or microfluidic systems. Recent advances in these platforms are reviewed by Shields et al. [8]. Studies involving MACS and/or FACS use either in-house, or supplier prevalidated reagents (antibodies or aptamers) specific to cell surface markers found in cell subpopulations, or markers accessible after cell fixation and permeabilization. Reagent validation usually takes the form of gene expression/surface marker analysis of sorted cells, cell function analyses, marker coexpression as observed histopathologically, by Western blotting, or by alternative means including physicochemical properties exhibited during flow cytometry [2]. The vast body of work involving cell sorting can be a very useful resource in implementing TDCS in in vivo pharmacology studies not only for lung disease but virtually for any indication with a substantial body of basic research involving cell sorting methods and appropriate validation of marker-specific reagents.

Using TDCS we were therefore able to show that oligonucleotide drugs dosed directly into mouse tracheas loaded at appreciable amounts only in airway/alveolar macrophages but with no statistically significant effect on a target gene, despite statistical power for measuring a 50% change exceeding 94% [2]. Histological and ADME follow-up experiments explained this outcome through the observation of rapid oligonucleotide transcytosis from the airway lumen into circulation, and elimination in urine in as little as 15 min after dosing. Tissues were obtained from animals in accordance with regulations and established guidelines and were reviewed and approved by an Institutional Animal Care and Use Committee or through an Ethical Review Board. Although our results were with modified short interfering RNA (siRNA) and third generation, short locked nucleic acid (LNA) drugs, the findings were in line with historical pharmacokinetic studies by Ionis pharmaceuticals on longer, second generation antisense oligonucleotides [9]. This suggested that more recent clinical measurements were not sensitive enough to measure circulatory and urine oligonucleotide levels in man [3]. Clinical efforts with naked siRNA and antisense oligonucleotides performed by a number of pharmaceutical companies were abandoned shortly afterward.

Presently, research on oligonucleotide drugs for respiratory diseases involves agents that work as toll like receptor agonists, splice modulating antisense, in vitro transcribed RNA therapeutics including long noncoding RNAs, mediators of DNA and RNA editing, and RNA interference modulators (microRNA mimics, siRNA, and microRNA inhibitors). This is on account of the recent regulatory approvals of the antisense drugs mipomersen (familial hypercholesterolemia), inotersen (hereditary transthyretin-mediated amyloidosis), nusinersen (spinal muscular atrophy; drugs developed by Ionis Pharmaceuticals), and eteplirsen (Duchenne's muscular dystrophy; developed by Sarepta Therapeutics), the siRNA drug patisiran (hereditary transthyretin-mediated amyloidosis; developed by Alnylam Pharmaceuticals), as well as unprecedented advances involving the development and use of an antisense drug for a single patient harboring a unique mutation, also known as "*n* of 1 medicine," as exemplified by milasen [10]. Crucially, all of these drugs effectively load onto disease-relevant target tissues and cells, either through first pass metabolism (targeting the liver) or by direct intrathecal injection to reach the central nervous system. Therefore, to achieve comparable success in the lung, with few exceptions, investigators are evaluating a cadre of nanoformulation approaches as drug delivery solutions to successfully transfect airways cells. Although the safety of particulate drug delivery to the lungs is still a substantial outstanding concern [3, 11, 12], the need remains for determining drug loading and effect in the lung cell types relevant to disease.

In this protocol we therefore detail the approach for processing an excised mouse lung to sort precise numbers of specific cell types for appropriate downstream analytics. We describe the steps needed to successfully prepare monocellular suspensions, and detail the approach for sorting three cell preparations, each consisting of 20,000 lung epithelial cells, macrophages, or nonepithelial/non-macrophage cells from a single lung lobe (Fig. 1). The two-stage sorting protocol first makes use of magnetic bead-based separation, followed by flow cytometric sorting using fluorochrome conjugated antibodies against cell surface markers of interest. This protocol is therefore an extension to a previously published method for in vivo RNA therapeutics pharmacology [1], and focuses exclusively on how to implement TDCS. In our hands, TDCS can be reliably followed up with transcriptomics, proteomics, and mass spectrometry, as well as subculturing (where cell division is naturally accommodated by the cell type of interest). With the emergence of single cell 'omics, the anticipated parallelization, and cost reduction of these newer bioanalytical approaches, we look forward to TDCS-based in vivo pharmacology delivering highly potent, safe, and targeted airway therapeutics.

2 Materials

2.1 Preparation of Monocellular Lung Suspension from a Mouse Lung Lobe

1. Digestion buffer: 2.5% v/v fetal bovine serum (FBS), 0.5 mM calcium chloride, 0.75 mM magnesium chloride and 1.5% w/v DNase I from bovine pancreas (lyophilized powder at >85% purity, >400 Kunitz units/mg protein; Sigma Aldrich, Dorset, UK; *see* **Note 1**) prepared in Dulbecco's Phosphate Buffered

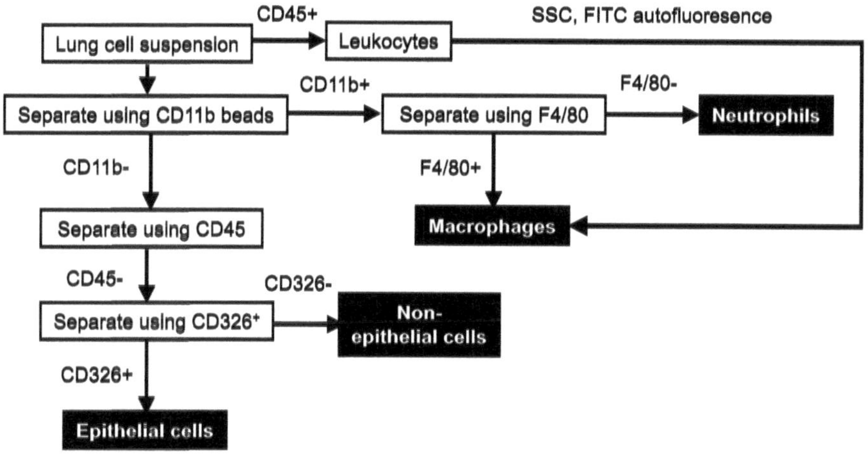

Fig. 1 Cell sorting strategy for the parallel isolation of lung epithelia, lung macrophages and remaining cells from a single mouse lung lobe digest. In addition to the previously published approach of obtaining macrophages (CD11b+; F4/80+), epithelia (CD11b−; CD45−; CD326+) and nonmacrophage/epithelial cells (CD11b−; CD45−; CD326−), the protocol is amenable to neutrophil isolation (CD11b+, F4/80−). For macrophage-focused work, a simple CD45+, side scatter (SSC) high, fluorescein isothiocyanate (FITC) autofluorescence high positive selection approach can be reliably implemented

Saline without calcium and magnesium (DPBS). Make fresh when needed.

2. Collagenase Buffer: 150 units/ml Collagenase 3 (Worthington Biochemical Corporation, Lakewood, NJ, USA) in digestion buffer; prepare the night before and keep at 4 °C or on ice until used (*see* **Note 1**).
3. Cell resuspension buffer: sterile 1× DPBS supplemented with 5% v/v FBS.
4. Oscillating platform incubator, set at 37 °C.
5. gentleMACS tissue dissociator (Miltenyi Biotec Ltd., Woking, UK).
6. gentleMACS C Tubes (purple), for tissue dissociation (Miltenyi Biotec Ltd.; *see* **Note 2**).
7. Sterile tissue vials such as 5 ml universals, 15 or 50 ml cell culture centrifugation tubes.
8. 50 ml sterile, cell culture centrifugation tubes.
9. Sterile 5 ml syringes.
10. Sterile 1× PBS.
11. 18 MΩ deionized water.
12. 3.6% w/v sodium chloride in sterile, deionized water.
13. Cell counting apparatus (hemocytometer and trypan blue or automated cell counter).

14. Desktop refrigerated centrifuge with bucket swing out rotor, for cell culture purposes.
15. 40 μm and 100 μm Cell Strainers.
16. Wet ice.
17. Serological pipettes (25 ml).
18. Serological pipette gun with variable speed control.
19. Sterile spatula(s) (*see* **Note 3**).

2.2 Isolation of Specific Cell Types from Digested Lung Tissue

1. autoMACS running buffer: 1× phosphate buffered saline supplemented with 2 mM EDTA, 0.5% w/v bovine serum albumin (BSA), and 0.09% w/v sodium azide, pH 7.2; stored at 4 °C for long-term use.
2. CD11b+ paramagnetic microbeads (Miltenyi Biotech).
3. Compensation beads: anti-rat IgG for the rat anti-mouse antibodies used in this protocol or alternative species as required.
4. BD Biosciences Accudrop beads: Drop delay set up beads (BD Biosciences, Crawley, UK).
5. Cytometer Setup and Tracking beads (CS and T beads) (BD Biosciences).
6. Stain buffer: 5% w/v BSA or similar in 1× PBS.
7. 2% BSA supplemented PBS: 2% w/v BSA or similar in 1× PBS.
8. Peridinin Chlorophyll Protein Complex (PerCP) anti-mouse F4/80 (Thermo Fisher Scientific).
9. Phycoerythrin (PE) anti-mouse CD326 (Biolegend, San Diego, CA).
10. Fluorescein isothiocyanate (FITC) anti-mouse CD45 (BD Biosciences).
11. 30 μm filter or cell strainer.
12. autoMACS Pro Separator (Miltenyi Biotec Ltd.; *see* **Note 4**).
13. Chilled collection blocks for autoMACS Pro (ensure chilled to 4 °C prior to use).
14. FACS tubes with 35 μm cell strainer cap.
15. Cell sorter capable of analysing four fluorochromes and depositing sorted cells into a 96-well plate (e.g., BD FACS Aria (BD Biosciences); *see* **Note 5**).
16. Uncoated, sterile, cell culture 96-well plates (round or flat bottom) appropriate to the downstream analytical approach to be used.

3 Methods

3.1 Preparation of Monocellular Lung Suspension from a Mouse Lung Lobe

1. Rinse the fresh, perfused mouse lung, with sterile PBS to eliminate any blood.
2. Transfer the lung lobe to 2 ml of digestion buffer in a sterile tissue vial (ensure full tissue submersion) and keep on ice until all lungs are harvested.
3. Transfer tissue into a gentleMACS C tube using a sterile spatula and add 5 ml of Collagenase Buffer per tube (*see* **Notes 6** and **7**).
4. Close the gentleMACS C tube using the provided impeller cap (*see* **Note 8**).
5. Mix by gentle inversion three times.
6. Keep on ice until all lungs are prepared.
7. Once all the lungs for your experiment are prepared, process them sequentially on the gentleMACS tissue dissociator by placing the tubes, inverted, onto the device, and running program m_lung_01.01 provided by the supplier, to disrupt the tissue.
8. Transfer the gentleMACS C tubes onto an oscillating platform incubator set at 37 °C and shake at 250 rpm for 30 min.
9. Return the gentleMACS C tubes onto the gentleMACS tissue dissociator and process the samples using program m_lung_02.01 to achieve monocellular suspensions.
10. Pulse-centrifuge the gentleMACS C tubes for 10 s at 400 × *g* to collect cells at the bottom of the tube.
11. Assemble a 50 ml centrifugation tube per lung lobe with a 40 μm cell strainer.
12. Pass the cells through the 40 μm cell strainer using a 5 ml syringe plunger.
13. Rinse the strainer with 3 × 1 ml of digestion buffer into the 50 ml centrifugation tube.
14. With the strainer still attached to the centrifuge tubes, centrifuge the cells at 400 × *g*, 4 °C for 10 min, to improve cell recovery rate.
15. Carefully remove and discard the supernatant without disturbing the cell pellet.
16. Resuspend the cells in 4 ml of cell resuspension buffer by gentle mixing using a 25 ml serological pipette, and keep on wet ice or at 4 °C.
17. Add 20 ml of deionized water; *quickly* cap the tube and invert to mix.

18. After 20 s make the solution isotonic by adding 8 ml of 3.6% w/v sodium chloride (*see* **Note 9**).
19. Centrifuge the cells at 400 × *g*, 4 °C for 10 min.
20. Carefully remove and discard the supernatant without disturbing the cell pellet.
21. Resuspend the cells in 5 ml cell resuspension buffer.
22. Count your cells, for example, by trypan blue exclusion assay on a hemocytometer (mix 25 μl of Trypan Blue with 25 μl of cell suspension and load onto the hemocytometer; count as per hemocytometer manufacturer instructions) or automated cell counting apparatus.
23. Store on ice or at 4 °C until cell sorting is carried out (*see* **Note 10**).

3.2 Isolation of Specific Cell Types from Digested Lung Tissue

Due to the high intrinsic autofluorescence of tissue resident macrophages which can make flow cytometric analysis more challenging and limit the choice of fluorochromes, a two-stage separation protocol is advised whereby macrophages and other myeloid cells are first removed in bulk using CD11b-specific paramagnetic beads, followed by flow cytometric staining and cell sorting (*see* **Note 11**; Fig. 1).

There are a large range of kits and reagents commercially available for the immune-magnetic isolation or depletion of particular cell types in a blood or tissue sample. Magnetic microbeads are coupled to antibodies specific for cell surface epitopes and when combined with a magnetic field, the desired cell type can be isolated or undesired cell types removed. This section describes the use of Miltenyi MACS reagents and equipment but the methods described could be carried out with equivalent reagents from other sources. Similarly, the fluorochromes used can be adapted to the capability of the cell sorter and fluorescent antibodies are available from a wide range of commercial suppliers. Table 1 summarizes antibody suppliers which have proven reliable in our hands when applying TDCS in pharmacological studies (all reagents were used at the manufacturer's recommended concentration).

3.2.1 Separation of CD11b+ Cells Using autoMACS Pro

1. Retain at least 0.5 ml of each digested lung sample and store at 4 °C. Run the remaining sample through the autoMACS Pro as described below.
2. Spin digested lung sample(s) at 400 × *g* for 5 min to pellet the cells and resuspend them in autoMACS running buffer at 10E7 cells per 80 μl.
3. Pass the sample through a filter to ensure a single cell suspension.
4. Add 20 μl of CD11b-specific microbeads per 10E7 cells and incubate at 4 °C for 15 min (*see* **Note 12**).

Table 1
Antibodies validated for compatibility with TDCS on live or fixed cells

Species	Target and clone	Supplier and cat. no.	Application
Mouse	CD105; 209701	BD Biosciences, R and D Systems FAB1320A	Endothelial cells or activated macrophages, positive selection; can discriminate the two populations by granularity
Mouse	CD45; 30-F11	BD Biosciences 557659, 557235	Type I epithelial cell negative selection; Leukocyte positive selection; Macrophage cell positive selection±
Mouse	F4/80; BM8	Invitrogen MF48021	Positive selection of macrophages in a CD11b− population; F4/80 negative selects for neutrophils
Mouse	CD144; 55-7H1	BD Biosciences 560411	Endothelial cell positive selection
Mouse	CD326; G8.8	Cambridge Biosciences 118205, Biolegend 118205	Epithelial cell positive selection in a CD45−, CD11b− population
Mouse	CD11b; M1/70	Miltenyi Biotech 130-049-601	Paramagnetic bead positive selection of macrophages, neutrophils, NK cells, granulocytes and dendritic cells (requires F4/80+ downstream for macrophage selection) and negative selection for epithelial cells (requires CD45−, CD326+ downstream)
Rat	ATP-binding cassette subfamily A member 3; 3C9	Abcam ab24751	Alveolar type II epithelial cells, positive selection[a]
Rat	EpCAM; polyclonal	Abcam ab71916	Epithelial cells, positive selection[a]
Rat	CD45; OX1	eBioscience 12-0461	Negative selection for epithelial enrichment[b]
Rat	CD68; ED1	Abcam ab31630	Macrophages, positive selection[b]
Rat	CD45; REA450	Miltenyi Biotec 130-109-682	Paramagnetic bead negative selection for epithelial enrichment against leukocytes and macrophages[b]
Mouse, rat	CD90.1; His51	Miltenyi Biotec 130-094-523	Paramagnetic bead positive selection for T cells[b]
Human	TLR2; TL2.1	Invitrogen 16203	Positive selection for epithelial cells[b]

±Include SSC and FITC channel autofluorescence in selection criteria
[a]Useful for paraformaldehyde-fixed and saponin-permeabilized cells only
[b]Validated on live cells only

5. If not done previously during the incubation, turn on and prime the autoMACS machine and ensure prechilled collection blocks are removed from the fridge.
6. Wash the samples with 1 ml ice-cold autoMACS running buffer and spin at 400 $\times g$.

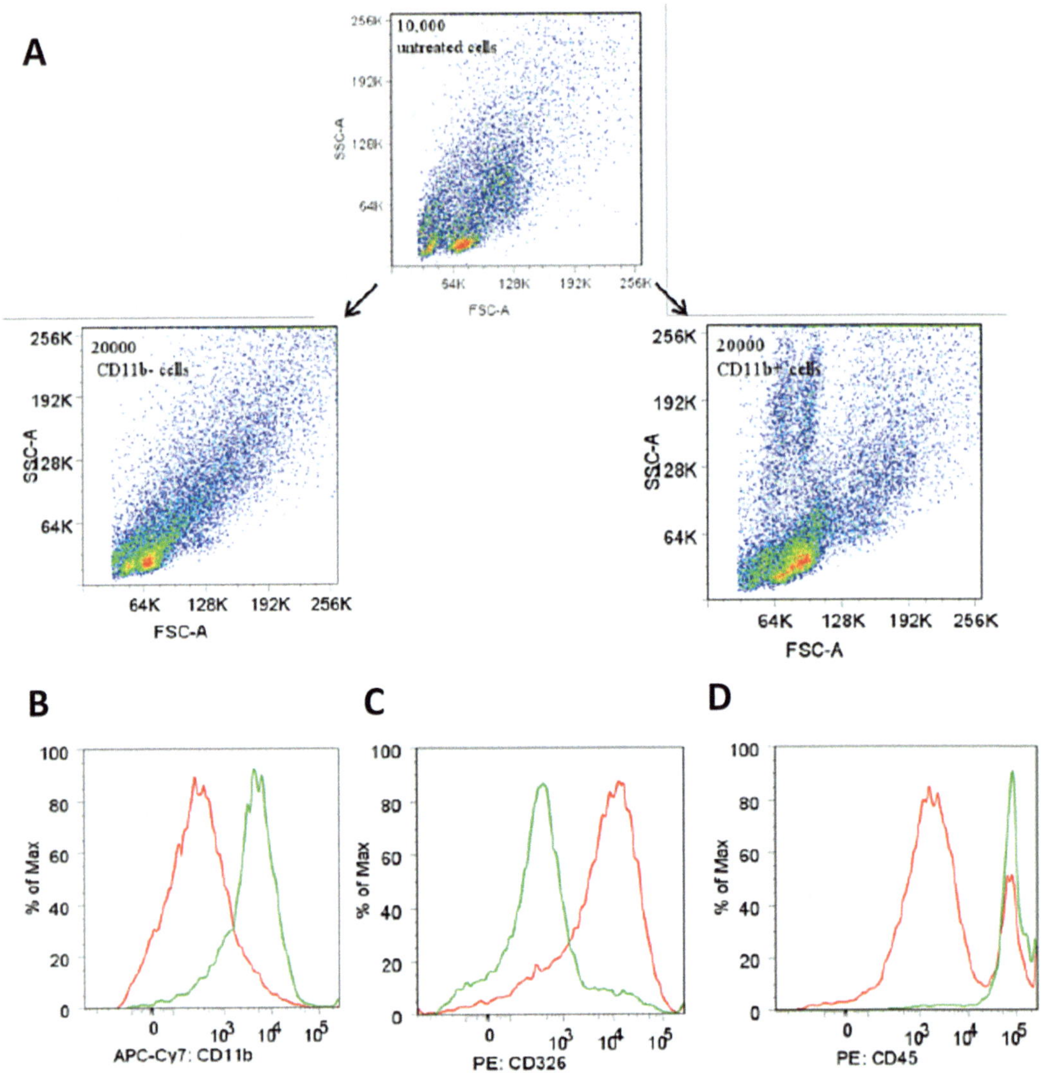

Fig. 2 (**a**) Representative scatter plots of digested lung samples prior to CD11b depletion and the CD11b− (left) or CD11b+ (right) fractions following separation. (**b–d**) Histograms comparing the CD11b− population to the CD11b+ population in terms of CD11b (**b**), CD326 (**c**), and CD45 (**d**) expression.

7. Discard the supernatant and resuspend in 500 μl autoMACS running buffer.
8. Run samples on the autoMACS, using the "deplete_s" program followed by a quick wash between each sample.
9. Both the CD11b+ and CD11b− fraction are collected into the prechilled collection block.
10. Spin samples down at 400 × *g* and resuspend in 100 μl stain buffer (*see* **Note 13**; *see* Fig. 2 for a typical forward scatter/side scatter (FSC/SSC) plot of the CD11b+ and CD11b− fractions).

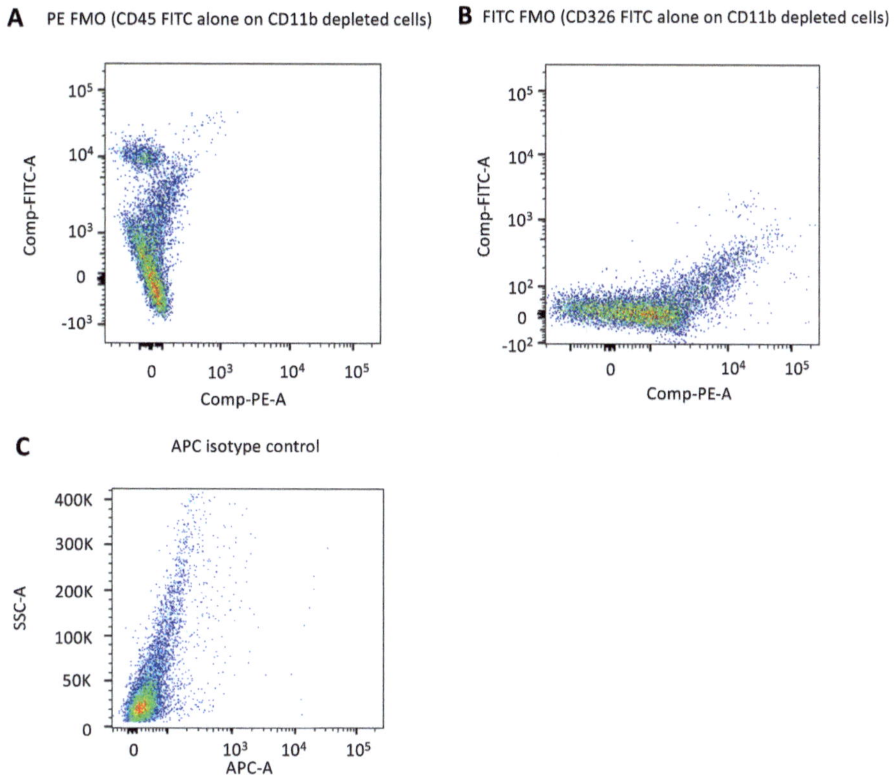

Fig. 3 Example of gating controls in flow cytometric analysis. CD11b− fractions were stained with two antibodies, making them appropriate for Fluorescence Minus One (FMO) controls. An example PE FMO (FITC antibody only) is shown in (**a**), and an example FITC FMO (PE antibody only) is shown in (**b**). The CD11b+ fraction was only stained with one antibody so here an FMO was not appropriate; instead, an APC conjugated isotype control was used as negative control to gate for F4/80 positive cells, with an example shown in (**c**)

3.2.2 Fluorescent Staining for Flow Cytometric Analysis and Sorting

Keep aside sufficient cells to set up appropriate controls as exemplified in Fig. 3 (*see* **Notes 14–16**).

1. Stain the fractions of CD11b− cells with anti-CD45 and anti-CD326 to identify leukocytes and epithelial cells (*see* Fig. 1).
2. Stain the fractions of CD11b+ cells with F4/80 to discriminate macrophages.
3. Use 20 μl of each antibody in a total volume of 100 μl cell resuspension buffer.
4. Incubate at 4 °C for 30 min.
5. At the same time, create single color controls for compensation by adding 1 drop of compensation beads to 100 μl cell resuspension buffer and incubate with 20 μl of one antibody for 30 min at 4 °C.
6. Wash samples and compensation beads with 1 ml stain buffer and spin at 400 × *g* for 5 min.

7. Resuspend the beads in 2 ml stain buffer and filter into a FACS tube to ensure a single cell suspension ready for analysis and sorting on the BD FACS Aria.
8. To allow accurate gating of populations, create an FMO (Fluorescence Minus One) control for each antibody used. For example, the PE FMO control will contain every antibody used *except* the PE antibody.

3.2.3 Sorting of Mixed Cell Populations, Macrophages, Epithelial Cells, and Nonepithelial Cells into 96-Well Plates for Downstream Assays

1. Set up the BD FACS Aria with a 70 μm nozzle and the pressure setting of medium drop drive frequency 60,000 with a "Purity" sort setting (e.g., 16-32-0; *see* **Note 17**).
2. Run BD CS&T beads to confirm Aria laser performance.
3. Run BD Accudrop beads to set up the drop delay and to align the 96-well plate.
4. Ensure SSC-W, SSC-H, FSC-W and FSC-H are enabled to allow doublet discrimination.
5. Add 100 μl of 5% BSA-supplemented PBS to each well of a 96-well plate.
6. Perform compensation using the single stained controls.
7. Take the third of the original sample that was not passed through the autoMACS Pro and spin at 400 × *g* to pellet.
8. Resuspend in 2 ml 2% BSA-supplemented PBS—this is the "mixed" population of cells and does not requiring any specific sorting but requires the correct number of live cells to be counted into the 96-well plate.
9. Gate the live, single cells on the basis of FSC/SSC. Sort 30,000 cells from within this gate into the appropriate well of a 96-well plate.
10. Run the CD11b+ population through the Aria and gate on live single cells and then on F4/80+ cells to sort 30,000 macrophages (Fig. 4a).

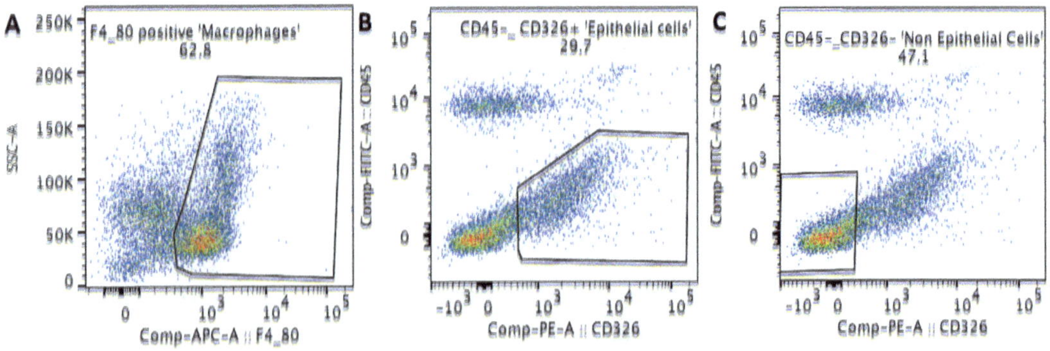

Fig. 4 Example of gating strategies for CD11b+, F4/80+ macrophage cells (**a**), CD11b− CD326+ epithelial cells (**b**), and CD11b− CD326− nonepithelial cells (**c**)

11. Run the CD11b− population through the Aria and gate on cells that are live/CD45−/CD326+ to sort 30,000 epithelial cells (Fig. 4b).
12. Continue to run the CD11b− population, gating on cells that are live/CD45−/CD326− to sort 60,000 nonepithelial cells (Fig. 4a) (*see* **Notes 18–20**; Figs. 3 and 4).

4 Notes

1. The source of DNase I, but more so collagenase, impacts significantly on process success and cell viability at completion of the TDCS process. This particular collagenase is sold as low protease activity which makes it also more appropriate for cell sorting applications. Although we have not tested the protease activity of the particular DNase I enzyme supplied from Sigma, we have not evaluated other enzymes in our workflow for impact on cell viability.
2. Important! Do not use the M tubes as these homogenize the tissue by vigorous mechanical shearing stress.
3. For infectious models/microbiome studies ensure that separate sterile spatulas are used per tissue.
4. The autoMACS Pro instrument was used to standardize multiple separations and help increase throughput but is not an absolute requirement. During method development, individual single use columns were used for some experiments and an acceptable throughput could be achieved in this manner with sufficient operators, although care would need to be taken to standardize technique.
5. The sorter used by the authors was a BD FACS Aria with 488 nm blue laser and 633 nm red laser. The laser and filter combinations available on any particular cell sorter will dictate the fluorochromes and combinations that can be used during cell sorting. If an instrument does not have a plate collection option, up to four populations can be sorted into tubes for later transfer to appropriate plates. It is worth bearing in mind though that at least one factor in the improved coefficients of variation observed with this method is the accurate deposition of defined cell numbers by the instrument—the equivalent of which is unlikely to be achieved manually.
6. For highly fibrous tissue (e.g., fibrosis models) it is advised to mince the tissue down into 1 mm^3 cubes first using a sterile scalpel and petri dish or an automated tissue chopping station before loading it into the gentleMACS C tube.

7. If a gentleMACS cell dissociator is not available, then skip **steps 3–11**; instead, process the tissue by mincing as described in the previous note, transfer it into a sterile vial, suspend in 5 ml digestion buffer/lung and incubate for 30 min on an oscillating platform incubator at 37 °C. Then triturate through a 5 ml syringe without a needle ~25 times and subsequently press the suspension through a 100 μm cell strainer using a sterile syringe plunger into a 50 ml cell centrifugation tube; push tissue clumps through the mesh if necessary. Proceed with **step 11**. This method is harsher and less reliable than the gentleMACS procedure in our experience.
8. Do not use normal cell centrifugation tube caps, as these will not allow the mechanic disruption to proceed.
9. **Steps 19** and **20** lyse any remaining red blood cells. This protocol is suited to other red blood cell lysis procedures (e.g., to obtain peripheral blood nucleated cells).
10. In our experience, cells will lose minimal viability (2–3%) over the next 48 h if kept at 4 °C and can even be safely shipped between sites within this timeframe if necessary.
11. CD11b is expressed on murine monocytes and macrophages but also on neutrophils, NK cells, dendritic cells and some subsets of activated lymphocytes. Using CD11b-specific magnetic separation is therefore not a purification, but an enrichment in one fraction and a reduction of autofluorescent cells in the other fraction. Further staining of the CD11b+ fraction allows for further discrimination of cell types of interest.
12. As only one sample can be processed by the machine at a time it is not recommended to stain all samples simultaneously as there will be a considerable lag time between staining and separation for the last samples processed. Subsequent samples can be stained and washed while previous ones are running through the machine. For this reason, it is useful (though not mandatory) to have two people carrying out this part of the protocol.
13. It is recommended to retain some of each fraction post magnetic separation to assess for viability and successful enrichment. A 100 μl sample can be stained with 2.5 μl of anti-CD11b antibody, incubated for 30 min and then washed with cell resuspension buffer. For viability, add 2 μl Sytox red, mix gently and proceed to analysis. Dead cells will stain positive in the APC channel and a % viability can be determined by gating on the negative cells.
14. Ideally, all steps will be completed in one day but it is possible to leave cells overnight at 4 °C at this stage for staining and sorting the following day. Viability was not affected and biomarker data showed that populations sorted on day 1 or day

2 were highly comparable, suggesting that sorting of a lung digest sample up to 24 h after preparation is an acceptable strategy when processing large numbers of mice. In our hands, the maximum throughput of lungs in one day was 12 and each sort (per animal) took approximately 30 min to achieve the required cell numbers.

15. Compensation controls will be required for most multicolor sorting experiments. With multilaser instruments it may be possible to select fluorochromes that avoid the need for compensation by being sufficiently spectrally separate or by being excited by different lasers. For example, on a four laser instrument, choosing one fluorochrome for each laser line may remove the requirement for compensation. However, this should always be checked initially with the appropriate single color controls. Compensation beads are most suitable in this instance due to the variable autofluorescence of cell populations in digested tissues. Unstained beads should be used for the unstained control, not unstained lung digest sample.

16. When first developing a panel, use irrelevant specificity isotype control antibodies to rule out nonspecific binding. Once confidence has been established in the antibodies to be used, isotype controls are not necessary for every experiment and Fluorescence Minus One (FMO) controls should be used to set population gates. For example, during method development, tests on ten different antibodies sold as luciferase-specific and compatible with sorting from a variety of suppliers failed to exhibit antigen specificity with this method; in stark contrast, no such issues were experienced with all other markers.

17. Depending on the cell type of interest and downstream application, a 100 μm nozzle might be more appropriate. The lower pressure and wider sort orifice causes less stress to sorted cells but in our hands resulted in poorer sort efficiency and fewer recovered cells. Viability staining of cells straight after sorting on a 70% nozzle showed the majority of the cells survived the sort and in our system those cells were assessed straight away, meaning that long term survival was not a concern. If downstream applications are to include culturing or functional studies, a 100 μm nozzle would be recommended. A purity sort mode was used in this protocol but each investigator should determine their own requirements of yield versus purity for specific applications. Efficiency on purity sort mode in our hands ranged from 79% to 95%.

18. The potential combination of cell surface markers and gating strategies for cell types in a digested mouse lung are very large. Since this method was developed there have been extensive studies published looking at full phenotypic characterization

of cell types in digested mouse lung—both hematological and structural. The populations identified with the antibodies described here are rather broad and can be added to or altered to more precisely identify numerous cell types depending on the investigator's specific interests. Staining for cell surface markers can be considerably more challenging in digested tissue than in blood due to the digestion process itself which may result in loss of cell surface epitopes. As an example, with the digestion protocol described herein, the authors had no success with a variety of anti-cytokeratin antibodies which had been described to bind strongly and specifically to epithelial cells which we hypothesize may be due to the loss of those markers during the digestion process itself.

19. "Fc block" (rat anti-mouse CD16/32) was trialed during development to prevent interaction of leukocyte Fc receptors with the Fc region of fluorescent antibodies but it made no difference compared to no Fc block controls so this was not continued. Other nonspecific binding was avoided by the presence of protein in the stain and sort buffers.
20. If fluorescence is being used to track delivery of oligonucleotides, the spectral profile of that dye will need to be considered in the panel design for cell sorting. For example, the use of Cy5-labeled oligonucleotides precluded the use of APC as a fluorochrome in this study.

References

1. Moschos SA, Spink KGG, Lindsay MA (2011) Measuring the action of CPP-siRNA conjugates in the lung. Methods Mol Biol 683:417–429
2. Moschos SAA, Frick M, Taylor B, Turnpenny P, Graves H, Spink KGG, Brady K, Lamb D, Collins D, Rockel TDD et al (2011) Uptake, efficacy, and systemic distribution of naked, inhaled short interfering RNA (siRNA) and locked nucleic acid (LNA) antisense. Mol Ther 19:2163–2168
3. Moschos SA, Usher L, Lindsay MA (2017) Clinical potential of oligonucleotide-based therapeutics in the respiratory system. Pharmacol Ther 169:83–103
4. Kumar M, Moschos SA (2017) Oligonucleotide therapies for the lung: ready to return to the clinic? Mol Ther. https://doi.org/10.1016/j.ymthe.2017.11.002
5. Morgan P, Van Der Graaf PH, Arrowsmith J, Feltner DE, Drummond KS, Wegner CD, Street SDA (2012) Can the flow of medicines be improved? Fundamental pharmacokinetic and pharmacological principles toward improving Phase II survival. Drug Discov Today 17:419–424
6. Cook D, Brown D, Alexander R, March R, Morgan P, Satterthwaite G, Pangalos MN (2014) Lessons learned from the fate of AstraZeneca's drug pipeline: a five-dimensional framework. Nat Rev Drug Discov 13:419–431
7. Morgan P, Brown DG, Lennard S, Anderton MJ, Barrett JC, Eriksson U, Fidock M, Hamrén B, Johnson A, March RE et al (2018) Impact of a five-dimensional framework on R&D productivity at AstraZeneca. Nat Rev Drug Discov 17:167–181
8. Shields CW, Reyes CD, López GP, López PGP (2015) Microfluidic cell sorting: a review of the advances in the separation of cells from debulking to rare cell isolation. Lab Chip 15:1230–1249
9. Nicklin PL, Bayley D, Giddings J, Craig SJ, Cummins LL, Hastewell JG, Phillips JA (1998) Pulmonary Bioavailability of a Phosphorothioate Oligonucleotide (CGP 64128A): Comparison with Other Delivery Routes. Pharm Res 15:583–591

10. Kaiser J (2018) A tailormade drug developed in record time may save girl from fatal brain disease. Science (80). https://doi.org/10.1126/science.aav7907
11. Alton EW, Boushey HA, Garn H, Green FH, Hodges M, Martin RJ, Murdoch RD, Renz H, Shrewsbury SB, Seguin R et al (2012) Clinical expert panel on monitoring potential lung toxicity of inhaled oligonucleotides: consensus points and recommendations. Nucleic Acid Ther 22:246–254
12. Forbes B, O'Lone R, Allen PP, Cahn A, Clarke C, Collinge M, Dailey LA, Donnelly LE, Dybowski J, Hassall D et al (2014) Challenges for inhaled drug discovery and development: Induced alveolar macrophage responses. Adv Drug Deliv Rev 71:15–33

Chapter 12

Delivery of Antisense Oligonucleotides Mediated by a Hydrogel System: In Vitro and In Vivo Application in the Context of Spinal Cord Injury

Pedro M. D. Moreno, Teresa Rodrigues, Marília Torrado, Isabel F. Amaral, and Ana P. Pêgo

Abstract

Biomaterials-based hydrogels are attractive drug-eluting vehicles in the context of RNA therapeutics, such as those utilizing antisense oligonucleotide or RNA interference based drugs, as they can potentially reduce systemic toxicity and enhance in vivo efficacy by increasing in situ concentrations. Here we describe the preparation of antisense oligonucleotide-loaded fibrin hydrogels exploring their applications in the context of the nervous system utilizing an organotypic dorsal root ganglion explant in vitro system and an in vivo model of spinal cord injury.

Key words Antisense oligonucleotides, Hydrogel, Fibrin, Gene silencing, Central nervous system, Spinal cord injury, Dorsal root ganglion

1 Introduction

Biomaterials-based hydrogels are three-dimensional networks with very high water content and currently under investigation for various biomedical purposes among which tissue-engineering and drug delivery show immense potential [1]. In the area of nerve regeneration, hydrogels can be seen as scaffolds able to provide not only a physical support but also a more permissive environment for axonal growth after injury, as well as serve as matrices to vectorize several components that can enhance the regenerative process [2, 3]. To this regard, antisense oligonucleotides (AONs) could be promising drugs to achieve enhanced regeneration through gene expression modulation. Single-stranded modified AONs have shown the capacity to be productively, albeit unspecifically, taken up by several cell types in vitro and in vivo [4–6], including neurons in the central nervous system (CNS) [7–10], and target their cognate RNA for gene expression modulation. Thus, combination of hydrogels with

Olof Gissberg et al. (eds.), *Oligonucleotide-Based Therapies: Methods and Protocols*, Methods in Molecular Biology, vol. 2036, https://doi.org/10.1007/978-1-4939-9670-4_12,

AONs could provide a platform for their controlled localization and presentation to the target tissue, augmenting their activity while potentially reducing systemic toxicity concerns.

An interesting biomaterial for hydrogel formation and application in the CNS is fibrin as it has been shown to act as a permissive bridging material for axonal regeneration improving functional recovery after spinal cord injury when applied to the lesion site [11–13]. Thus, we here demonstrate the setup of an AON-loaded fibrin hydrogel platform to explore hydrogel-assisted AON delivery in two nervous system settings: the organotypic dorsal root ganglion (DRG) explant culture; and the rat spinal cord hemisection in vivo model system. Of notice is the fact that the organotypic DRG explant culture allows for the maintenance of the neuronal network and extracellular microenvironment creating an interesting and flexible in vivo-mimicking system on which to study AON-nerve cell interaction, uptake and silencing efficiency [14]. We have recently demonstrated that the fibrin-AON system provides an efficient platform for the local application of AONs inside the lesioned area of the spinal cord (in a rat spinal cord hemisection model) where AONs spread throughout the entire lesioned area achieving efficient gene silencing activity [14].

2 Materials

Unless mentioned otherwise all reagents are of analytical quality. Diligently follow all waste disposal regulations when disposing of waste materials.

Animal procedures need to follow ethically acceptable institutionally approved procedures and national and international regulations as well as be performed by personnel trained in laboratory animal procedures.

2.1 Preparation and Characterization of AON-Loaded Fibrin Hydrogels

1. Tris-buffered saline (TBS, 10× concentration): 1370 mM NaCl; 27 mM KCl; 330 mM Tris, pH 7.4, in Type 2 (pure) water. Sterilize by filtration (0.22 μm).
2. Fibrinogen solution: 30 mg/mL fibrinogen, 1× TBS pH 7.4. Add 0.250 g of plasminogen-free fibrinogen from pooled human plasma containing factor XIII (F4883, Sigma-Aldrich) (*see* **Note 1**) to a 50 mL conical centrifuge tube containing 10 mL of Type I (ultrapure) water (resistivity of 18.3 MegaΩ·cm at 25 ° C) and place it in a water bath at 37 °C for 4 h to allow solubilization, stirring gently every hour (final concentration: 25 mg/mL). Prepare one Spectra/Por® 7 standard regenerated cellulose dialysis tubing (8 kDa MWCO, Spectrum®) by previously immersing it in water for 30 min to remove the preservative solution, and dialyze the fibrinogen

against 5 L of 1× TBS pH 7.4 at RT during 24 h. Transfer to a conical centrifuge tube and sterilize by filtration (0.22 μm) using a low protein binding filter. Determine the concentration of fibrinogen using a NanoDrop™ UV-Vis spectrophotometer (or alternatively, a UV-Vis spectrophotometer and a quartz cuvette) (*see* **Note 2**). Concentrate the fibrinogen solution in a Sartorius Vivaspin® 20 mL centrifugal concentrator (50 or 100 kDa MWCO) (*see* **Note 3**) accordingly to the expected fibrinogen final concentration—30 mg/mL (if dilution is needed after concentration use 1× TBS, pH 7.4).

3. Alexa Fluor 488-labeled human fibrinogen: (1.5 mg/mL) fibrinogen from human plasma—Alexa Fluor™ 488 Conjugate (ThermoFisher Scientific, #F13191).
4. Thrombin stock solution at 100 National Institute of Health standard (NIH) U/mL in TBS pH 7.0. Thaw a vial with thrombin from human plasma (T7009, Sigma-Aldrich) on ice. Add slowly sterile TBS pH 7.0 directly into the thrombin flask (use a syringe with a needle to penetrate the rubber closure on the vial) to dissolve thrombin to a final concentration of 100 NHI units/mL (*see* **Note 4**). Place the thrombin flask on an orbital shaker at 4 °C and mix at a slow speed for 2 h. Sterilize the thrombin solution by filtration (0.22 μm) using a low protein binding filter. Prepare aliquots (25–50 μL) on ice (*see* **Note 5**) and store them at −20 °C. After thawed, aliquots may be stored at 4 °C for 1 week.
5. $CaCl_2$ stock solution at 50 mM in TBS pH 7.4. Dissolve 55.49 mg of $CaCl_2$ (102,378, Merck) in 10 mL of 1× TBS pH 7.4 and sterilize the solution by filtration (0.22 μm). Prepare 200 μL aliquots and store them at −20 °C. After thawed, aliquots may be stored at 4 °C.
6. Aprotinin stock solution at 5 mg/mL in 1× Phosphate buffered saline (PBS, 1×) pH 7.4. Dissolve 10 mg of aprotinin (A3428, Sigma-Aldrich) in 2 mL of 1× PBS and sterilize the solution by filtration (0.22 μm) using a low protein binding filter). Prepare 20 μL aliquots and store them at −20 °C; after thawed, aliquots may be stored at 4 °C for 1 week.
7. AONs: 50 μM Full phosphorothioate linked, 2′*O*-methyl-RNA single stranded oligonucleotide (Cy5-*mC*mC*mU*mC*mU*mU*mA*mC*mC*mU*mC*-mA*mG*mU*mU*mA*mC*mA) (*see* **Note 6**).
8. Phosphate buffered saline solution (PBS, 1×) (137 mM NaCl, 2.7 mM KCl, 10 mM Na_2HPO_4, 2 mM K_2HPO_4).
9. Microcentrifuge tubes (0.6 mL), Maxymum Recovery (Axygen).
10. 15-well μ-slide Angiogenesis (IBIDI).
11. Laser scanning confocal microscope.

2.2 Culture of Dorsal Root Ganglion (DRG) Explants Within AON-Loaded Fibrin Hydrogels

1. Timed pregnant (E18) 3-month-old female Wistar rats.
   All animals maintained under a 12-h/12-h light/dark cycle and fed with regular rodent's chow and tap water ad libitum.
2. Hanks's balanced salt solution (GIBCO).
3. DMEM/F12-P/S medium: DMEM/F12 with GlutaMAX™ (GIBCO), 1% (v/v) Penicillin/Streptomycin (P/S) (Biowest).
4. Supplemented DMEM/F-12 medium: DMEM/F12 with GlutaMAX™ (Gibco), 2% (v/v) B-27 (Thermo Fisher Scientific), 1% (v/v) P/S, 1.25 mg/mL amphotericin B (Capricorn Scientific), 30 ng/mL nerve growth factor (NGF) (Millipore), and 10 mg/mL aprotinin (Sigma-Aldrich).
5. Dumont 55 fine forceps.
6. Stereomicroscope with a digital camera.
7. 15-well μ-Slide Angiogenesis plates (IBIDI).
8. Microcentrifuge tubes (0.6 mL), Maxymum Recovery (Axygen).
9. mirVana miRNA Isolation Kit (Ambion).
10. Standard qPCR kits (one or two-step) and equipment.

2.3 Local Application of AON-Loaded Hydrogel in the Rat Hemisection Spinal Cord Injury Model

1. Anesthesia machine (isoflurane—IsoVet®—system).
2. Buprenorphine solution 0.3 mg/mL (Bupaq®).
3. Ophthalmic solution (Siccafluid®).
4. Humid food.
5. Glycosylated isotonic serum (BRAUN VET®).
6. EtOH 70% (v/v).
7. Iodopovidone solution 7.5% (m/v) (Braunol®).
8. Surgical equipment (scalpel, scissors, scraper, bone trimmer or rongeurs, forceps, sterile surgical compresses).
9. Digital scale.
10. Shaving machine.
11. Heating pads.
12. Materials for fibrin gel preparation as in Subheading 2.1.
13. Poly(trimethylene carbonate-co-ε-caprolactone) (P(TMC-CL)) patch (preparation of which is described in [15] and [16]) (*see* **Note** 7).
14. RNAlater (Thermofisher).
15. 1.5 mL glass tissue grinder (Wheaton).
16. Standard qPCR kits (one or two-step) and equipment.

3 Methods

3.1 Preparation of AON-Loaded Fibrin Hydrogels and Characterization by Confocal Microscopy

1. Take the purified fibrinogen solution at 30 mg/mL stored at −80 °C and thaw it in a 37 °C water bath keeping it at room temperature until use. Thaw an aliquot of Alexa-Fluor-488-labeled human fibrinogen (1.5 mg/mL) on ice and keep it covered from light.
2. Thaw the aliquots containing thrombin, $CaCl_2$, and aprotinin on ice.
3. Finally take the Cy5-labeled AON at initial 50 μM concentration (in nuclease-free water) and place it on ice and covered from light.
4. To prepare a 20 μL AON-loaded fibrin gel drop for characterization, the fibrinogen solution containing 0.14 mg/mL (i.e., 1% of total amount of unlabeled fibrinogen) of Alexa Fluor 488-labeled human fibrinogen is mixed in an 0.6 mL maximum recovery tube, with an equal volume of a thrombin working solution in 1× TBS pH 7.4 prepared from the stock solutions of thrombin, $CaCl_2$ and aprotinin. The final concentration of fibrin components is of 14 mg/mL fibrinogen, 2 NIH U/mL human thrombin, 2.5 mM $CaCl_2$, and 10 μg/mL aprotinin.
5. Incorporate the AONs (at 6 μM final concentration) into the fibrinogen solution before mixing with the thrombin working solution. Homogenize the polymerizing solution with the help of a 10 μL micropipette by pipetting three times up and down before transferring it to 15-well μ-slide Angiogenesis. Readily incubate it for 30 min at 37 °C in a 5% CO_2 humidified incubator to allow fibrin cross-linking by factor XIIIa.
6. Before imaging in a laser scanning confocal microscope, check gelation visually and hydrate the gel with 40 μL PBS.
7. AONs were previously observed to integrate into the fibrin network being closely colocalized with the fibrin fibers and not freely diffusing in the aqueous portion of the gel, while also leading to an increase in the average pore area of the fibrin network (Fig. 1) (*see* **Note 8**).

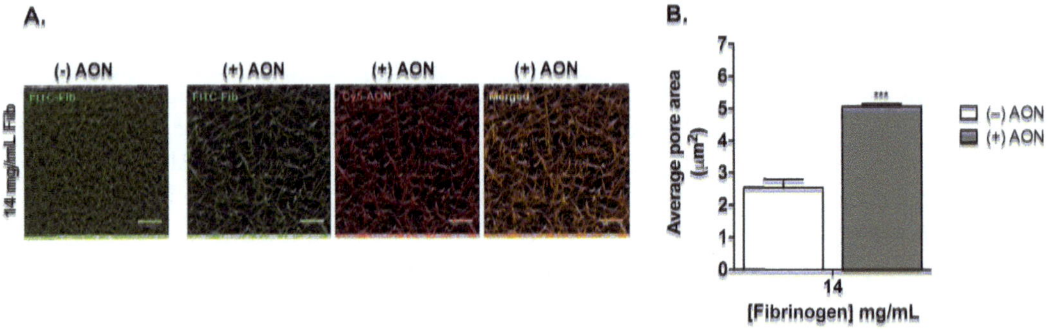

Fig. 1 Characterization of fluorescently labeled fibrin hydrogels using confocal microscopy. (**a**) Representative maximum Z-projections of confocal stack images of the corresponding fibrin gels (at fibrin concentrations of 14 mg/mL containing 1% (w/w) FITC- Fibrinogen). Complete association (colocalization) of Cy5-AONs with fibrin fibers (FITC-Fib) is observed. Scale bars, 10 μm. (**b**) Analysis of average pore area using confocal microscopy images taken from the fibrin gels. Maximum Z-projections were used to calculate the average pore area per image field using MATLAB. Two-way ANOVA, followed by Bonferroni post hoc test, was used for statistical analysis (mean ± standard deviation, $n = 3$ image fields per gel; $****p < 0.0001$; $***p = 0.0001$). Adapted from [14] and used with permission from the American Society of Gene & Cell Therapy

3.2 Gene Silencing in Dorsal Root Ganglion (DRG) Explants Mediated by AON-Loaded Fibrin Hydrogels

3.2.1 Rat DRG Explant Isolation

1. Sacrifice a pregnant adult Wistar rat (E18, considering E0.5 at the morning when a vaginal plug is detected) by CO_2 asphyxiation. Place the animal in the induction chamber set to 7 min of induction and 2 min of dwell time. To assure death, do an incision in the jugular vein. Confirm death by absence of heart beat.
2. Harvest embryos by caesarean section. For that, disinfect all the abdomen with 70% (v/v) ethanol and perform a C-cut in the skin, along the inguinal area. Then, to avoid damage of the uterus, lift the abdominal wall and cut through in the same manner. Gently pull the gravid uterus and collect it by cutting the uterine veins and arteries and separating it from the vagina.
3. Place the entire uterus inside a falcon containing sterile ice-cooled HBSS and leave it on ice for at least 10 min in order to anesthetize embryos.
4. Carefully, open the uterus wall with a scissors and collect all embryos to a petri dish with the same cold medium.
5. Under a stereomicroscope, sacrifice embryos by decapitation. Place the remaining body in their prone position in a petri dish containing DMEM/F12-P/S medium.
6. Separate the tail from the body and do an incision throughout the midline of the spinal column using fine forceps.
7. Gently pull away the spinal cord, leaving the DRGs exposed. At E18 the spinal cord should separate easily, leaving the DRGs in their cavities.

8. Finally, with Dumont 55 fine forceps, collect DRGs with extremely care to maintain their entire structure and conserve them in a petri dish with ice-cold DMEM/F12-P/S medium until further use (*see* **Note 9**).

3.2.2 Embedding and Culture of DRGs in Hydrogel

1. Inside a laminar flow chamber for sterile conditions and with the help of a stereomicroscope with a digital camera, plate a DRG explant in the center of a well of a 15-well μ-Slide Angiogenesis plate, using Dumont 55 fine forceps (*see* **Note 10**).
2. Prepare 20 μL fibrin gels as described in Subheading 3.1 except:
   (a) No fluorescently labeled fibrinogen is used.
   (b) A 6 μM final concentration of AON (LNA-based, fully phosphorothioated gapmers) against the gene target of interest is used (in our previous work [14] an LNA-AON gapmer (LNA 6624) was used to down-regulate GSK3b: +C* + A* + T*g*a*t*c*t*g*g*a* + G* + C* + T, and as control an LNA-AON gapmer (LNA 6424) against GFP:+T*+G*+G*c*c*g*t*t*t*a*c*+G*+T*+C (*see* **Note 6**).

   Each mixture should be done just before plating, as it polymerizes fast.
3. Quickly, add the polymerizing fibrin gel to the previous platted DRG, making sure that it stays as centered as possible. After a few seconds the gel should turn opaque indicating that fibrinogen polymerization has started.
4. Repeat the same procedure with the other wells and place the plate in a 37 °C, 5% CO_2 humidified incubator for 30 min to allow fibrin cross-clinking by factor XIIIa.
5. After that time, add 40 μL of supplemented DMEM/F-12 medium to each well and place it back in the incubator.
6. Culture DRG explants for up to 7 days, changing the medium every 3 days of culture. For that, remove half volume of the medium in each well and add new supplemented DMEM/F-12 medium.
7. After 7 days of culture, collect DRGs to Maxymum recovery microcentrifuge tubes (0.6 mL) containing 300 μL of lysis solution of the mirVana miRNA Isolation Kit and preserve it at −80 °C until analysis (*see* **Note 11**).
8. Proceed with RNA isolation following the manufacturer's protocol. After, a one-step qPCR kit can be used for quantitative real-time PCR for gene expression analysis. An example result is shown in Fig. 2.

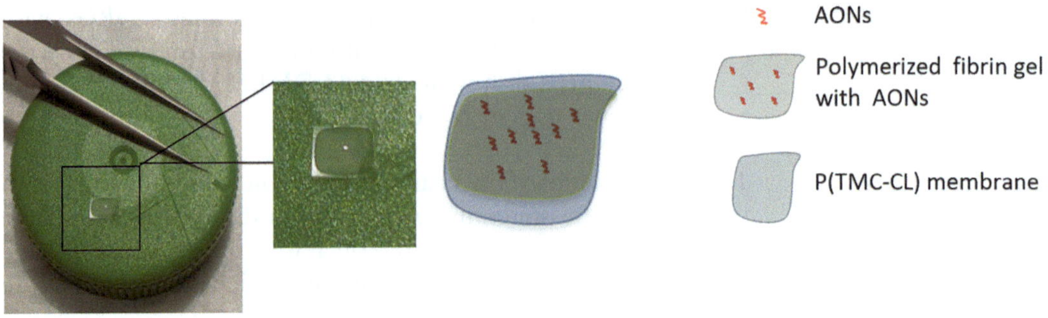

Fig. 2 View of pTMC-CL polymer patch with a drop of AON-containing gel formed on top. The patch is transferred to the lesion site with the gel side contacting the spinal cord. The schematic drawing shows the system as it is transferred to the lesion site, composed by the pTMC-CL membrane patch, then below the prepolymerized fibrin gel containing the AONs which will contact the lesion

3.3 Gene Silencing by Local Application of AON-Loaded Hydrogel in the Rat Hemisection Spinal Cord Injury Model

First of all, the animals are handled to accustom them to experimental manipulation and recognize the experimenter, in order to minimize stress. After animals' habituation, the surgery is performed and for its success the operating environment is cleaned, the instruments are sterilized, the animal is prepared (asepsis) and lastly the surgeon is prepared.

3.3.1 Application of AON-Loaded Hydrogel After Spinal Cord Hemisection

1. Weigh the animal.
2. Anaesthetize the animal with isoflurane, with induction rate of 5% and maintenance rate ranging between 1.5% and 3% (*see* **Note 12**).
3. Shave the animal fur from T10 vertebra until the ears and clean: 3 times with EtOH 70% (v/v) and iodopovidone solution intercalated.
4. Inject buprenorphine solution and glycosylated serum (3 mL) subcutaneously.
5. Perform a single incision between T10 vertebrae and approximately above the shoulder blade. Insert the retractor. Cut the fat (scissors), remove the muscle (scraper) and cut the muscle right above the T7–T9 vertebrae. Clean the vertebrae T7 and T8 using the scraper. Cut the bone (bone trimmer or rongeur) right under the vertebrae T8 and remove the vertebrae (laminectomy). Spinal cord will be immediately visible.
6. With the microscissors cut the spinal cord dorsally, approximately 2–3 mm in depth with one single cut (*see* **Note 13**).
7. Using the procedures for hydrogel preparation as in Subheading 3.1 (except here, to achieve a faster gelation time, 25 U/mL of final thrombin concentration and 25 μg/mL of final aprotinin concentration) are used for in vivo experimentation as well as AON at an initial concentration of 5 mM) the gel (5 μL) is prepared inside a clean maximum recovery 0.6 mL

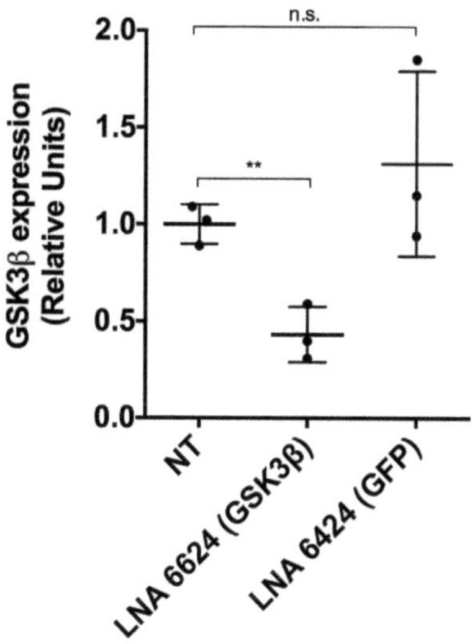

Fig. 3 Downregulation of GSK3β in DRG explants mediated by an AON-loaded fibrin hydrogel. Relative RNA quantification by qRT-PCR after a 7-day exposure to LNA AONs. LNA AONs against an irrelevant sequence (LNA6424-GFP) were used as controls. Each point represents an independent experiment where RNA from a pool of 10–15 independently treated DRG explants was used per condition and per independent experiment for qPCR quantification. Results indicate mean ± SD. One way-ANOVA with Dunnett's multiple comparison test (versus nontreated [NT]) was used where indicated ($*p < 0.05$; $**p < 0.01$; n.s., not significant). Adapted from [14] and used with permission from the American Society of Gene & Cell Therapy

microtube. After mixing both component mixtures, the gel (5 μL, containing 5 nmol of AON) is quickly transferred to the top of a pTMC-CL patch of around 0.5 cm length and 0.3 cm wide (methods for the preparation of pTMC-CL fiber patch are reported elsewhere in [15] and [16]) and set it aside to polymerize (Fig. 3).

A second 5 μL drop is then made in another tube and pipetted into the lesioned site of the spinal cord just as it starts to turn into gel (it should take less than 1 min) (*see* **Note 14**). Let stabilize for 1 min and then transfer the patch with the initial 5 μL drop onto the top of the lesion such that the gel drop is underneath the patch and in contact with the lesion (this gives a total amount of 10 nmol of AONs applied to the lesion site, however other AON quantities can be tested). A schematic picture of the test system is shown in Fig. 4a.

8. Suture the musculature and subcutaneous tissue closed and lastly suture the skin, using PGA (polyglycolic acid) surgical suture thread (*see* **Note 15**).

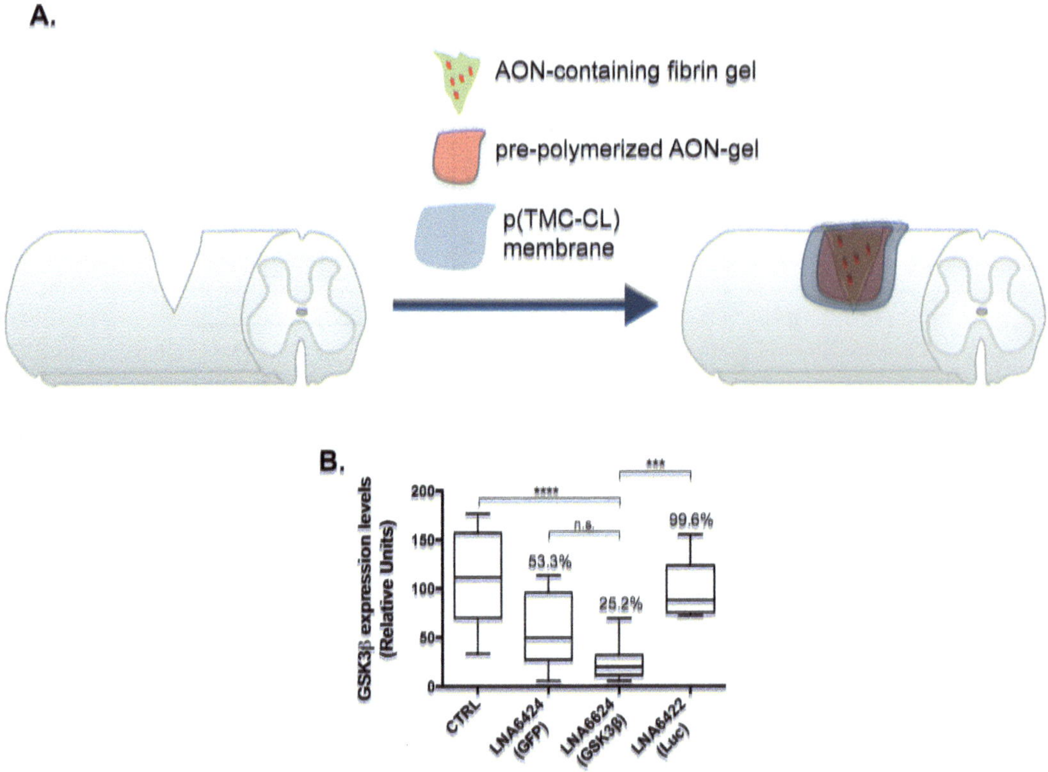

Fig. 4 Overview of the gene silencing hydrogel system locally applied to the injured spinal cord (rat spinal cord hemisection model system). (**a**) Schematic representation of the AON-hydrogel system for local downregulation of gene targets in the lesioned spinal cord. (**b**) Functional activity of LNA AONs after local application of the AON-loaded fibrin gel delivery system, evaluated 5 days postlesion. Fibrin gel with no AONs was applied in the lesion of control group rats (CTRL). LNA AONs against GFP or Luciferase (LNA6424-GFP and LNA6422-Luc) were also used as additional controls. Relative quantification of GSK3**β** RNA levels by qRT-PCR is indicated. Values above box plots refer to GSK3b expression levels as relative mean percentages. Error bars represent minimum–maximum (min-max), with line at median (control, $n = 9$; LNA6624, $n = 11$; LNA6424, $n = 11$; LNA6422, $n = 7$). One-way ANOVA, with Tukey multiple comparison, was used for statistical analysis ($***p < 0.001$, $****p < 0.0001$; n.s., not significant). Adapted from [14] and used with permission from the American Society of Gene & Cell Therapy

3.3.2 Spinal Cord Extraction for Gene Expression Analysis

1. Five days post-SCI, euthanize the animals using a CO_2 chamber (to assure death, cut the first spinal cord segments, immediately caudal to the occipital bone).
2. Sprinkle the animal fur with EtOH 70% (v/v) and using a tissue scissors, cut the skin over the vertebral column from the hip to the head.
3. Using a bone scissors, cut the vertebrae dorsally and delimit your region of interest. After that, cut muscle and bone, laterally in both sides along the vertebral column. At this point, the vertebral column should be separated from the body.

4. Gently remove each vertebra, cutting with a bone trimmer or rongeurs in both sides laterally to the dorsal lamina. The vertebral canal is open and the spinal cord exposed.
5. Using a tissue scissors, cut the nerve roots along the spinal cord segments and carefully remove the spinal cord from the ventral bone using a scraper.
6. Spinal cord is then put into a centrifuge tube with chilled RNAlater in a volume enough to cover it entirely (*see* **Note 16**).
7. The portion of the spinal cord including the lesion (around 0.5 cm to each side centered at the lesion) is cut with a clean scalpel and weighed.
8. Tissue is then chopped into smaller pieces for RNA extraction using miRvana miRNA Isolation Kit. A 1 mL tissue grinder on ice was used for tissue homogenization before proceeding with remaining of RNA extraction protocol following the manufacturer's protocol.
9. Quantitative RT-PCR can then be used for analysis of gene silencing results (Fig. 4b).

4 Notes

1. Fibrinogen (as received) is stored at −20 °C. Prior to weighing fibrinogen, allow it to equilibrate at RT.
2. To determine the concentration of fibrinogen:
   (a) Dilute fibrinogen solution 1:40 in 1× TBS 7.4 in a microcentrifuge tube; prepare 3 replicates;
   (b) At the NanoDrop™, apply 2 μL of 1× TBS 7.4 onto the measurement pedestal to measure the blank; pipette an aliquot (2 μL) of each sample onto the pedestal and measure the absorbance at 280 nm and at 320 nm;
   (c) Determine fibrinogen concentration (mg/mL) according to the following equation, where ε corresponds to the mass extinction coefficient of a solution of 1 mg/mL of fibrinogen at 280 nm (1.51 L g^{-1} cm^{-1}); calculate the mean and multiply by the dilution factor (40) to obtain the concentration of the purified fibrinogen solution.

$$\frac{(A_{280} - A_{320})}{\varepsilon} = [\text{Fibrinogen}]$$

3. For concentration of fibrinogen, first sterilize the body of the Vivaspin® device with 70% (v/v) ethanol; incubate for 20 min, centrifuge at 3000 × *g* for 2 min and discard the ethanol; repeat the procedure twice with sterile water to remove any traces of ethanol; Transfer the fibrinogen solution to the concentrator

and centrifuge at 3750 × *g* for 15 min at RT until reaching the desired volume; Check again the concentration of fibrinogen in the NanoDrop and if needed adjust the concentration to 30 mg/mL with sterile 1× TBS pH 7.4 in the LFC; Prepare 200 μL aliquots and store them at −80 °C. After thawed, aliquots may be stored at 4 °C for 1 week.

4. Thrombin is diluted in 1× TBS pH 7.0 since thrombin activity is reduced at pH > 7.

5. Thrombin aliquots are prepared in microcentrifuge tubes previously coated with 0.1% (w/v) bovine serum albumin (BSA). For BSA coating, weight 100 mg of BSA (Albumin fraction V, 1.12018.0025, Merck) and transfer it to a conical centrifuge tube containing 10 mL of 1× TBS pH 7.0. Sterilize 1% (w/v) BSA by filtration (0.22 μm) with a low protein binding filter into a new conical centrifuge tube and heat inactivate it at 70 °C for 5 min (1% w/v BSA stock solution may be stored at −20 °C). Dilute 1% (w/v) BSA stock solution with sterile 1× TBS pH 7.0 to obtain 0.1% (w/v) BSA. Pipette 100 μL of 0.1% (w/v) BSA into 1.5 mL microcentrifuge tubes and incubate them at 37 °C for 1 h in orbital shaker at 100 rpm. Carefully aspirate the BSA solution before use.

6. DNA bases are written in small letters; 2′-*O*-methyl RNA bases are written as mN (*N*, nucleotide), phosphorothioate linkages are indicated by an asterisk. Oligonucleotides should always be HPLC purified. Several oligonucleotide synthesis companies are available for ordering such oligonucleotides. When received, oligonucleotides (lyophilized) are diluted in nuclease-free water (non-DEPC treated, Qiagen) aliquoted and stored at −20 °C.

7. The poly(trimethylene carbonate-co-ε-caprolactone) (P(TMC-CL)) patch does not influence the fibrin inserted in the lesion site, however it can be used to further increase the amount of AONs being released into the lesion as it serves as a barrier for outward diffusion by helping to contain and isolate the lesion site.

8. To measure the pore size area of fibrin gel the following specifications are recommended when acquiring the photos: use a Plan-Apochromat ×63/1.4NA Oil objective and acquire images of ten optical sections covering a depth of 10 μm. In MatLab software, and using a 2D projection of the previously taken optical sections, pores can then be segmented and areas computed.

9. Despite being a time-consuming procedure, DRG isolation should be done as quickly as possible to maintain the explants integrity and cell viability.

10. To help transferring the DRG to the center of the well, add a drop of medium (approx. 2 μL) before plating it.
11. With the mirVana RNA extraction kit around ten DRGs need to be pulled together for RNA extraction in order to have good quality RNA at enough amounts for subsequent analysis. However, other methods of RNA isolation can in principle be used if RNA from single DRGs is desirable.
12. To guarantee that animals are fully anaesthetized, postural, tail and paw reflexes are analyzed and procedures are only carried out when no response from the animals is observed (e.g., loss of posture and absence of tail pinch and pedal withdrawal reflexes). Use an ophthalmic solution (SiccaFluid) in order to avoid injuries of cornea and electrical heating pads to maintain body temperature during surgery and throughout the recovery period.
13. Control any bleeding that appears after the lesion using cotton swabs or hemostatic gauze to make sure the gel is transferred only when bleeding has stopped.
14. To help identifying when the gel is being formed adjust the pipette with a volume higher than the volume you are transferring. Then keep gently pushing the pipette piston up and down just enough that you see the gel solution descending to the tip. You should notice a higher resistance to the pipetting of the solution building up. Just when you start noticing this effect immediately transfer the "about to" polymerize gel into the lesion site. Take care not to push too much the pipette tip into the lesion site.
15. Make available humid/soft food and reestablish water access after surgery. It is important the frequent bladder management (empty the animals' bladder twice a day and immediately after the surgery) and maintain the animals on a heat pad during 24 h post injury. Also administer buprenorphine for 3 days (twice a day, subcutaneously). Assess the animals' physical appearance and wounds daily, as well as record their weight variations. In case problems emerge with the health status of the animal evaluate possible humane ending point (euthanasia).
16. The extracted spinal cord can be stored in RNAlater at 4 °C overnight before continuing with the RNA extraction protocol or before freezing at −80 °C for long-term storage.

Acknowledgments

This work was supported by Fundação para a Ciência e a Tecnologia (FCT, Portugal) in the framework of the Harvard-Portugal

Medical School Program [HMSP-ICT/0020/2010]; Project NORTE-01-0145-FEDER-000008, supported by Norte Portugal Regional Operational Programme (NORTE 2020), under the PORTUGAL 2020 Partnership Agreement, through the European Regional Development Fund (ERDF), Fundo Europeu de Desenvolvimento Regional funds through the COMPETE 2020—Operacional Program for Competitiveness and Internationalization (POCI), Portugal 2020; by Portuguese funds through FCT/Ministério da Ciência, Tecnologia e Ensino Superior in the framework of the project "Institute for Research and Innovation in Health Sciences" (POCI-01-0145-FEDER-007274); Santa Casa da Misericordia de Lisboa—Prémio Neurociências Mello e Castro (MC-1068-2015) and the fellowships SFRH/BPD/108738/2015 (FCT) to P.M.D.M and Infarmed (FIS-FIS-2015-01_CCV_20150630-88) to M.T.

References

1. Chai Q, Jiao Y, Yu X (2017) Hydrogels for biomedical applications: their characteristics and the mechanisms behind them. Gels 3:6–15. https://doi.org/10.3390/gels3010006
2. Pêgo AP, Kubinova S, Cizkova D et al (2012) Regenerative medicine for the treatment of spinal cord injury: more than just promises? J Cell Mol Med 16:2564–2582. https://doi.org/10.1111/j.1582-4934.2012.01603.x
3. Carballo-Molina OA, Velasco I (2015) Hydrogels as scaffolds and delivery systems to enhance axonal regeneration after injuries. Front Cell Neurosci 9:13. https://doi.org/10.3389/fncel.2015.00013
4. Stein CA, Hansen JB, Lai J et al (2010) Efficient gene silencing by delivery of locked nucleic acid antisense oligonucleotides, unassisted by transfection reagents. Nucleic Acids Res 38:e3. https://doi.org/10.1093/nar/gkp841
5. Straarup EM, Fisker N, Hedtjärn M et al (2010) Short locked nucleic acid antisense oligonucleotides potently reduce apolipoprotein B mRNA and serum cholesterol in mice and non-human primates. Nucleic Acids Res 38:7100–7111. https://doi.org/10.1093/nar/gkq457
6. Crooke ST, Wang S, Vickers TA et al (2017) Cellular uptake and trafficking of antisense oligonucleotides. Nat Biotechnol 35:230–237. https://doi.org/10.1038/nbt.3779
7. Passini MA, Bu J, Richards AM et al (2011) Antisense oligonucleotides delivered to the mouse CNS ameliorate symptoms of severe spinal muscular atrophy. Sci Transl Med 3:72ra18. https://doi.org/10.1126/scitranslmed.3001777
8. Kordasiewicz HB, Stanek LM, Wancewicz EV et al (2012) Sustained therapeutic reversal of Huntington's disease by transient repression of Huntingtin synthesis. Neuron 74:1031–1044. https://doi.org/10.1016/j.neuron.2012.05.009
9. Khorkova O, Wahlestedt C (2017) Oligonucleotide therapies for disorders of the nervous system. Nat Biotechnol 35:249–263. https://doi.org/10.1038/nbt.3784
10. Smith CIE, Zain R (2018) Therapeutic oligonucleotides: state of the art. Annu Rev Pharmacol Toxicol. https://doi.org/10.1146/annurev-pharmtox-010818-021050
11. Johnson PJ, Parker SR, Sakiyama-Elbert SE (2009) Controlled release of neurotrophin-3 from fibrin-based tissue engineering scaffolds enhances neural fiber sprouting following subacute spinal cord injury. Biotechnol Bioeng 104:1207–1214. https://doi.org/10.1002/bit.22476
12. King VR, Alovskaya A, Wei DYT et al (2010) The use of injectable forms of fibrin and fibronectin to support axonal ingrowth after spinal cord injury. Biomaterials 31:4447–4456. https://doi.org/10.1016/j.biomaterials.2010.02.018
13. Sharp KG, Yee KM, Steward O (2014) A re-assessment of long distance growth and connectivity of neural stem cells after severe spinal cord injury. Exp Neurol 257:186–204. https://doi.org/10.1016/j.expneurol.2014.04.008

14. Moreno PMD, Ferreira AR, Salvador D et al (2018) Hydrogel-assisted antisense LNA Gapmer delivery for in situ gene silencing in spinal cord injury. Mol Ther Nucleic Acids 11:393–406. https://doi.org/10.1016/j.omtn.2018.03.009
15. Pires LR, Rocha DN, Ambrosio L, Pêgo AP (2015) The role of the surface on microglia function: implications for central nervous system tissue engineering. J R Soc Interface 12:20141224–20141224. https://doi.org/10.1098/rsif.2014.1224
16. Pires LR, Lopes CDF, Salvador D et al (2017) Ibuprofen-loaded fibrous patches-taming inhibition at the spinal cord injury site. J Mater Sci Mater Med 28:157. https://doi.org/10.1007/s10856-017-5967-7

Chapter 13

Evaluation of Cell-Penetrating Peptide Delivery of Antisense Oligonucleotides for Therapeutic Efficacy in Spinal Muscular Atrophy

Suzan M. Hammond, Frank Abendroth, Michael J. Gait, and Matthew J. A. Wood

Abstract

Antisense oligonucleotides (ASOs) are a widely used form of gene therapy, which is translatable to multiple disorders. A major obstacle for ASO efficacy is its bioavailability for in vivo and in vitro studies. To overcome this challenge we use cell-penetrating peptides (CPPs) for systemic delivery of ASOs. One of the most advanced clinical uses of ASOs is for the treatment of spinal muscular atrophy (SMA). In this chapter, we describe the techniques used for in vitro screening and analysing in vivo biodistribution of CPP-conjugated ASOs targeting the survival motor neuron 2, *SMN2*, the dose-dependent modifying gene for SMA.

Key words Cell-penetrating peptides, Oligonucleotide delivery, Spinal muscular atrophy, Survival motor neuron, Splice switching oligonucleotides

1 Introduction

The primary obstacle for clinical translation of antisense oligonucleotide therapies is bioavailability. A widely used technique for improving bioavailability of antisense oligonucleotides (ASOs) is the use of cell-penetrating peptides (CPPs). One of the first to develop this technique was the Langel group who demonstrated that the coupling of CPPs to mRNA improved uptake in vitro and in vivo [1]. Historically, direct conjugation of a CPP was limited to neutral ASOs such as peptide nucleic acid (PNA) and phosphorodiamidate morpholino oligomer (PMO) chemistries. CPPs for delivery of charged ASOs are available through complexation (reviewed in [2]). However, many more recent designs have become available which are able to directly conjugate CPPs to negatively charged ASOs [3]. CPP delivery of ASOs has been widely used in many disease models including Duchenne muscular dystrophy and spinal muscular atrophy (SMA)

Olof Gissberg et al. (eds.), *Oligonucleotide-Based Therapies: Methods and Protocols*, Methods in Molecular Biology, vol. 2036, https://doi.org/10.1007/978-1-4939-9670-4_13,

[4–7]. To dramatically improve delivery of charge neutral ASOs, the Wood and Gait labs have developed the Pip peptide advanced delivery technology. Pip peptides, PMO internalizing peptides, are covalently conjugated to PMOs [8, 9] and capable of delivery to a variety of adult tissues including liver, kidney, skeletal muscles, diaphragm, heart, and central nervous system of adult mice [4–8].

Spinal muscular atrophy (SMA) is a leading genetic cause of infant mortality primarily due to lower α-motor neuron degeneration and progressive muscle weakness. SMA results from loss of the ubiquitous survival motor neuron 1 gene, *SMN1* [10, 11]. Humans have a second nearly identical copy, *SMN2*, whose expression differs from *SMN1* due to a single translationally silent nucleotide transition within exon 7 leading to generation of an alternative exon 7-excluded transcript [12–15]. As a result, the majority of *SMN2* transcripts lack exon 7 (Δ7*SMN2*), resulting in truncated and partially functional protein [16]. Only a small percentage of transcripts include exon 7 (FL*SMN2*) and generate fully functional SMN protein. *SMN2* therefore fails to compensate for loss of *SMN1* unless sufficient copies are present to generate functional levels of FL*SMN2* transcripts [11]. In this chapter, we will focus on analysis of the *SMN* mRNA. Details on western blotting can be found in Groen et al. [17].

A genetic therapy-based approach for SMA utilizes single-stranded, splice-switching oligonucleotides (SSOs) to enhance *SMN2* pre-mRNA exon 7 inclusion via steric block of splice regulatory pre-mRNA elements [18]. Targeting the splice silencer N1 (ISS-N1) site within intron 7 by deletion or ASO steric blockage improves exon 7 inclusion [19, 20]. ISS-N1 targeted ASOs developed by IONIS and Biogen partnership have received US Food and Drug Administration (FDA) and European Medicines Agency (EMA) approval and shown great promise for patients with SMA [21]. However, these ASOs do not cross the blood–brain barrier and therefore have to be delivered directly to the spinal cord via intrathecal administrations. Further, while ASO targeting to central nervous system (CNS) is essential, not all canonical SMN roles are neuron-specific and there is evidence that treating peripheral as well as CNS tissues will be essential for high efficacy ASO therapy [22–31]. This chapter describes a methodology for screening peptide-conjugated morpholinos in vitro and evaluating Peptide-PMOs distribution in vivo.

2 Materials

2.1 Preparation of Peptide-PMO

1. PMO: 25mer sequence for splice modification of *SMN2*, targeting intronic splice suppressor N1 region ISSN1 [32]: 5′-GTAAGATTCACTTTCATAATGCTGG-3′.

2. Peptide-PMO (*see* **Note 1**).
3. Sonicator.
4. ddH_2O.

2.2 In Vitro Transfection

1. SMA type II patient-derived fibroblasts, three copies of *SMN2* gene (Coriell Institute GM03813).
2. T75 Flask.
3. 96-well plate.
4. 0.25% trypsin–EDTA solution.
5. Dulbecco's phosphate-buffered saline (PBS).
6. Fibroblast Growth Medium: DMEM-5%FBS: Dulbecco's Modified Eagle Medium, 5% fetal bovine serum.
7. Peptide-PMO (Gene Tools LLC, PepGen).
8. CO_2 incubator set to 37 °C.

2.3 In Vitro Peptide-PMO Screening: Direct RNA to qRT-PCR Protocol

1. Lysate buffer: 10 mM Tris pH 8, 1% Triton X-100, 3 mM $MgCl_2$, 1 mM EDTA, 1 mM $CaCl_2$.
2. DNase I, RNase free, 10,000 μ/ml.
3. Proteinase K, RNase free (20 mg/ml).
4. DEPC-treated RNase-free water.
5. Multichannel pipette.
6. PCR thermo cycler.
7. TaqMan™ Gene Expression Assays for Probe and Primer Sets (Table 1) [33].
8. twin.tec 96-Well plate (Eppendorf™).
9. MicroAmp, Optical Adhesive Film.
10. SuperScript III Platinum One-Step qRT-PCR Kit: SuperScript® III/Platinum® Taq Mix and 2× Reaction Mix.
11. qRT-PCR TaqMan compatible real-time PCR Thermocycler.
12. Reaction Mix, 20 μl per well: 0.5 μl SuperScript™ III RT/Platinum™ Taq Mix, 10 μl 2× Reaction Mix, 1 μl 20× Primer Mix including probes (final concentrations listed in Table 1), 2 μl Cell lysate, 6.5 μl DEPC-treated water.

2.4 Intravenous Administration

1. Weighing scale.
2. Warm air system.
3. Rodent restrainer.
4. 70% ethanol.
5. Peptide-PMO Solution in 0.9% saline.
6. 0.3–0.5 ml syringe with 29 G needle 12 mm long.

Table 1
Probe and primers for direct RNA to qRT-PCR protocol

Primer/ probe	Sequence	Exon/Exon junction	Final concentration
SMN2 FL Forward Primer	5'-GCTCACATTCCTTAAATTAAGGAGAAA-3'	Ex7-Ex8	400 nM
SMN2 Reverse Primer	5'-TCCAGATCTGTCTGATCGTTTCTT-3'	Ex8	400 nM
SMN2 Forward Probe	5'-FAM-CTGGCATAGZAGCAGCACTAAATGACACCAC–BFQ-3'	Ex8	150 nM
SMN2 Δ7 Forward Primer	5'-TGGCTATCATACTGGCTATTATATGGAA-3'	Ex6-Ex8	400 nM
SMN2 Reverse Primer	5'-TCCAGATCTGTCTGATCGTTTCTT-3'	Ex8	400 nM
SMN2 Forward Probe	5'-FAM-CTGGCATAGZAGCAGCACTAAATGACACCAC–BFQ-3'	Ex8	150 nM
hGAPDH Forward Probe	5'-Hex-CGCCTGGTCZACCAGGGCTGCT–BFQ-3'	Ex3	75 nM
hGAPDH Forward Primer	5'-CAACGGATTTGGTCGTATTGG-3'	EX2-Ex3	100 nM
hGAPDH Reverse Primer	5'-TGATGGCAACAATATCCACTTTACC-3'	Ex3	100 nM
Z = Zen™ modification Fam = 6-Carboxyfluorescein Hex = Hexachlorofluorescein BFQ = 3 Iowa Black™ FQ			
Naryshkin et al., [33]			

FLSMN2 and Δ7SMN2 transcripts amplified in separate wells using specific forward primers and common reverse primers and probe sets. hGAPDH probe and primers used for normalization

Z = Zen™ modification
Fam = 6-Carboxyfluorescein
Hex = Hexachlorofluorescein
BFQ = 3 Iowa Black™ FQ
Naryshkin et al. [33]

7. Cryovials.
8. Liquid nitrogen.
9. Dewar flask.
10. Dissection scissors.
11. Dissection forceps.

2.5 RNA Extraction and Single Stranded cDNA Preparation from Tissues

1. TRIzol reagent (Invitrogen).
2. Chloroform.
3. Isopropanol.
4. 75% ethanol.
5. Nuclease-free water.
6. Microcentrifuge tubes.
7. Tissue Homogenizer (Precellys®24—Bertin Corp).
8. Lysing kit beads and tubes (Precellys®—Bertin Corp).
9. NanoDrop spectrophotometer.
10. cDNA Reverse Transcription Kit.
11. PCR thermal cycler.

Table 2
Probe and primers for in vivo analysis of total *SMN2*, FL*SMN2* and Δ7*SMN2* transcripts

Primer/ probe	Sequence	Exon/Exon junction	Final Concentration
SMN2 FL Reverse Primer	5'-TCGTTTCTTTAGTGGTGTCATTTAG-3'	Ex8	500 nM
SMN2 FL Forward Primer	5'-TATCATACTGGCTATTATATGGGTTTT-3'	Ex6-Ex7	500 nM
SMN2 FL Probe	5'-FAM-AAGGAGAAAZTGCTGGCATAGAGCAGC-BFQ-3'	Ex7-Ex8	250 nM
SMN2 Δ7 Reverse Primer	5'-TCCAGATCTGTCTGATCGTTTCTT-3'	Ex8	500 nM
SMN2 Δ7 Forward Primer	5'-TGGCTATCATACTGGCTATTATATGGAA-3'	Ex6-Ex8	500 nM
SMN2 Δ7 Probe	5'-FAM-CTGGCATAGZAGCAGCACTAAATGACACCAC–BFQ-3'	Ex8	250 nM
SMN2(12) Reverse Primer	5'-TCAGTGCTGTATCATCCCAAATG-3'	Ex2a	500 nM
SMN2(12) Forward Primer	5'-CAGGAGGATTCCGTGCTGTT-3'	Ex1	500 nM
SMN2(12) Probe	5'-HEX-CGGCACAGGZCCAGAGCGATG–BFQ-3'	Ex1-Ex2a	250 nM
Z = Zen™ modification Fam = 6-Carboxyfluorescein Hex = Hexachlorofluorescein BFQ = 3 Iowa Black™ FQ			
d'Ydewalle et al., [34]			

Z = Zen™ modification
Fam = 6-Carboxyfluorescein
Hex = Hexachlorofluorescein
BFQ = 3 Iowa Black™ FQ
d'Ydewalle et al. [34]

2.6 Quantitative PCR from Tissues, TaqMan™ Based Assays

1. TaqMan™ Fast Advanced Master Mix which includes a proprietary mix of AmpliTaq® Fast DNA Polymerase, uracil-*N* glycosylase (UNG), dNTPs with dUTP, ROX™ dye, and optimized buffer components (Applied Biosystems™).
2. Microcentrifuge tubes.
3. Single stranded cDNA.
4. TaqMan™ Gene Expression Assays, for Probe and Primer Sets (Table 2) [34].
5. qRT-PCR TaqMan compatible Real-Time PCR Thermocycler.

2.7 Perfusion and Tissue Preparation

1. Pentobarbital (200 mg/ml).
2. 4% paraformaldehyde (PFA) chilled to 4 °C.
3. 1× PBS chilled to 4 °C.
4. 30% sucrose in PBS.
5. Dissecting scissors.
6. Dissecting forceps.
7. 27 gauge needle.
8. 1 ml syringe.
9. Fixative tubing.

10. Hemostat.
11. Tubing pump (*see* **Note 2**).
12. 15 ml tubes.
13. OCT medium.
14. Dry ice.

2.8 Immunohistochemistry

1. Cryostat.
2. Microscope slide superfrost.
3. Hydrophobic pen.
4. Humidified slide staining tray (*see* **Note 3**).
5. 1× PBS.
6. 0.1% Triton X-100 in 1× PBS.
7. Blocking buffer: 1% Triton X-100, 4% BSA in 1× PBS.
8. Purified anti-neurofilament H (NF-H), nonphosphorylated antibody (BioLegend).
9. DAPI mounting medium.

3 Methods

The method for testing Peptide-PMOs in vitro is different from the methods we use for testing Peptide-PMOs in vivo. Our in vitro designed assays were developed to minimize the time between RNA extraction and quantitative PCR analysis and allow testing of multiple peptide-PMOs. Most in vitro assays are performed on patient-derived fibroblasts. However, any cell line expressing human *SMN2* can be applied (*see* **Note 4**).

3.1 Preparation of Peptide-PMOs

1. Suspend peptide-PMOs in ddH_2O to desired concentration. Store at −20 °C until ready to use (*see* **Note 5**).
2. Thaw peptide-PMO at room temperature and incubate for 30 min at 37 °C.
3. Sonicate for 30 s with a probe sonicator or 5 min with a water bath sonicator, briefly vortex and pulse spin.

3.2 In Vitro Transfection for Screening of Peptide-PMO

1. Expand patient-derived fibroblasts into T75-flask in fibroblast growth medium.
2. When cell are around 80% confluency, wash once with 1× PBS.
3. Aspirate PBS and trypsinize (2 ml trypsin–EDTA) cells for 5 min at 37 °C.
4. Add 2 ml DMEM-5% FBS and count cells.

5. Dilute cells to 50,000 cells/ml in DMEM-5% FBS medium and dispense 100 µl/well in 96-well plate. Incubate overnight at 37 °C and 5% CO_2.
6. The next day add 10 µl of test compound in PBS into each well (at least three replicates per compound) and again incubate overnight.

3.3 In Vitro Peptide-PMO Screening: Direct RNA to qRT-PCR Protocol (See Note 6)

1. Add 20 µl DNase I per ml of Lysate buffer and incubate at room temperature for at least 5 min.
2. Aspirate media from 96-well plate and wash once with 1× PBS, making sure to remove most of the PBS.
3. To the freshly prepared Lysate buffer containing DNase I, add 10 µl Proteinase K per ml.
4. Add 30 µl of Lysate buffer containing DNase I and Proteinase K to each well using a multichannel pipette, and incubate for 5–10 min at room temperature.
5. Preheat PCR Thermocycler to 75 °C.
6. Transfer the lysate into an Eppendorf twin.tec 96-Well plate, seal the plate with optical adhesive film and incubate for 15 min at 75 °C in a preheated PCR-Thermocycler (*see* **Note 7**).
7. Immediately cool down lysate to 4 °C and use for qRT-PCR experiments within 30 min.
8. Set up 18 µl reaction mix per well and mix well with pipette: 10 µl 2× Reaction Mix, 0.5 µl SuperScript™ III RT/Platinum™ Taq Mix, 1 µl 20× TaqMan™ Gene Expression Assay, 6.5 µl nuclease-free water.
9. To run samples in triplicate wells, dilute 6.6 µl cell lysate with 59.4 µl reaction mix.
10. Pipet 20 µl reaction mix with cell lysate per well, spin down plate.
11. Run on real-time thermocycler using the following cycle conditions: 48 °C 15 min, 95 °C 120 s, 40 cycles of: 95 °C 15 s, 60 °C 45 s.
12. Calculate relative gene expression by using $\Delta\Delta$Ct method normalized to untreated or peptide-PMO scrambled sequence treated cells. *hGAPDH* probe and primers are used as internal controls. (An example is shown in Fig. 1.)

3.4 In Vivo Intravenous Administration in Adult Mice (Over 3 Weeks of Age) (See Notes 8 and 9)

1. Weigh mice and prepare the injection volume (maximum 10 µl/g bodyweight) of peptide-PMO in 0.9% saline (*see* **Note 10**).
2. Warm the mice in the heat box at 39 °C for 5–10 min.
3. Place one mouse at the time into the restrainer, with tail accessible.

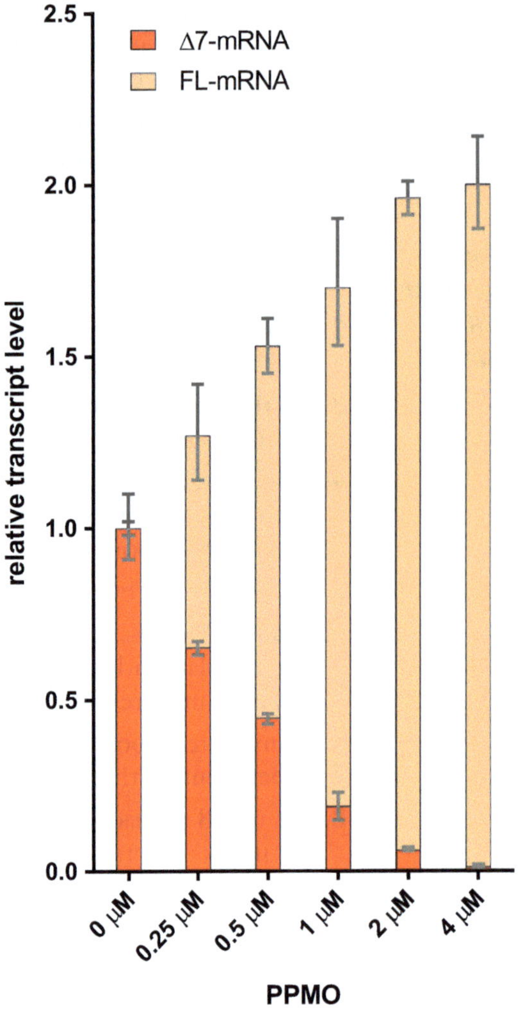

Fig. 1 SMA fibroblasts were treated with 0–4 μM concentration of PPMO in 96-well plate. Direct RNA to qRT-PCR analysis of FLSMN2 and Δ7SMN2 transcripts following peptide-PMO (PPMO) dosing. qRT-PCR was analyzed using ΔΔCt method and normalized to untreated cells

4. Spray or wipe the injection site with 70% ethanol.
5. Administer the intravenous injection to the tail vein using a 29 G needle with the bevel side up.
6. Release the mouse from the restrainer and gently compress injection site with a paper towel or tissue until bleeding has ceased. Place mice in a recovery cage for observation before returning them to the home cage (*see* **Note 11**).
7. Seven days post administration kill animals and harvest the tissues (*see* **Note 12**).
8. Place tissues in labeled and weighed cryovials and flash freeze in liquid nitrogen for RNA extraction. Store at −80 °C.

3.5 RNA Extraction and Single Stranded cDNA Preparation from Tissues

1. Weigh out 15–25 mg tissue and place in Precelly's bead tubes.
2. Add 1 ml TRIzol® Reagent.
3. Homogenize tissues in the homogenizer.
4. Follow RNA extraction using TRIzol® Reagent manufacturer's instructions.
5. Measure the RNA concentration on a spectrophotometer and resuspend the samples to 200 ng/μl in RNase free water.
6. Store RNA at −20 °C or −80 °C.
7. Using 1.0 μg RNA in 20 μl reaction volume, prepare cDNA using ABI High Capacity cDNA Reverse Transcription Kits.
8. Dilute cDNA 1:5 after synthesis with 80 μl ddH_2O to give a final concentration 10 ng/μl.
9. Store cDNA at −20 °C.

3.6 Quantitative PCR from Tissues, TaqMan™ Based Assays (See Note 13)

1. Remove cDNA from freezer and thaw on ice.
2. Set up 19.8 μl reaction mix per well and mix well with pipette: 11 μl 2™ TaqMan™ Fast Advanced Master Mix, 1.1 μl 20× TaqMan™ Gene Expression Assay, 7.7 μl nuclease-Free water (*see* **Note 14**).
3. To run samples in triplicate wells, dilute 6.6 μl cDNA with 59.4 μl reaction mix.
4. Pipet 20 μl reaction mix with cDNA per well.
5. Spin down plate.
6. Run on Real-Time PCR machine using the following cycle conditions: 50 °C for 2 min then 95 °C for 20 s holding stages, followed by 40 cycles of 1 s at 95 °C and 20 s at 60 °C (*see* **Note 15**).
7. Analyze results using ΔΔCt method (*see* **Note 16**).

3.7 Perfusion Fixation and Tissue Preparation for Immuno-histochemistry

1. Administer peptide-ASO tagged with fluorescent tag such as Cy5 and perform perfusion fixation 24 h post-administration.
2. Set up apparatus for perfusion fixation. Fixative tubing should run through tubing pump. Attach one end of fixative tubing to back end of 1 ml syringe without plunger and place the opposite end of the tubing into container of ice-cold 1× PBS. Attach needle to syringe. Prime tubing with 1× PBS to remove air bubbles. Perfusion fixation should be done on a surgical stage or platform to allow drainage.
3. Administer 45 mg/kg pentobarbital via intraperitoneal injection, wait until the mouse has no response to foot, and tail pinch (*see* **Note 17**).
4. Pin mouse loosely to dissecting board and open the chest cavity by cutting through the rib cage to expose the heart. Do not cut

the rib cage off completely but pin them out of the way. Cut right atrium to remove blood. Insert a needle into the left ventricle and secure its position with a hemostat.

5. Perfuse ice-cold PBS through the body under low pressure, about 0.75 ml/min, until liquid runs clear from the right atrium. If liquid comes out of the mouth and nose the blood vessels have been destroyed (*see* **Note 18**).
6. Once liquid runs clear from the animal replace PBS with ice-cold 4% PFA and continue perfusion using 50–100 ml per animal. Animals should become stiff and may move during the 4% PFA perfusion.
7. Isolate brain and spinal cord and soak in 4% PFA at 4 °C for 3–4 h in 15 or 50 ml tubes. Spinal cord can be isolated from spinal column before soaking in 4% PFA or just before washes.
8. To isolate spinal cord from the spinal column first clean muscle and fibrotic tissue from the spinal column and pin to a dissecting board dorsal side up. Start from the cranial part of the column by transecting the vertebral arches at both sides with fine angled scissors (i.e., 10 mm cutting edge). Pull away the dorsal processes while cutting. Gently transect the ventral roots and tease the spinal cord out of the column with forceps.
9. Wash tissues 4 times for 30 min with 1× PBS. Cryopreserve the tissues by leaving them in a 15 ml tube with 30% sucrose in PBS for 3 days at 4 °C. Tissues will sink to the bottom of tube when they have become saturated with sucrose.
10. Cut brain and spinal cord into required segments and embed tissues in OCT medium. Freeze on dry ice and store at −80 °C until ready to section for slides.

3.8 Immunohistochemistry

For direct observation of Peptide-PMOs in the brain and spinal cord, it is recommended to use compounds labeled with a fluorescent tag, such as Cy5. In this protocol, we stain the neurofilament to image neurons. The protocol can be modified to include other cell specific staining. However, if you are costaining with Neuro-Trace Nissl it is important that the Nissl is the last step of the staining.

1. Tissues frozen in OCT should be taken from freezer and placed into cooled cryostat to acclimate for 30 min.
2. Cut sections at 20 μm and collect on slides.
3. Leave slides at room temperature (RT) until dry, approximately 30 min. Store the slides at −80 °C until ready to stain.
4. Thaw slides to RT. All the following steps are performed in slide staining tray without rotation or rocking.

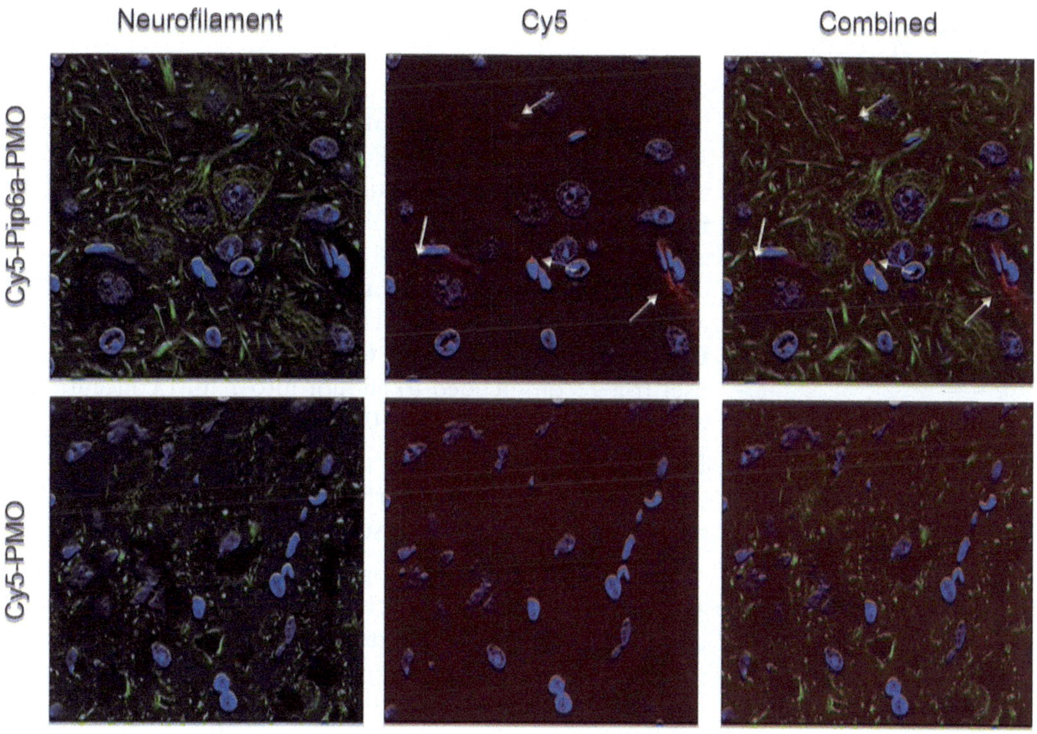

Fig. 2 Immunohistochemistry on adult SMN2 transgenic mouse spinal cord treated with Cy5 labeled Pip6a-PMO and PMO. Five-week-old mice were given an IV administration of 20 mg/kg Pip6a-Cy5-PMO or Cy5-PMO. Slides were stained with anti-neurofilament H. Images were captured on a Zeiss 880 Airyscan high resolution laser scanning confocal microscope, 40×. Cy5 represents the localization of Cy5 labeled compounds

5. Circle the tissue sections on the slides with the hydrophobic pen and allow to dry.
6. Rehydrate the tissue sections with 1× PBS for 40 min at RT.
7. Permeabilize the tissue with 0.1% Triton X-100 in PBS for 10 min at RT then wash twice for 5 min with 1× PBS.
8. Add blocking buffer and incubate overnight at 4 °C in a humidified chamber.
9. Remove the blocking buffer and add anti-neurofilament antibody diluted 1:2500 in blocking buffer. Leave overnight at 4 °C in a humidified chamber.
10. Wash three times for 5 min with 1× PBS. Remove excess PBS from slide and allow drying at RT for 1 h.
11. Mount with DAPI mounting medium and store slides at 4 °C. Image tissues on confocal microscope. For an example *see* Fig. 2.

4 Notes

1. Peptides are directly conjugated to PMOs with or without a labeled tag element through companies like Cambridge Research Biochemicals and PepGen. The protocol for biogenesis and conjugation of peptides has been published [4]. The neutral nature of the PMO allows for direct conjugation with charged peptides without the peptides interacting with the oligonucleotides. Generate small aliquots of peptide-PMO and store in −20 °C freezer to minimize freeze-thaw cycles. Concentration and volume will depend on the experimental use. It is recommended to aliquot into 1 mM concentrations for in vitro experiments or 40 μg/μl for in vivo studies.
2. Either a pump or gravity driven system can be used for controlling flow during perfusions. Gravity systems reduces the chances of excessive pressure which may destroy capillaries.
3. A light protected slide staining tray can be purchased, however, any system in which slides are laid flat on a raised surface (i.e., across two serological pipettes) within a closed and covered (i.e., aluminum foil) container will work. We lay moist paper towels in the chamber alongside the slides to create a moisture rich environment, which keeps the antibody solution from drying out.
4. Any human cell line containing *SMN2* can be used with this protocol. Although typically performed in patient fibroblasts, we have also performed screens of peptide-PMOs in human neuroblastoma cell line SH-SY5Y cells. However, in most cases, the amplification of exons 1–2a will encompass both *SMN1* and *SMN2* transcripts. This may provide different levels of "activity" between cell types or animal models. It is important to know the genetic background of these systems including deletion areas.
5. Morpholinos—sequence design followed by extensive testing has given us the ISSN1 sequence [20]. Morpholinos have different binding properties than other oligo chemistries. As such the oligo sequence needed to be modified for the PMO chemistry binding [32]. To avoid solubility issues, PMOs should be diluted to 1 mM or less in ddH_2O.
6. The mRNA levels of *SMN2* Δ7, *SMN2*-FL and *GADPH* are quantified using Taqman based RT-qPCR. For screening purpose, only the mRNA levels of *SMN2* Δ7 and GADPH are quantified, as they are the most abundant.
7. Incubation for 15 min at 75 °C deactivates of Proteinase K and DNase I.

8. We perform our in vivo analysis with intravenous administrations as it works best for delivery to the central nervous system. However, Peptide-PMOs may be administered via intraperitoneal or subcutaneous injection if only treating peripheral tissues. Analysis of biodistribution and efficacy following various modes of delivery have been described in the Duchenne muscular dystrophy mouse model, mdx [5, 35].
9. We generally harvest tissues 7 days post administration although PMOs are known to maintain a high level of activity in SMA mice for at least 4 weeks.
10. Peptide-PMOs will often generate an adverse effect in mice if given at high doses. Unless the peptide-PMO has been previously tested we recommend performing a single dose escalation study starting at a low dose (i.e., 10 mg/kg) and careful observation up to 1 h after administration.
11. Unless the mouse has a severe adverse effect or drops in body temperature, they tend to recover better in a recovery cage rather than a heat box.
12. Brain and spinal cord should be subdivided into its segments as needed during harvest. For details into dissection please *see* [36, 37]. Division of the spinal cord is easiest while still in the spinal column. Once each segment is separated, the spinal cord is isolated by individually removing vertebra with curved forceps until spinal cord is exposed.
13. We have tested multiple SYBR-green and Taqman Assays. To date the best probe/primers sets we have discovered comes from d'Ydewalle et al. [34]. Even with this system, we have found the delta7 transcript assay can result in low efficiency when analysing liver samples.
14. This will generate a 22 μl final volume per well to give 10% extra per well for pipetting error.
15. Real-Time PCR machine using the following cycle conditions are optimized for StepOne™ Real-Time PCR machine. Optimized conditions for other Real-Time PCR machines can be found in product literature for TaqMan Fast Advanced Master Mix (ThermoFisher Scientific).
16. The reaction efficiency can be determined by running multiple standard curves or via running the Real-time PCR Data Markup Language (RDML) file through a LinReg program. The primers described here fall between 1.8 and 2.0 in efficiency.
17. There is a large variation in drug responses between mice of different strains, sex and environments. When using pentobarbital for the first time it is advisable to anesthetize one or two animals and carefully observe their response before embarking on a large-scale study [38].

18. When blood vessels have been destroyed, it is no longer recommended to continue with perfusion. However, if this occurs during 4% PFA perfusion but not during 1× PBS perfusion then it is still advisable to extract tissues and immerse them in 4% PFA for 3–4 h.

References

1. Pooga M, Soomets U, Hallbrink M, Valkna A, Saar K, Rezaei K et al (1998) Cell penetrating PNA constructs regulate galanin receptor levels and modify pain transmission in vivo. Nat Biotechnol 16(9):857–861. https://doi.org/10.1038/nbt0998-857
2. Boisguerin P, Deshayes S, Gait MJ, O'Donovan L, Godfrey C, Betts CA et al (2015) Delivery of therapeutic oligonucleotides with cell penetrating peptides. Adv Drug Deliv Rev 87:52–67. https://doi.org/10.1016/j.addr.2015.02.008
3. Jirka SMG, t Hoen PAC, Diaz Parillas V, Tanganyika-de Winter CL, Verheul RC, Aguilera B et al (2018) Cyclic peptides to improve delivery and exon skipping of antisense oligonucleotides in a mouse model for Duchenne muscular dystrophy. Mol Ther 26(1):132–147. https://doi.org/10.1016/j.ymthe.2017.10.004
4. Betts C, Saleh AF, Arzumanov AA, Hammond SM, Godfrey C, Coursindel T et al (2012) Pip6-PMO, a new generation of peptide-oligonucleotide conjugates with improved cardiac exon skipping activity for DMD treatment. Mol Ther 1(8):e38
5. Betts CA, Saleh AF, Carr CA, Muses S, Wells KE, Hammond SM et al (2015) Implications for cardiac function following rescue of the dystrophic diaphragm in a mouse model of duchenne muscular dystrophy. Sci Rep 5:11632. https://doi.org/10.1038/srep11632
6. Hammond SM, Hazell G, Shabanpoor F, Saleh AF, Bowerman M, Sleigh JN et al (2016) Systemic peptide-mediated oligonucleotide therapy improves long-term survival in spinal muscular atrophy. Proc Natl Acad Sci U S A 113(39):10962–10967. https://doi.org/10.1073/pnas.1605731113
7. Yin H, Saleh AF, Betts C, Camelliti P, Seow Y, Ashraf S et al (2011) Pip5 transduction peptides direct high efficiency oligonucleotide-mediated dystrophin exon skipping in heart and phenotypic correction in mdx mice. Mol Ther 19(7):1295–1303
8. Jearawiriyapaisarn N, Moulton HM, Buckley B, Roberts J, Sazani P, Fucharoen S et al (2008) Sustained dystrophin expression induced by peptide-conjugated morpholino oligomers in the muscles of mdx mice. Mol Ther 16(9):1624–1629. https://doi.org/10.1038/mt.2008.120
9. Lebleu B, Moulton HM, Abes R, Ivanova GD, Abes S, Stein DA et al (2008) Cell penetrating peptide conjugates of steric block oligonucleotides. Adv Drug Deliv Rev 60(4–5):517–529. https://doi.org/10.1016/j.addr.2007.09.002
10. Lefebvre S, Burglen L, Reboullet S, Clermont O, Burlet P, Viollet L et al (1995) Identification and characterization of a spinal muscular atrophy-determining gene. Cell 80(1):155–165
11. Wirth B (2000) An update of the mutation spectrum of the survival motor neuron gene (SMN1) in autosomal recessive spinal muscular atrophy (SMA). Hum Mutat 15(3):228–237
12. Cartegni L, Krainer AR (2002) Disruption of an SF2/ASF-dependent exonic splicing enhancer in SMN2 causes spinal muscular atrophy in the absence of SMN1. Nat Genet 30(4):377–384. https://doi.org/10.1038/ng854
13. Kashima T, Manley JL (2003) A negative element in SMN2 exon 7 inhibits splicing in spinal muscular atrophy. Nat Genet 34(4):460–463. https://doi.org/10.1038/ng1207
14. Lorson CL, Hahnen E, Androphy EJ, Wirth B (1999) A single nucleotide in the SMN gene regulates splicing and is responsible for spinal muscular atrophy. Proc Natl Acad Sci U S A 96(11):6307–6311
15. Monani UR, Lorson CL, Parsons DW, Prior TW, Androphy EJ, Burghes AH et al (1999) A single nucleotide difference that alters splicing patterns distinguishes the SMA gene SMN1 from the copy gene SMN2. Hum Mol Genet 8(7):1177–1183
16. Le TT, Pham LT, Butchbach ME, Zhang HL, Monani UR, Coovert DD et al (2005) SMNDelta7, the major product of the

centromeric survival motor neuron (SMN2) gene, extends survival in mice with spinal muscular atrophy and associates with full-length SMN. Hum Mol Genet 14(6):845–857. https://doi.org/10.1093/hmg/ddi078
17. Groen EJN, Perenthaler E, Courtney NL, Jordan CY, Shorrock HK, van der Hoorn D et al (2018) Temporal and tissue-specific variability of SMN protein levels in mouse models of spinal muscular atrophy. Hum Mol Genet 27 (16):2851–2862. https://doi.org/10.1093/hmg/ddy195
18. Hammond SM, Wood MJ (2011) Genetic therapies for RNA mis-splicing diseases. Trends Genet 27(5):196–205. https://doi.org/10.1016/j.tig.2011.02.004
19. Hua Y, Vickers TA, Baker BF, Bennett CF, Krainer AR (2007) Enhancement of SMN2 exon 7 inclusion by antisense oligonucleotides targeting the exon. PLoS Biol 5(4):e73. https://doi.org/10.1371/journal.pbio.0050073
20. Singh NK, Singh NN, Androphy EJ, Singh RN (2006) Splicing of a critical exon of human survival motor neuron is regulated by a unique silencer element located in the last intron. Mol Cell Biol 26(4):1333–1346
21. Walke DW, Blackley A (2014) Isis pharmaceuticals reports data from ISIS-SMN Rx phase 2 studies in infants and children with spinal muscular atrophy. Ionis pharmaceuticals webpage
22. Araujo A, Araujo M, Swoboda KJ (2009) Vascular perfusion abnormalities in infants with spinal muscular atrophy. J Pediatr 155 (2):292–294
23. Bowerman M, Swoboda KJ, Michalski JP, Wang GS, Reeks C, Beauvais A et al (2012) Glucose metabolism and pancreatic defects in spinal muscular atrophy. Ann Neurol 72 (2):256–268. https://doi.org/10.1002/ana.23582
24. Braun S, Croizat B, Lagrange MC, Warter JM, Poindron P (1995) Constitutive muscular abnormalities in culture in spinal muscular atrophy. Lancet 345(8951):694–695
25. Davis RH, Miller EA, Zhang RZ, Swoboda KJ (2015) Responses to fasting and glucose loading in a cohort of well children with spinal muscular atrophy Type II. J Pediatr 167 (6):1362–1368 e1361. https://doi.org/10.1016/j.jpeds.2015.09.023
26. Fischer U, Liu Q, Dreyfuss G (1997) The SMN-SIP1 complex has an essential role in spliceosomal snRNP biogenesis. Cell 90 (6):1023–1029
27. Hayhurst M, Wagner AK, Cerletti M, Wagers AJ, Rubin LL (2012) A cell-autonomous defect in skeletal muscle satellite cells expressing low levels of survival of motor neuron protein. Dev Biol 368(2):323–334. https://doi.org/10.1016/j.ydbio.2012.05.037
28. Liu Q, Fischer U, Wang F, Dreyfuss G (1997) The spinal muscular atrophy disease gene product, SMN, and its associated protein SIP1 are in a complex with spliceosomal snRNP proteins. Cell 90(6):1013–1021
29. Pellizzoni L, Yong J, Dreyfuss G (2002) Essential role for the SMN complex in the specificity of snRNP assembly. Science 298 (5599):1775–1779. https://doi.org/10.1126/science.1074962
30. Rajendra TK, Gonsalvez GB, Walker MP, Shpargel KB, Salz HK, Matera AG (2007) A *Drosophila melanogaster* model of spinal muscular atrophy reveals a function for SMN in striated muscle. J Cell Biol 176(6):831–841. https://doi.org/10.1083/jcb.200610053
31. Rudnik-Schoneborn S, Vogelgesang S, Armbrust S, Graul-Neumann L, Fusch C, Zerres K (2010) Digital necroses and vascular thrombosis in severe spinal muscular atrophy. Muscle Nerve 42(1):144–147
32. Zhou H, Janghra N, Mitrpant C, Dickinson RL, Anthony K, Price L et al (2013) A novel morpholino oligomer targeting ISS-N1 improves rescue of severe spinal muscular atrophy transgenic mice. Hum Gene Ther 24 (3):331–342. https://doi.org/10.1089/hum.2012.211
33. Naryshkin NA, Weetall M, Dakka A, Narasimhan J, Zhao X, Feng Z et al (2014) Motor neuron disease. SMN2 splicing modifiers improve motor function and longevity in mice with spinal muscular atrophy. Science 345 (6197):688–693. https://doi.org/10.1126/science.1250127
34. d'Ydewalle C, Ramos DM, Pyles NJ, Ng SY, Gorz M, Pilato CM et al (2017) The antisense transcript SMN-AS1 regulates SMN expression and is a novel therapeutic target for spinal muscular atrophy. Neuron 93(1):66–79. https://doi.org/10.1016/j.neuron.2016.11.033
35. Godfrey C, Muses S, McClorey G, Wells KE, Coursindel T, Terry RL et al (2015) How much dystrophin is enough: the physiological consequences of different levels of dystrophin in the mdx mouse. Hum Mol Genet 24 (15):4225–4237. https://doi.org/10.1093/hmg/ddv155
36. Harrison M, O'Brien A, Adams L, Cowin G, Ruitenberg MJ, Sengul G et al (2013)

Vertebral landmarks for the identification of spinal cord segments in the mouse. NeuroImage 68:22–29. https://doi.org/10.1016/j.neuroimage.2012.11.048

37. Li KW (2011) Neuroproteomics: deciphering brain function and disorders. NeuroMethods 57:3–9. https://doi.org/10.1007/978-1-61779-111-6_1

38. Lovell DP (1986) Variation in pentobarbitone sleeping time in mice. 1. Strain and sex differences. Lab Anim 20(2):85–90. https://doi.org/10.1258/002367786780865142

Chapter 14

Injection and Infusion of Compounds to the Central Nervous System

Margherita Zamboni

Abstract

The present protocol describes in detail the steps necessary for executing two highly versatile and minimally invasive surgical approaches for localized delivery of compounds to the central nervous system. The procedures have been designed for use on laboratory mice but can also be tailored for experimentations involving other small rodent models. Following the instructions outlined below, treatments can either be administered through single injections or infused over a longer period of time, at locations identified through stereotaxic coordinates, which ensure efficient targeting of the brain region of interest, as well as increased reproducibility between surgeries. Although the surgical interventions are well tolerated by laboratory animals, it is recommended to closely monitor the mice postoperatively for a few days, and take the necessary measures to prevent stress and discomfort.

Key words Intracranial injection, Intraventricular injection, Osmotic pump, Mouse, Central nervous system

1 Introduction

The present protocol outlines two surgical procedures for achieving intracranial delivery of compounds to manipulate brain function and treat neurological diseases modelled in laboratory mice and other small rodents. The approaches described below are highly versatile and can be tailored to different experiments by adapting stereotaxic coordinates, volumes, and rates of injection of the drug under investigation. Intracranial delivery can be useful whenever one intends to achieve a localized effect of the treatment, or when compounds are not expected to cross the blood-brain barrier. Administration can, in one case, be performed through a single injection, which may be directed to the lateral ventricles, as well as to other regions of the brain parenchyma through identification of appropriate stereotaxic coordinates. This approach can, for instance, be employed for stable labeling and recombination of cells through virus-mediated transduction [1] or plasmid

Olof Gissberg et al. (eds.), *Oligonucleotide-Based Therapies: Methods and Protocols*, Methods in Molecular Biology, vol. 2036, https://doi.org/10.1007/978-1-4939-9670-4_14,

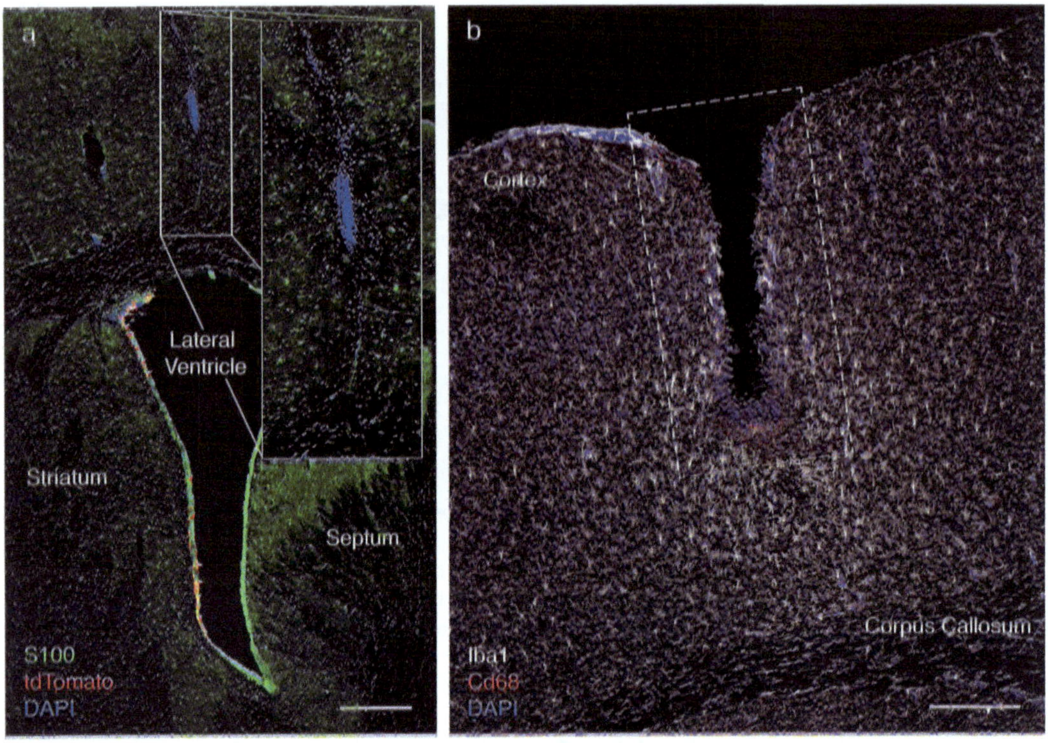

Fig. 1 Intracranial injection and minipump-mediated delivery of treatments are versatile and marginally invasive techniques for targeting the central nervous system. A wide range of substances (e.g., oligonucleotides) can be delivered to the brain through a single injection directed to the brain parenchyma or the ventricular system. Depicted in panel **a** is one example of application that requires intracranial injection. In this context, a plasmid was delivered to cells lining the lateral ventricle to induce expression of a fluorescent reporter (tdTomato). Injections typically cause minor damage to the tissue (magnified picture in **a**) and recruit cells to build a glial scar, as highlighted by a dense DAPI staining at the injection site. Depicted in panel **b** is the characteristic lesion derived by the cannula from a minipump implanted in the mouse cortex for delivery of a treatment over a period of 4 weeks. Immune cells expressing Iba1 and Cd68 are recruited to the infusion site to mount a mild inflammatory reaction in response to the penetrating injury. Scale bars: (**a**) 400 μm, (**b**) 150 μm

electroporation [2] (Fig. 1a), as well as for treatments, for which a single exposure is sufficient to achieve the desired effects. Alternatively, compounds can be infused into the brain over a longer period of time [3, 4], which ranges from 1 day up to 6 weeks [5]. This is achieved via implantation of an osmotic minipump, positioned subcutaneously on the animal's back, that steadily supplies the solution to the brain by means of a cannula fixed onto the skull. A major advantage of the minipump is that it allows for sustained delivery without the need for repeated injection, which in turn helps preventing unnecessary stress in the experimental mouse. The damage to the brain parenchyma is, however, slightly more pronounced when employing an osmotic pump, as opposed to a single injection (Fig. 1b), because the needles used for the two approaches differ in size, and the cannula from the pump remains implanted in the parenchyma during the entire duration of treatment. Despite a larger lesion size derived from the cannula, animals tolerate the implantation of a minipump well and do not normally display signs of discomfort or neurological damage.

The surgical interventions presented here share some of the materials and procedures, such as those related to identifying stereotaxic coordinates, as well as preoperative and postoperative care. Steps common to both operations are described in the same sections, whereas practices specific to one approach are outlined separately. Throughout the procedures, it is important to work in aseptic conditions, and follow recommendations specified by local entities for the use of laboratory animals.

2 Materials

Given below is a list of compounds and equipment needed to perform the surgical procedures that may be shared between techniques or specific to each of the methods outlined. All surgical equipment shall be sterilized (e.g., autoclaved) upon entering the surgical facility. In between procedures, instruments need to be cleaned of blood and sanitized using heat (e.g., with a glass bead sterilizer) or soaked in a disinfectant. Allow instruments to cool down before using on animals, if sanitized with heat. Rinse the tools with sterile saline after using chemical disinfection.

2.1 Preparing the Microinjection System

1. Microinjection apparatus with delivery system to be mounted onto the arm of the stereotaxic frame.
2. 10 μL syringe (e.g., NanoFil) with 33 G needle (5 mm-long tip)
3. Test substance.

2.2 Loading the Osmotic Minipump

1. Alzet® Osmotic minipump (*see* **Note 1**).
2. Brain Infusion Kit (*see* **Note 1**).
3. Test substance.
4. Falcon tube filled with sterile Dulbecco's PBS.
5. Sterile tweezers.
6. Disposable 1 mL syringes.
7. Incubator set at 37 °C.

2.3 Surgical Procedures

1. Adult mouse brain atlas [6].
2. Isoflurane (store at room temperature in a ventilated cabinet).
3. Anesthesia unit with vaporizer.
4. Ethanol 70%.

5. Betadine®: 100 mg/mL Betadine®.
6. Sterile wipes.
7. Ophthalmic ointment (e.g., Vaseline).
8. Sterile saline.
9. Injectable analgesic drug: 50 mg/mL Carprofen.
10. Electrical razor.
11. Stereotaxic apparatus with anesthesia mask and holders for syringes.
12. Homeothermic system for body temperature control.
13. Surgical pen with a fine tip.
14. Tissue scissors.
15. Fine forceps.
16. Sterile absorption spears.
17. High speed drill (e.g., dental drill with a 1.4 mm burr).
18. Hemostat.
19. Scalpel.
20. Bone wax.
21. Tissue adhesive (e.g., Vetbond).
22. Silk 5–0 sutures.
23. Local anesthetic, such as Lidocaine: 5%.

3 Methods

Carry out procedures in a suitable surgical room, taking care of sanitizing tools and gloves according to specifications provided by the local facility for experimental animals. Intracranial injection and implantation of the osmotic pumps follow the same procedures for calculating the stereotaxic coordinates, animal preparation and postoperative care, and are therefore described in the same sections. Steps that are specific to each of the procedures are outlined in separate sections, labeled as "Injection" or "Minipump," respectively.

3.1 Preparing the Microinjection System

1. Load the test substance to be injected into the microsyringe following the manufacturer's specifications. If the compound is dissolved in a thick solution, backfilling of the syringe may be necessary. It is advisable to load the syringe with enough compound to inject multiple animals.
2. Latch the plunge of the microsyringe onto the delivery system from the microinjection apparatus.

3. Adjust the settings of the microinjection system following the manufacturer's instructions. Set the appropriate volume of compound to be administered (*see* **Note 2**). Specify the rate of delivery (e.g., 50 to 200 nL/min, *see* **Note 3**).

3.2 Loading the Osmotic Minipump

1. Perform this procedure 24 to 48 h prior to the operation.
2. Assemble the parts making up the Brain Infusion Kit following the manufacturer's instructions.
3. Cut the catheter connecting the infusion cannula to the pump to the desired length (e.g., 3 cm is typically a suitable length for mice weighting 25–30 g, *see* **Note 4**).
4. Attach the infusion cannula to the catheter and glue adapters to the cannula, if needed (*see* **Note 5**).
5. Load the Brain Infusion Kit with the test compound from the catheter. Make sure not to create air bubbles within the tubing system and ensure that the cannula is not obstructed by allowing a drop of the compound to flow through the needle.
6. Following the manufacturer's guidelines, assemble the osmotic pump, being careful not to touch the semipermeable membrane with your hands. It is recommended to hold the pump with tweezers instead.
7. Fill the pump using a disposable 1 mL syringe and a blunt 25 G needle provided in the kit. Keep the pump's chamber upright and load the compound until it overflows. This will ensure the absence of air bubbles within the reservoir.
8. Keeping the pump in an upright position, slowly insert the flow moderator through the pump's chamber and remove the cap.
9. Attach one end of the catheter to the flow moderator.
10. Place the assembled minipump in a 50 mL Falcon tube filled with sterile saline and place in an incubator set at 37 °C, for 24 to 48 h (*see* **Note 6**).

3.3 Surgical Procedures

3.3.1 Calculate Stereotaxic Coordinates (Injection and Minipump)

1. Use a mouse brain atlas [6] (Fig. 2) to determine the stereotaxic coordinates to target the region of interest (e.g., lateral ventricle for intracerebroventricular injection or specific structures in the brain parenchyma for intracranial injection, *see* **Note 7**).
2. Rostrocaudal and mediolateral coordinates shall be calculated from Bregma, which is the point on the skull that is formed by the intersection between coronal and sagittal sutures. Dorsoventral coordinates shall be determined from the skull or from the dura (i.e., when the needle is directly in contact with the cortical surface, after piercing the cranium).
3. Determine the rostrocaudal distance from Bregma first. For intracerebroventricular delivery, levels between +1 and

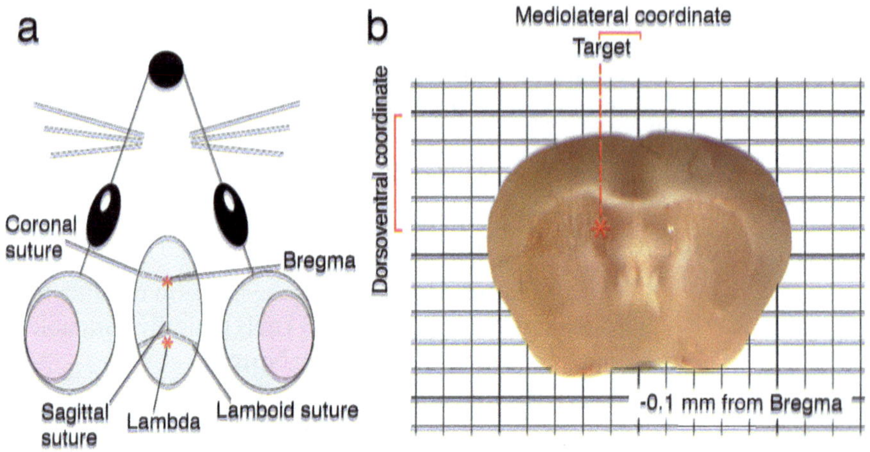

Fig. 2 Stereotaxic coordinates for the injection (or infusion) site are calculated based on the distance from Bregma. Upon exposure of the dorsal surface of the skull (**a**), it is possible to identify the major landmarks used for calculation of the stereotaxic coordinates. Bregma is the point at which coronal and sagittal sutures intersect. To reach the target site for injection, first bring the needle of the syringe to Bregma and move it, thereafter, to the desired location using the stereotaxic arms. Rostrocaudal, mediolateral, and dorsoventral coordinates of the target brain region can be identified on a mouse (or rat) brain atlas (**b**)

−1 mm from Bregma are appropriate. It is recommended to select a level at which lateral ventricles are larger, to ensure effective targeting of the brain structure (e.g., 0.1 mm caudal to Bregma can be a suitable rostrocaudal plane).

4. Determine the mediolateral distance from Bregma based on the selected rostrocaudal plane. If you have selected 0.1 mm caudal to Bregma as the rostrocaudal level, opt for a position that is 0.75 mm lateral to the midline.
5. Determine the depth for the injection/infusion. Calculate the dorsoventral coordinate from the skull or from the dura. If you have selected a position at −0.1 mm rostrocaudal and 0.75 mm lateral from Bregma, the needle can be place 3 mm deep from the skull (or 2.5 mm from the brain surface).

3.3.2 Prepare Animals for Surgery (Injection and Minipump)

1. Fill the isoflurane unit according to the manufacturer's specifications and turn on the instrument. Set the concentration of isoflurane to 4%, with air delivered at a rate of 400 mL/min.
2. Remove the animal from its cage and place it in the isoflurane chamber for induction of anesthesia.
3. Inspect the animal's consciousness level without removing it from the chamber (*see* **Note 8**).
4. Remove the animal from the isoflurane chamber upon induction of anesthesia and test suppression of paw reflex by pinching the hind paw.

5. If the reflexes are suppressed and the animal is unconscious, administer Carprofen solution (5 mg/kg) subcutaneously into the animal's flank.
6. Position the animal on the heating pad and place the rectal probe into the mouse's anus, to allow regulation of body temperature throughout the procedure.
7. Fix the animal's head on the stereotaxic apparatus. Stereotaxic injections require a three-point fixation, where the animal's head is mounted on the frame by the teeth and the ears.
8. First, position the teeth into the mouth bar.
9. Next, insert both ear bars and tighten them making sure that the head is immobilized and breathing is not suppressed (excessive tightening of the bars may block the trachea and impede proper breathing).
10. Ensure that the head is immobilized and straight along the rostrocaudal, mediolateral, and dorsoventral axes.
11. Lower isoflurane concentration to 2.5% and airflow to 200 mL/min (*see* **Note 8**).
12. Apply ointment on the mouse's eyes.
13. Shave the head and remove the hair with sterile wipes.
14. Disinfect with sterile wipes. Use two alternating rounds of ethanol 70% and Betadine®.

3.4 Intraventricular Delivery of the Compound (Injection)

1. Using sharp scissors, perform a small incision (<5 mm) on the animal's head, along the midline.
2. Clean the skull of blood using sterile absorption spears.
3. Find the desired location for the injection by first placing the tip of the syringe at Bregma and then moving rostrocaudally and mediolaterally with the stereotaxic arms.
4. Mark the position with a surgical pen.
5. Use the fine tip of a drill to thin the skull at the desired location. The bone should not be perforated by the drill to avoid damage to the cortical surface, but it should be slim enough to be pierced by the needle of the microsyringe.
6. Lower the syringe through the thinned skull and to the desired dorsoventral coordinates.
7. Let rest in that position for 2 min.
8. Begin infusion of the compound with the microinjection apparatus.
9. Let the needle rest in position for 5 min before retracting it slowly.

10. Once the needle has been removed from the brain, cover the small hole on the skull with a small amount of bone wax.
11. Apply 100 μL Lidocaine 5% solution at the surgical wound.
12. Reclose the incision with a drop of tissue adhesive. To do so, hold the edges of skin together with forceps and apply a small volume of glue.

3.5 Minipump Implantation (Minipump)

1. Using sharp scissors, perform a 10 mm-long incision on the mouse's head, along the midline.
2. Clean the skull of blood using sterile absorption spears.
3. Prepare a subcutaneous pocket for placement of the osmotic pump on the animal's back. Lift the skin of the head from the caudal edge of the surgical wound and insert the hemostat through the incision. Keep the hemostat parallel to the animal's back and open a pocket lateral to its spine. The subcutaneous space may be widened to accommodate the pump through opening and closing of the jaws of the hemostat. Avoid making the pocket to large, to prevent a prolonged healing process.
4. On the skull, determine the stereotaxic coordinates for the infusion cannula and mark with the surgical pen.
5. Carefully drill a hole at the desired location (*see* **Note 9**).
6. Insert the minipump in the subcutaneous pocked and latch the infusion cannula onto the holder of the stereotaxic arm.
7. Move the cannula with the stereotaxic arm to the desired site of infusion and carefully lower the needle through the hole that had been performed on the animal's skull. Lower the cannula enough to allow the needle to penetrate through the brain parenchyma, but allow approximately 1 mm of space between the skull and the plastic rim of the cannula.
8. Immobilize the cannula onto the skull using adhesive. Place a small drop of glue on the skull underneath the cannula and lower the cannula until it contacts the skull. Let the assembly rest for 1 min, or until the glue has solidified (*see* **Note 10**).
9. Test for a correct immobilization of the cannula by gently pulling the assembly upward.
10. If the brain infusion kit is correctly fixed onto the animal's skull, separate the plastic holder from the cannula with a scalpel.
11. Apply local anesthetic to the surgical field.
12. Close the surgical wound. The cannula mounted on the animal's head will create some tension on the skin, which may prolong healing time and may cause the incision to reopen. It is recommended, for this procedure, to use both tissue adhesive and sutures to close the incision. First, perform three or four

loose stitches that will help relieving tension on the overlaying tissue. Next, cover the surgical incision with a small amount of glue that will allow the edges of the wound to adhere.

3.6 Postoperative Care (Injection and Minipump)

1. After the procedure, carefully remove the animal from the stereotaxic apparatus.
2. Place the animal in a clean cage and monitor it until it has regained consciousness (*see* **Note 11**). The time required for the animal to recover varies depending on the procedure, with minipump implantation typically requiring slightly longer time, and based on the duration of the surgical intervention.
3. Closely monitor the animals for the next postoperative days and check for signs of discomfort (*see* **Note 12**). Analgesic drugs may be administered for a few days following the procedure, if deemed necessary. It is advisable to contact the responsible veterinary to discuss the most appropriate pain relief strategy.
4. At the end of the treatment, it is possible to validate the correct positioning of the injection and minipump ex vivo (*see* **Note 13** for intracerebroventricular injection and **Note 14** for minipump-mediated delivery).

4 Notes

1. Alzet® offers several models of implantable minipumps and brain infusion kits suitable for use on laboratory rats and mice, as well as other experimental animals. The pumps come in three different sizes, with differing reservoir volumes (2 mL, 200 μL, and 100 μL), and can deliver treatments up to 6 weeks at differing rates of infusion (between 0.11 and 10 μL/h). The Brain Infusion kits differ in gauge (30 or 28) and length (3 or 5 mm) of the implantable needle. Selection of the model will depend on the application, such as the model animal and the brain region to be targeted. Please review Alzet® website (www.alzet.com) for a complete overview of minipumps and infusion kits.
2. When compounds are to be delivered to the lateral ventricle, volumes up to 5 μL can be infused. Smaller volumes (<1 μL) are recommended when targeting the brain parenchyma to avoid overflow of the drug or potential complications due to increased intracranial pressure.
3. Rate of delivery during intracerebroventricular or intracranial injections may vary depending on the target region to be injected. It is advised to test with a pilot experiment the best rate of injection that prevents overflowing of the compound,

while keeping the duration of administration as short as possible.

4. Catheter length is calculated based on the desired infusion site, and it is measured from the location on the skull to the subcutaneous position for the osmotic pump (typically below the animal shoulder). Furthermore, the catheter should be approximately 25% longer than the calculated distance, to avoid tension and obstruction of movement of the animal's head and neck.
5. Brain Infusion Kits provide 0.5 mm-thick spacers that allow placement of the needle of the cannula to the desired depth. If adapters are required to adjust the penetration depth, glue each spacer to the plastic rim of the cannula using cyanoacrylate adhesive. Avoid applying glue to the opening of the needle to avoid obstruction of the flow. Adapters are in most cases not necessary for intraventricular delivery, when using Alzet® Brain Infusion Kit 3.
6. The delivery rate of the osmotic minipump is not stable when the compound is first loaded into the reservoir. It is, therefore, recommended to prime the pump with a 24 to 48 h incubation at 37 °C. This will ensure a consistent flow of the compound upon implantation of the osmotic pump.
7. There may be small neuroanatomical differences between mouse strains. Therefore, it is recommended to run a pilot experiment to identify the appropriate stereotaxic coordinates that target the desired brain regions.
8. Monitor respiration throughout the induction of anesthesia, as well as during the surgical procedure, making sure that breathing has slowed down but is never suppressed. Longer operations may pose some strain on the animal, which may display some respiratory depression. Adjust the concentration of isoflurane accordingly: Lower the concentration to 1.5 to 2% if breathing slows down excessively.
9. As an alternative to piercing the skull, it is also possible to use the drill to thin the bone and then pierce it with the cannula. A drawback of this approach is the risk of obstructing the lumen of the cannula with small pieces of bone, which may in turn interfere with infusion of the test substance.
10. Fixation of the infusion kit using adhesive works well in all applications and prevents the cannula from moving or detaching from the animal's skull. In alternative, you may consider fixating the implant with dental cement, which can be anchored to the skull by means of a surgical screw positioned in proximity of the plastic rim of the infusion kit. This procedure may provide further stability to the implant, but it is technically more challenging and not recommended for use on mice.

11. Consider whether mice should be housed separately. Sometimes mice bite stitches off their cage mates, thereby reopening the surgical wound and exposing the silicon catheter from the Brain Infusion Kit. In turn, the tubing may easily be severed and cause disconnection of the osmotic pump. If animals are housed together, carefully monitor their behavior to prevent breaking of the minipump assembly.
12. Mice typically tolerate well the procedures outlined in the present chapter. It is, nevertheless, advisable to check regularly on the operated animals and make sure the surgical wound remains sealed. Additionally, it is important to ensure that the animal does not feel discomfort from the minipump. For instance, the animal may scratch the head, at the infusion site, or the back, around the subcutaneous pocket. In this case, consider applying local anesthetics and consult the veterinary for expert advice. Careful monitoring of the animal is also necessary in case there is reason to suspect that symptoms will arise following administration of the specific treatment being investigated.
13. When brains are collected and sectioned, it is possible to validate the correct placement of the needle during the injection. Typically, the injection tract will be visible under the microscope using a simple Hoechst staining to label cell nuclei. Cells will appear more densely packed along the site of injection due to a reactive response mounted by immune cells as a consequence of the penetrating lesion caused by the needle.
14. The site of minipump implantation will likely be visible in brain slices under a dissection microscope due to the relatively large lesion caused by the cannula implanted in the brain throughout the duration of treatment. In addition, it is recommended to validate that the compound contained in the reservoir had been delivered throughout the experiment. For this purpose, remove the osmotic pump from the subcutaneous pocket of a euthanized animal and separate the flow moderator from the reservoir. With a 1 mL syringe and a blunt 25 G needle, draw the compound left in the inner chamber of the pump to estimate the volume that had been delivered during the experiment. Look for presence of sedimentation: You can assume that the treatment has been delivered if the reservoir is empty (or contains a smaller volume of solution) and if there is no precipitation of the compound at the bottom of the reservoir.

References

1. Yamazaki Y, Hirai Y, Miyake K, Shimada T (2014) Targeted gene transfer into ependymal cells through intraventricular injection of AAV1 vector and long-term enzyme replacement via the CSF. Sci Rep 4:5506. https://doi.org/10.1038/srep05506

2. Barnabe-Heider F, Meletis K, Eriksson M, Bergmann O, Sabelstrom H, Harvey MA, Mikkers H, Frisen J (2008) Genetic manipulation of adult mouse neurogenic niches by in vivo electroporation. Nat Methods 5(2):189–196. https://doi.org/10.1038/nmeth.1174
3. Sztainberg Y, Chen HM, Swann JW, Hao S, Tang B, Wu Z, Tang J, Wan YW, Liu Z, Rigo F, Zoghbi HY (2015) Reversal of phenotypes in MECP2 duplication mice using genetic rescue or antisense oligonucleotides. Nature 528 (7580):123–126. https://doi.org/10.1038/nature16159
4. Schoch KM, DeVos SL, Miller RL, Chun SJ, Norrbom M, Wozniak DF, Dawson HN, Bennett CF, Rigo F, Miller TM (2016) Increased 4R-tau induces pathological changes in a human-tau mouse model. Neuron 90 (5):941–947. https://doi.org/10.1016/j.neuron.2016.04.042
5. Grathwohl SA, Jucker M (2013) Replacement of osmotic minipumps to extend the intracerebral infusion time of compounds into the mouse brain. BioTechniques 55(2):75–78. https://doi.org/10.2144/000114064
6. Keith BJ, Franklin M, Paxinos G (2008) The mouse brain in stereotaxic coordinates, compact: the coronal plates and diagrams. Elsevier Science

Chapter 15

In Vitro Assessment of the Hepatotoxicity Potential of Therapeutic Oligonucleotides

Sabine Sewing, Tanja Minz, and Franziska Boess

Abstract

The mechanisms of antisense oligonucleotide-induced liver toxicity are still poorly understood. Assessment of the hepatic safety profile is currently mostly investigated directly in rodent studies. A predictive preclinical in vitro model that is capturing liver liabilities of antisense oligonucleotides can be of great help to be used as a first filter in the screening process of therapeutic oligonucleotides. We describe here an in vitro cytotoxicity assay using freshly isolated mouse hepatocytes or cryopreserved human hepatocytes that recapitulates the hepatotoxic profile of antisense oligonucleotides previously observed in rodents and can be used for the prioritization of molecules prior to in vivo testing.

Key words Antisense oligonucleotide, In vitro hepatotoxicity, Liver perfusion, Cytotoxicity, Hepatocytes, 3R

1 Introduction

Antisense oligonucleotides (AONs) become an emerging therapeutic modality that allows modulation of target proteins that cannot be targeted by small molecules or therapeutic antibodies. Critical steps in the development of therapeutic AONs involve identification of a selective oligonucleotide, guaranteeing sufficient stability, delivery to the right organ, and finding a favorable safety profile. The major adverse effects caused by AONs in vivo can be summarized as accumulation and toxicity in liver and kidney as well as inflammatory reactions at the site of injection and flu like-symptoms [1]. Treatment of mice and rats with toxic AONs resulted in significantly increased plasma aminotransferase levels (ALT and AST) and histopathological evidence for necrosis and apoptosis in liver and kidney [2, 3].

We describe here an in vitro screening assay to profile AONs for liver liability before any animal studies are initiated. The procedure involves isolation of primary mouse hepatocytes after liver perfusion and the use of cryopreserved human hepatocytes. After

Olof Gissberg et al. (eds.), *Oligonucleotide-Based Therapies: Methods and Protocols*, Methods in Molecular Biology, vol. 2036, https://doi.org/10.1007/978-1-4939-9670-4_15,

plating, the cells are treated with oligonucleotides without assistance of delivery technology, and cellular toxicity is assessed by quantification of secreted lactate dehydrogenase and intracellular ATP concentration. These experimental conditions successfully recapitulated the well-described in vivo hepatotoxic profile of a panel of test AONs [4]. Thus the assay allows a rapid, early in vitro assessment of a key liability of AONs and can be used to prioritize lead series before initiation of animal studies. It has the potential to significantly reduce the hepatotoxicity risk during AON development and contributes to the principles of the 3R in animal experimentation by a reduction of animal use for liver safety testing.

2 Materials

2.1 Mouse Liver Perfusion

1. One pair of straight forceps.
2. One pair of angled forceps.
3. One pair of scissors (one tip rounded).
4. One pair of ophthalmic scissors.
5. Vessel clips.
6. Scalpel.
7. 1 ml syringe and 0.33 × 12.7 mm cannula (29 G).
8. Cotton pads.
9. Plastic tray and wax board (approx. 20 × 25 cm).
10. Tape.
11. Timer.
12. Peristaltic pump with flow adjusted to 7 ml/min.
13. Silicon rubber tubing (ID 3 mm).
14. Gavage needle Luer 0.6, attached to tubing.
15. Water bath set at 37 °C.
16. Gas mix 5% CO_2/95% O_2, tubing connected to gas bottle.
17. Autoclaved glassware (100 ml and 500 ml bottles).
18. 150 ml sterile filter.
19. Sterile petri dishes Ø100 mm.
20. Pentobarbital-solution 50 mg/ml in 0.9% NaCl.
21. Ice.
22. 70% ethanol.
23. 50 mM EGTA stock solution: 1.903 g EGTA dissolved in ~80 ml ddH_2O, adjusted pH to 7.4 with 10 N NaOH, and added up to 100 ml with ddH_2O.

24. 1 M HEPES stock solution: 23.83 g HEPES dissolved in ~80 ml ddH_2O, adjusted pH to 7.4 with 10 N NaOH, and added up to 100 ml with ddH_2O.
25. HBSS: Hank's balanced salt solution w/o Ca^{++}, w/o Mg^{++}, w/o phenol red.
26. 10× Preperfusion solution (PPS): 250 ml HBSS 50 ml 1 M HEPES stock solution, and 25 ml 50 mM EGTA stock solution.
27. PPS: 10 ml 10× PPS diluted with 100.0 ml HBSS (*see* **Note 1**).
28. 10× Perfusion solution I (PS I): 19.66 g $NaHCO_3$ dissolved in 1000 ml HBSS.
29. PS I: 15 ml 10× PS I diluted with 150 ml HBSS (*see* **Note 1**).
30. Perfusion solution II (PS II): 57.5 mg bovine serum albumin (BSA) and 63.8 mg $CaCl_2$ dissolved in 15 ml HBSS (*see* **Notes 1** and **2**).
31. 0.2 U/ml Collagenase solution: 35 mg Collagenase Type 2 (Worthington), kept in an Eppendorf tube on ice) freshly dissolved in 15 ml PS II and after dissolution mixed with 165 ml PS I (*see* **Note 3**).

2.2 Mouse Hepatocyte Isolation

1. Nylon meshes (40- and 70-μm mesh size).
2. WME medium: William's Medium E w/o phenol red.
3. Hank's balanced salt solution w/o Ca^{++}, w/o Mg^{++}, w/o phenol red.
4. 10× DPBS w/o Ca^{++}, Mg^{++}.
5. Percoll Solution: 500 ml 100% Percoll, diluted with 55.5 ml 10× DPBS.
6. Collagen-coated 96-well plates.

2.3 Oligonucleotide Treatment in Hepatocyte Cultures

1. Complete WME medium: WME medium without phenol red, 10% fetal calf serum, 100 U/ml penicillin, 0.1 mg/ml streptomycin, and 2 mM glutamine.
2. WME incubation medium: William's Medium E w/o phenol red, 100 U/ml penicillin, 0.1 mg/ml streptomycin, and 2 mM glutamine, no serum.
3. Thawing medium: cryopreserved hepatocytes recovery medium (CHRM; Thermo Fisher).
4. PBS.
5. Cryopreserved human hepatocytes or freshly prepared mouse hepatocytes.
6. Collagen-coated 96-well plates.

2.4 Cytotoxicity Determination

1. 96-well transparent polypropylene U-shaped plates.
2. PBS.
3. Cytotoxicity Detection Kit (Roche Diagnostics GmbH).
4. CellTiter-Glo® Luminescent Cell Viability Assay (G9242, Promega Corporation, Madison WI, USA).
5. WME medium: William's Medium E w/o phenol red.
6. Opaque white 96-well plates.

3 Methods

3.1 Mouse Liver Perfusion

1. Primary mouse hepatocytes are isolated from 10- to 13-week-old male C57Bl6 mice by a retrograde two-step collagenase liver perfusion (*see* **Note 4**).
2. Place PPS and PS I into a water bath at 37 °C, keep PS II on ice. Introduce the gas tubing (gas mix of 5% CO_2/95% O_2) to the bottle containing PS I to bubble 5% CO_2/95% O_2 through PS I (*see* **Note 5**).
3. Check and adjust flow rate of the pump to be 7 ml/min, and then use to rinse tubing with attached gavage needle with 70% ethanol followed by distilled water. Then start circulation of PPS through the tubing and discard the first 15 ml. Stop the Pump.
4. Anaesthetize the mouse with 0.05–0.1 ml pentobarbital solution i.p. Check the deepness of the anesthesia by hind leg reflex testing once the mouse has fallen asleep (*see* **Note 6**).
5. Once the anesthesia is deep (hind leg reflex no longer present), fix the anesthetized animal with tape ventral side up on the wax board. The latter is placed in the plastic tray to collect waste liquids.
6. Moisten the ventral fur of the mouse with 70% ethanol and detach the skin from the abdominal wall by a cut from the pelvis to the sternum and two deep incisions at right angle to the first cut.
7. Open the abdominal wall and cut along the linea alba (*care has to be taken not to injure any organ*) and apply two cuts at right angle to the first one to enable flipping the two flags over the thoracic cage.
8. Displace intestine, stomach etc. to the right in order to expose the vena cava caudalis and portal vein.
9. Open the diaphragm and cut ribs to allow flipping of the thoracic cage upward and expose lungs and heart (*see* **Note 7**). Lay open the heart and the vena cava caudalis by displacing the lungs and adjacent tissue.

10. Hold the right ventricle carefully with forceps and incise the right atrium using a pair of ophthalmic scissors.
11. Insert the gavage needle through the incision and via the right atrium into the vena cava (care has to be taken to enter far enough into the vena cava without disrupting it but not to enter the needle into the liver; stop shortly before the liver) and fix the needle with a vessel clip.
12. Ligate the vena cava caudalis distal to the junction with vena hepatica with another vessel clip.
13. Cut the portal vein and simultaneously turn on the peristaltic pump. Upon switching on the pump, the liver should turn pale and become blown up a little bit.
14. Perfuse the liver for 5 min with PPS.
15. In the meantime dissolve the collagenase in PS II and add the collagenase/PS II solution to PS I (collagenase solution).
16. After 5 min perfusion with PPS, stop the pump shortly, allowing transfer of the tube from the PPS bottle to the bottle with collagenase solution and then restart the pump again (*see* **Note 8**).
17. Perfuse the liver with the collagenase solution for 12 min.
18. After the end of the perfusion, remove the vessel clips and gavage needle, and carefully detach the liver from surrounding tissue, lift it out and place it into a petri dish. Add some few milliliters of remaining perfusion solution to cover the liver.

    The excised perfused liver should now be transferred (transport on ice) into a laminar flow bench for further work up and cell isolation.

3.2 Mouse Hepatocyte Isolation and Seeding

1. Wash he perfused liver in chilled WME and transfer it into another sterile petri dish, filled up with 10 ml of chilled WME.
2. Mechanically open the liver capsule by cutting the tissue at many spots with a sterile scalpel, and release the liver cells into the chilled WME by holding the liver with sterile forceps at the portal vein and gently shaking the tissue (*see* **Note 9**).
3. Place a 70 μm nylon mesh into a 50 ml tube and strain cell suspension through it. Repeat this step, but strain the cell suspension through a 40 μm nylon mesh.
4. Wash the meshes with chilled WME to harvest residual cells, resulting in a final total volume of 50 ml cell suspension.
5. Incubate the cell suspension for 20 min at room temperature to allow hepatocytes to sediment, then remove the supernatant and resuspend cells in 25 ml chilled WME.
6. Remove dead cells in the cell suspension by a Percoll centrifugation step (Percoll density: 1.06 g/ml), by mixing 90% Percoll

solution with the cell suspension in a ratio of 1:1 and centrifugation at 50 × *g* for 10 min. Remove and discard dead cells and debris floating on top as well as the Percoll solution, leaving the pellet of hepatocytes at the bottom of the tube.

7. Wash cells with 50 ml chilled WME to remove residual Percoll, and centrifuge for 5 min at 50 × *g*.
8. Discard supernatant and resuspend the hepatocyte pellet in 20 ml complete WME culture medium. Go to Subheading 3.3, **step 2**.

3.3 Oligonucleotide Treatment of Cultured Hepatocytes

For tests in mouse hepatocyte cultures go directly to **step 2**.

1. Thaw one vial of cryopreserved human hepatocytes in 50 ml thawing medium, centrifuge cells at 90× *g* for 10 min (*see* **Note 10**) and suspend cells in 10 ml complete WME medium at a density of approx. 1 × 10^6 cells/ml.
2. Count hepatocytes using a method of your choice (*see* **Note 11**).
3. Dilute further in complete WME medium to appropriate concentration (*see* **Note 11**) and seed hepatocytes into collagen-coated 96-well plates into a final volume of 100 μl (*see* **Note 11**).
4. Incubate plates at 37 °C and 5% CO_2 for 3–4 h for attachment.
5. Prepare oligonucleotide dilutions in WME incubation medium (*see* **Note 12**).
6. Remove seeding medium from the cells and replace by addition of 90 μl WME incubation medium and 10 μl of oligonucleotide solutions to the cell culture. Prepare triplicates for each condition (potential plate layout is shown in Fig. 1).
7. Incubate for 66 h at 37 °C and 5% CO_2.

3.4 Determine LDH in the Cell Culture Supernatant

Lactate dehydrogenase (LDH) released into the culture medium is determined using a Cytotoxicity Detection Kit according to the manufacturer's protocol:

1. Prepare LDH standard dilution series into a 96-well transparent PP U-shape plate from the stock solution provided in a 1.5 ml Eppendorf tube, by serial dilution in PBS, using a dilution factor of 2. Prepare 100 μl/plate of each 9 concentrations (LDH1-LDH9) ranging from 75 mU/ml to 0.3 mU/ml and one blank (PBS). Standards are pipetted into the two bottom rows of the 96-well LDH_plate (*see* Fig. 2 for layout).
2. Remove cell culture plates from the incubator and transfer 2–5 μl of cell culture supernatant from each well of the assay plate into the LDH_plate.
3. Add PBS to each well to get a final volume of 100 μl.

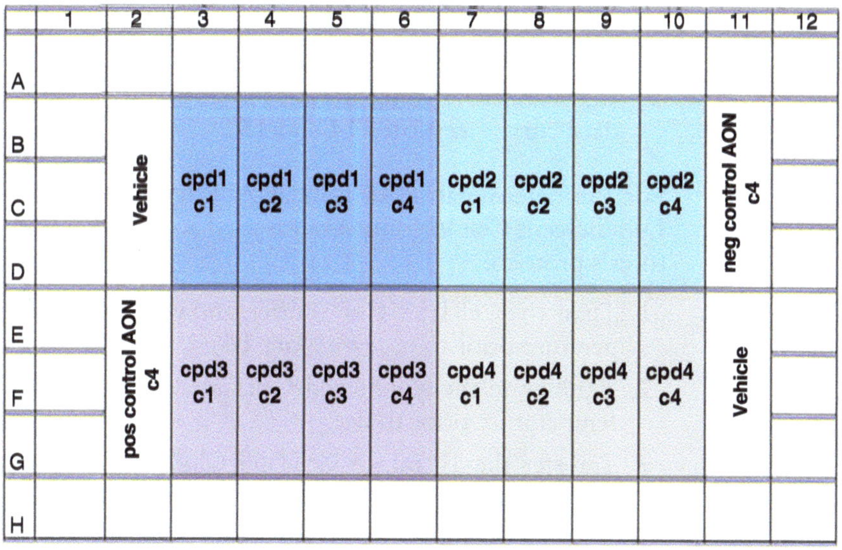

Fig. 1 Plate layout for oligonucleotide treatment: four test AONs (here cpd 1–4) in four concentrations (c1–c4) plus vehicle as well as positive and negative control AONs at the highest concentration (c4) in triplicates

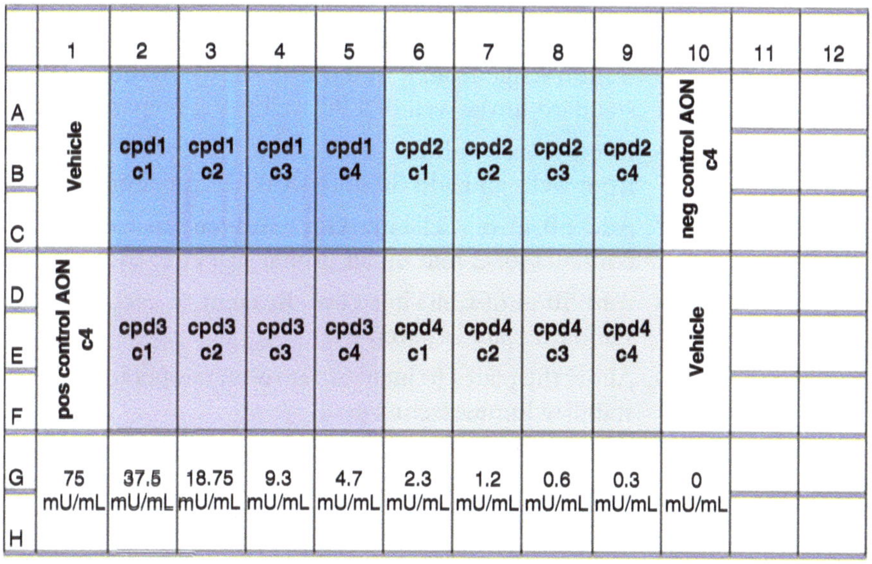

Fig. 2 Plate layout for Lactate dehydrogenase determination (LDH_plate): LDH standard curve is prepared on each test plate in rows G and H in duplicates covering 0–75 mU/ml. Samples are transferred from incubation plate (*see* Fig. 1) as outlined

4. Prepare Reaction mixture shortly before use by diluting the catalyst in the dye solution (1:46; both reagents provided in the kit), mix well and add 100 µl of the Reaction mixture to each well (including standard curve).
5. Mix for 30 s on an orbital shaker or mix with tips (*see* **Note 13**).

6. Allow the plate to incubate at room temperature for 30 min.
7. Record at OD 490 nm.
8. Calculate LDH concentrations in (mU/ml) according to standard curve (*see* **Notes 14** and **15**).

3.5 Determine Intracellular ATP

For the determination of cellular ATP levels the CellTiter-Glo® Luminescent Cell Viability Assay is used according to the manufacturer's protocol.

1. Thaw the CellTiter-Glo® Buffer, and equilibrate to room temperature prior to use (*see* **Note 16**).
2. Equilibrate the lyophilized CellTiter-Glo® Substrate to room temperature prior to use.
3. Transfer the 10 ml, of CellTiter-Glo® Buffer into the amber bottle containing CellTiter-Glo® Substrate to reconstitute the lyophilized enzyme–substrate mixture. This forms the CellTiter-Glo® Reagent.
4. Mix by gently vortexing, swirling or inverting the contents to obtain a homogeneous solution (*see* **Note 17**).
5. Prepare ATP standard dilutions by serial three-fold dilutions starting with 8 μM ATP in WME medium to obtain a concentration range from 8 to 0 μM (9 steps). Add 50 μl of each ATP standard into a well of a 96-well plate; prepare duplicates.
6. Remove cell culture plates from incubator, aspirate medium from wells and add 50 μl fresh WME medium to each well.
7. Add 50 μl of CellTiter-Glo® Reagent to each well and mix contents for 2 min on an orbital shaker to induce cell lysis.
8. Add 50 μl of CellTiter-Glo® Reagent to each well of the ATP standard plate (*see* **step 5**).
9. Allow the plates to incubate at room temperature for 10 min to stabilize luminescent signal.
10. Transfer 70 μl from each well of the plates including the standard plate to an opaque white 96-well plate and record luminescence on a luminescence plate reader for 1 s (*see* **Note 18**).
11. Calculate intracellular ATP concentrations according to the standard curve (*see* **Notes 14** and **15**).

4 Notes

1. PPS, PS I and PS II are sterile filtered and put into sterile glass bottles.
2. Addition of calcium chloride only on the day of the experiment.

3. Collagenase solution needs to be freshly prepared immediately before use (*see* Subheading 3.1, **step 15**).
4. Make sure permission for animal studies from the local regulatory agencies/authorities are available, and all study protocols are in compliance with the respective guidelines.
5. Gas should only produce small bubbles in the liquid.
6. Deepness of anesthesia is tested by the hind leg withdrawal reflex. The animal's hind limb is slightly extended and the interdigital webbing of the foot is firmly pinched by use of an atraumatic forceps. A clear attempt to withdraw the limb is indicating that the anesthesia is not (yet) deep enough to guarantee, that the mouse will not experience any pain upon the surgical procedure. In case the hind leg reflex is still there, either wait a bit longer and test again and/or increase the dose of the anesthetics by a second low volume injection of pentobarbital injection ip.
7. Upon opening of the diaphragm the following steps have to be performed as quickly as possible in order to get a well perfused liver.
8. When changing the perfusion buffer, assure that no air bubble is getting into the tubing, as it may block smaller vessels when reaching the liver tissue.
9. Avoid any rough treatment of the tissue to avoid damaging the cells.
10. Not all batches of cryopreserved human hepatocytes efficiently take up AONs into the productive compartment under the described conditions without delivery assistance. Therefore it is recommended to test initially different batches of cryopreserved human hepatocytes to identify a "responder" batch, that is, a batch of cells showing knockdown efficacy with a given test AON and changes in ATP and LDH levels with a well described toxic control AON.
11. Count cells either with a Neubauer Cell chamber or an automated Cell counter (Life technologies after standard stain with trypan blue). Seed mouse hepatocytes at a density of 2.5×10^4 cells/well and human hepatocytes at a density of 4×10^4 cells/well in the 96-well plate. Only use the inner 60 wells of a 96-well plate for AON treatment—fill the outer wells with PBS during incubation (*see* Fig. 1).
12. Oligonucleotides are diluted in WME incubation medium to generate stock solutions that are tenfold higher concentrated than the planned final concentration on the cells, that is, to obtain a final concentration of 30 μM a stock solution of 300 μM is prepared.

ALT conc. in mice	1	2	3	4	5	6	7
	64 U/lL	59 U/L	67 U/L	1889 U/L	2368 U/L	1890 U/L	ND

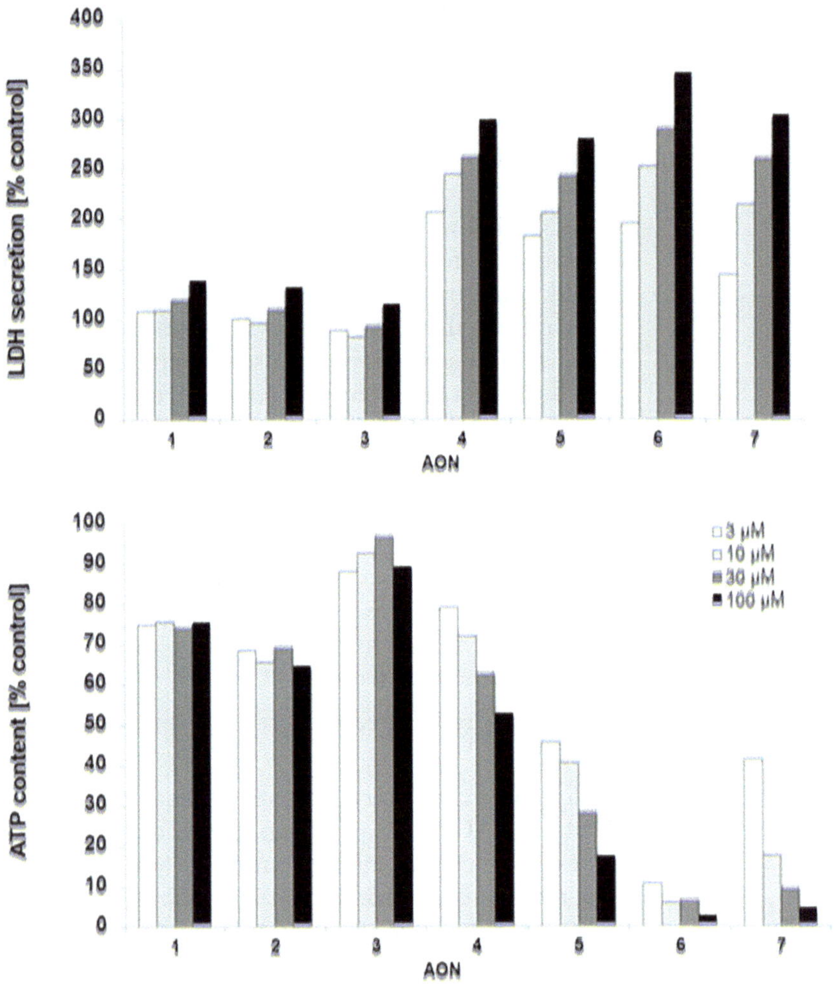

Fig. 3 Changes in intracellular ATP and secreted LDH from freshly isolated mouse hepatocytes after 66 h treatment with indicated concentrations of antisense oligonucleotides 1–7 (AON). Data are plotted as percentage of vehicle control. Data table on top shows in vivo hepatotoxicity of test AONs (indicated by increases in plasma ALT levels): AONs 1–3 were not hepatotoxic in mice while AONs 4–7 showed clear elevations of plasma ALT levels in mice (for details *see* ref. 4)

13. Avoid generating bubbles when mixing sample with the LDH reaction mixture. Bubbles will interfere with absorbance measurement.

14. To be able to compare data from different experiments it is useful to normalize the results: calculate the concentrations of ATP and LDH in relation to the vehicle control values to obtain changes as [% of control] (*see* Fig. 3).

15. Include a positive (toxic) and a negative (nontoxic) oligonucleotide control on each plate as quality control, that allow to relate the toxicity parameters for each AON to the respective assay window on each plate. Calculate as follows:

$$(\text{Value sample} - \text{Value negative control})/$$
$$(\text{Value positive control} - \text{Value negative control}) \times 100$$

In case the assay window is not large enough (i.e., changes in ATP or LDH between safe and toxic control are smaller than factor 2–3), the experiment should be repeated.
16. For convenience the CellTiter-Glo® Buffer may be thawed and stored at room temperature for up to 48 h prior to use.
17. The CellTiter-Glo® Substrate should go into solution easily in less than 1 min.
18. ATP standards are kept on a separate plate. For the ATP luminescence readout: Instrument settings depend on the manufacturer. An integration time of 0.25–1 s per well should serve as a guideline.

Acknowledgments

We thank E. Durr and N. Schaub for their excellent support.

References

1. Frazier KS (2015) Antisense oligonucleotide therapies: the promise and the challenges from a toxicologic pathologist's perspective. Toxicol Pathol 43:78–89
2. Burdick AD, Sciabola S, Mantena SR et al (2014) Sequence motifs associated with hepatotoxicity of locked nucleic acid-modified antisense oligonucleotides. Nucleic Acid Res 42:4882–4891
3. Stanton R, Sciabola S, Salatto C et al (2012) Chemical modification study of antisense gapmers. Nucleic Acid Ther 22:344–359
4. Sewing S, Boess F, Moisan A et al (2016) Establishment of a predictive in vitro assay for assessment of the hepatotoxic potential of oligonucleotide drugs. PLoS One 11:e0159431

Chapter 16

Identifying Suitable Target Regions and Analyzing Off-Target Effects of Therapeutic Oligonucleotides

Lykke Pedersen, Peter H. Hagedorn, and Troels Koch

Abstract

Antisense oligonucleotides (AONs) that promote degradation of complementary RNA are being developed as therapeutics. Here, we describe a simple computational workflow for identification of the regions on an RNA that are suitable for targeting with such AONs. The workflow is based on the statistical programming language R, and the calculations and data processing can be carried out on a desktop computer. Our workflow integrates well-established data resources and RNA structure-prediction tools and can be modified easily and expanded as new resources become available.

Key words Antisense oligonucleotides, Target regions, Off-target effects, Computational prediction, Ribonuclease H

1 Introduction

It is a goal for drug discovery to address unmet clinical needs by developing chemical compounds that are efficacious, well-tolerated, and interact specifically with their intended biomolecular targets [1–3]. A major strength of the antisense oligonucleotide (AON) drug-technology platform is that it enables use of information on nucleic-acid sequences and transcriptomics to identify and evaluate suitable target regions on an RNA molecule of interest as well as to analyze for hybridization-based off-target effects [4, 5].

Here, we focus on the computational methods for such analyses for the class of AONs designed to promote ribonuclease H (RNase H)-mediated cleavage of complementary RNAs [6]. Since the cleaved RNA fragments are subsequently degraded by endogenous exonucleases, this class of AONs can be used for targeted RNA knockdown. Specifically, we focus on the AONs designed as high-affinity gapmers, that is, in which a central region of DNA nucleotides that recruits RNase H are flanked by regions of chemically modified nucleotides. An example of such modified nucleotides is locked nucleic acids (LNAs), which confers increased binding

Olof Gissberg et al. (eds.), *Oligonucleotide-Based Therapies: Methods and Protocols*, Methods in Molecular Biology, vol. 2036, https://doi.org/10.1007/978-1-4939-9670-4_16, © Springer Science+Business Media, LLC, part of Springer Nature 2019

affinity and nuclease resistance to the gapmer [7]. Transcriptomics methods for target-region identification and analyses of off-target effects have been reviewed elsewhere [4, 8].

Single-stranded gapmers can, in principle, be designed to bind with full complementarity to any sequence region on a primary RNA target of interest using classical Watson–Crick base-pairing rules for hybridization [9]. Depending on the length of the primary transcript and the lengths chosen for the target regions, the total number of possible target regions will often be on the order of hundreds of thousands [10]. Studies evaluating up to hundreds of regions across a target suggest that some regions are much more suitable for targeting with gapmers than others [11, 12]. Mechanistically, these differences between regions can be ascribed to several factors which can influence gapmer properties. This includes factors intrinsic to the gapmer itself (like self-folding), as well as factors arising from the interaction between the gapmer and the surrounding environment (like binding to the RNA target or to proteins). If some of these factors can be predicted computationally based on the nucleobase sequence, such computational analyses can help guide the selection of the target regions most suitable for experimental evaluation in a drug-discovery project.

With respect to activity, some factors are well understood and prediction methods have been devised based on thermodynamic or statistical models. These include: the hybridization between target and gapmer [13, 14]; the accessibility of the target region on the RNA [15]; the secondary structure of the gapmer [16, 17]; and the sequence preferences of the RNase H enzyme [18]. Other factors, such as the propensity of gapmers to bind to proteins [19, 20], have not yet been characterized and are not understood to an extent that allows for the development of computational models. However, gapmer–protein interactions govern uptake and retention in tissues and cells [21], subcellular distribution [22], and endosomal trafficking and release and, therefore, impact activity as well.

Other considerations can also rank some sequence regions in preference over others. For example, many drug-discovery projects rely on studies in rodents and nonhuman primates for pharmacodynamic evaluation of target engagement and the downstream effects thereof [23]. In such projects, the preferred target regions could be limited to those conserved across the species of interest [11]. Similarly, one could exclude target regions containing known sites of high-frequency polymorphisms, since gapmers designed to such regions would not match perfectly in patients expressing the gene variants from one or both alleles. Also, some target regions are found more than once on the RNA target, and it has been shown that gapmers binding to such repeated regions can be more potent [24]. To manage off-target effects, identical or nearly identical regions found in many different RNA molecules can be identified in the RNA target of interest and avoided. This would be expected to reduce the chance of the gapmer binding to unintended, perfectly or partially matched sequence regions in nontarget RNAs, and therefore reduce off-target effects [4, 5]. All of these factors can be predicted by well-established sequence analysis methods using publicly available information on nucleic-acid sequences [25].

Finally, certain sequence motifs in gapmers have been associated with activation of immune cells [26] or increased hepatotoxic potential [27, 28]. Such motifs can be modified chemically in the gapmers, or the complementary motifs in the RNA target can be identified by sequence analysis and deselected [11].

Taken together, many factors related to the sequence of the RNA target or the sequence and chemical modification pattern of the gapmer can influence gapmer properties. Some of these factors can be confidently predicted with sequence- or more general structure-based models and can, therefore, be included when selecting target regions and designing gapmers computationally [29–31]. Other factors are less well-understood presently. With more experimental and modelling work, these factors may become possible to predict computationally in the future. With enough data one may even be able to skip modelling mechanistic factors individually and instead train machine-learning algorithms to predict properties directly from the chemical structure of the gapmer and RNA target [28, 32, 33].

In this chapter we describe a simple computational workflow for enumerating all possible target regions for a given RNA target of interest. Relevant properties, such as those described above, are predicted for each region and organized in a table. In this data table, rows represent target regions, columns represent various calculated properties and predictions, and the numbers in each cell characterize the predicted value of the particular target region for the particular property. This table allows ranking and selection of the target regions judged overall most suitable for gapmer design. The workflow is based on the statistical programming language R [36] and all calculations and data processing can be carried out on a standard desktop computer. Sequence information is queried and retrieved from public data resources using well-established and community-maintained database interfaces. Well-validated and publicly available RNA structure-prediction tools are also integrated in the workflow. Basic R programming skills will allow any user to expand the workflow based on individual needs and preferences. The workflow can also easily be adjusted as new databases and RNA prediction tools are developed.

In our experience, libraries of gapmers targeting regions selected by consideration of predicted properties demonstrate higher hit rates and lower attrition rates compared with libraries of gapmers in which target regions have been selected randomly. When deciding on the number of suitable target regions to evaluate experimentally, we recommend careful statistical analysis based on estimated predictive accuracies [11, 34]. In a nutshell, not all predictions will be correct, and therefore, if only a few regions are chosen, one risk missing the regions that would in reality have been ideal for target engagement. Depending on resources, choosing between 50 and 500 target regions will usually be adequate.

As a final note, when gapmers are developed for therapeutics, identification of hits in suitable target regions is just the first step in the discovery process. As for all therapeutic modalities, substantial efforts in medicinal chemistry and drug design are needed to turn hits into chemically optimized lead molecules with good drug-like properties [10, 35].

2 Materials

The computational workflow is based on the R programming language for statistical computing [36] with selected data-analysis packages [37, 38] and Bioconductor packages [39–41] for retrieval and analysis of nucleic-acid sequences. All commands that should be executed in the R console are shown in courier font (*see* **Note 1**). Key features of the code are mentioned as a note after each code box.

2.1 Set Up the Programming Environment

1. Retrieve and install R from the Comprehensive R Archive Network: cran.r-project.org.
2. Execute the following commands in the R console to retrieve and install the relevant packages:

```
source("https://bioconductor.org/biocLite.R")
# Install and update Bioconductor packages
library(BiocInstaller)
# Human genome
biocLite("BSgenome.Hsapiens.NCBI.GRCh38")
# Making and working with genome annotations
biocLite("GenomicFeatures")
# Memory efficient string storage and manipulation of
sequences
biocLite("Biostrings")
# Interface to biomart.org
biocLite("biomaRt")
# Annotation Database Interface
biocLite("AnnotationDbi")
# Data analysis and visualization
install.packages("tidyverse")
# Data clustering
install.packages("cluster")
```

See **Note 2**.

2.2 Organize All Human pre-mRNA Sequences and the Target of Interest

1. Define the directory path where annotation data are to be stored:

```
path = "Path to directory where annotation will be
stored"
```

2. Get human transcript annotations:

```
library(GenomicFeatures)
library(AnnotationDbi)

txdb_hsa = makeTxDbFromBiomart(
  biomart="ENSEMBL_MART_ENSEMBL",
  dataset="hsapiens_gene_ensembl",
   taxonomyId=9606)
  saveDb(txdb_hsa,paste0(path, "txdb_hsa_biomart.
db"))
```

The function `makeTxDbFromBiomart()` creates a local transcript database from BioMart, in this case for human transcripts as annotated in Ensembl [25]. However, any other transcript annotation could have been chosen.

3. Store all human pre-mRNA sequences from the 23 standard chromosomes in a DNAStringSet object:

```
library(BSgenome.Hsapiens.NCBI.GRCh38)
txdb_hsa = loadDb(paste0(path,"txdb_hsa_biomart.db"))
gdb_hsa = genes(txdb_hsa)
chr_to_keep = c(as.character(1:22),'X','Y','MT')
Hsapiens@user_seqnames <- setNames(chr_to_keep,
chr_to_keep)
Hsapiens@seqinfo <- Hsapiens@seqinfo[chr_to_keep]
gdb_hsa = gdb_hsa[seqnames(gdb_hsa) %in% chr_to_keep]
HS = getSeq(Hsapiens, gdb_hsa )
```

The human genome is stored in the BSgenome object `Hsapiens` after loading of the BSgenome.Hsapiens.NCBI.GRCh38 package. The human genome is trimmed to only contain the 23 standard chromosomes by resetting the sequence names using `setNames()` and the sequence information in `seqinfo`. Human pre-mRNA sequences are then extracted by applying the `getSeq()` function on `Hsapiens` and using the genomic positional information stored in the Granges object `gdb_hsa`.

4. As an example for this workflow, the Target of myb1 membrane trafficking protein (*TOM1*), with Ensembl ID

ENSG00000100284, is chosen as the RNA target of interest. For this target collect the pre-mRNA sequence as follows:

```
ensembl_ID = 'ENSG00000100284'
RNA_target = HS[names(HS)==ensembl_ID]
```

5. To prepare for analysis of polymorphisms (*see* Subheading 2.4), organize chromosomal coordinates:

```
target_ranges = gdb_hsa[names(gdb_hsa)==ensembl_ID]

chr_coord = c(
    chr=as.numeric(as.character(seqnames(targe-
t_ranges))),
  start=start(target_ranges),
  end=end(target_ranges),
  strand=ifelse(strand(target_ranges)=='+',1,-1))
```

See Note 3.

2.3 Organize Ortholog pre-mRNA Sequences for the RNA Target in Other Species

1. Obtain the mouse ortholog of the human RNA target:

```
library(biomaRt)
library(Biostrings)
martMM = useMart(biomart="ensembl",
                 dataset="mmusculus_gene_ensembl")

martHS = useMart(biomart="ensembl",
                 dataset="hsapiens_gene_ensembl")
ortho_ENS = getBM(attributes = "mmusculus_homolog_en-
sembl_gene",
                 filters = "ensembl_gene_id",
                 values = ensembl_ID, mart = martHS,
                 bmHeader = FALSE)

RNA_target_mouse = DNAStringSet(
  getBM(attributes = c("gene_exon_intron", 'ensembl_-
gene_id'),
        filters = "ensembl_gene_id",
        values =
ortho_ENS$mmusculus_homolog_ensembl_gene,
        mart = martMM)$gene_exon_intron)
```

See Note 4.

2.4 Organize Polymorphism Information

1. Obtain all human polymorphisms for the RNA target:

```
library(tidyverse)

PMs = getBM(attributes = c("minor_allele_freq",
                           "chromosome_start"),
            filters = "ensembl_gene_id",
            values = ensembl_ID,
            mart = martHS) %>%
  as_tibble() %>%
  arrange(chromosome_start,
          desc(minor_allele_freq)) %>%
  filter(!is.na(minor_allele_freq),
         !duplicated(chromosome_start)) %>%
  rename(chr_start=chromosome_start,
         PM_freq=minor_allele_freq)
```

Here the `getBM()` function retrieves the minor allele frequencies for human polymorphisms and their chromosomal position. The retrieved attributes are arranged in a data frame by the `as_tibble()` function and sorted according to chromosomal position and descending allele frequencies. Next, duplicated chromosome positions are filtered out along with NA entries in the data frame. The operator `%>%` pipes an R object into a function or an expression call.

2.5 Organize Prediction of AON and RNA Secondary Structures

For all structure predictions, we use algorithms implemented in the ViennaRNA package [17] (*see* **Note 5**).

2.5.1 Install ViennaRNA Package

1. Follow the instructions on https://www.tbi.univie.ac.at/RNA/documentation.html to install the ViennaRNA package locally.
2. Once installed, check the installation by running the commands below in a terminal window. These commands display the version of the installed functions.

```
RNAplfold -V
RNAduplex -V
RNAfold -V
```

2.5.2 Predict Accessibility for an RNA Target

1. The function below defines a wrapper for the RNAplfold algorithm. The algorithm computes the probability that a region of length *1* to `u.in` is unpaired with any other bases in a window

of size `W.in` on the RNA transcript `seq.char`. The parameter `L.in` is the maximum distance allowed between two base pairs (*see* **Note 6**):

```
RNAplfold_R = function(seq.char, L.in = 40,
                              W.in = 80, u.in = 16){
  cmmnd2 = paste("RNAplfold -L", L.in, "-W", W.in, "-u",
u.in)
  seq.char = as.character(seq.char)
  cat(seq.char, file = paste("|", cmmnd2, sep = ""))
  acc.tx = read.delim("plfold_lunp", as.is = T, skip = 2,
                          header = F, row.names = 1)
  acc.tx = acc.tx[, colSums(is.na(acc.tx)) !=
nrow(acc.tx)]
  colnames(acc.tx) = 1:ncol(acc.tx)
  file.remove("plfold_lunp")
  file.remove("plfold_dp.ps")
  return(acc.tx)
}
```

The function `cat()` pipes the RNA sequence `seq.char` to RNAplfold by a system call within R. The output of RNAplfold is two files: `plfold_lunp`, containing the pair probabilities, and `plfold_dp.ps`, which is a dot plot with averaged pair probabilities. The wrapper above outputs a data frame with computed pair probabilities for different lengths of regions in separate columns. The function will overwrite the two output files if they already exist in the working directory.

2.5.3 Predict Duplex Formation and Self-Folding for Oligonucleotides

1. The functions below provide wrappers for the RNAduplex and RNAfold algorithms (*see* **Note 7**). These algorithms predict the minimum free energy of duplex formation and self-folding, respectively:

```
RNAduplex_R = function(seqs){
  sys_cmd = system('RNAduplex',input = c(seqs,seqs),
                        intern = TRUE)
  as.numeric(sapply(
    strsplit(sys_cmd, "\s+", perl = T), function(x){
      gsub("\\(|\\)", "", tail(x, n=1) )
    }))
}
```

```
RNAselffold_R = function (seqs) {
   output = system('RNAfold --noPS', input=c(seqs),
intern = T)
  output = unlist(strsplit(output[grepl('[0-9]', out-
put)], '[(]'))
   as.double(gsub(' |[)]', '', output[grepl('[0-9]',
output)]))
}
```

System calls can be performed within R using the `system ()` function. In the code above, it is used for calls to RNAduplex and RNAfold to obtain data frames with energies for duplex formation and self-folding of RNA sequences.

3 Methods

After executing the commands shown above in Materials, the following data objects should be in the R-environment:

- `HS`, a DNAStringSet object with all human pre-mRNA sequences.
- `RNA_target`, a DNAStringSet object with the pre-mRNA sequence of the RNA target.
- `chr_coord`, a vector with chromosomal coordinates for the RNA target,
- `PMtab`, a table with the polymorphism frequencies for the RNA target.
- `RNA_target_mouse`, a DNAStringSet object with the mouse ortholog of the RNA target.

3.1 Construct All Target Regions Using the RNA Target Sequence

The purpose of this code section is to construct a data frame (`target_annotation`) containing sequences of target regions of different lengths together with their positional information relative to the RNA target sequence from which they are derived.

1. Split the RNA target into target regions (here subsequences of lengths from 14 to 20 nucleobases) and annotate each target region with a start and end position on the RNA target and a length:

```
l = width(RNA_target)

oligo_lengths = 14:20

target_annotation = lapply(oligo_lengths, function(i){
  tibble(start=1:(l-i+1),length=i)}) %>%
  bind_rows() %>%
  mutate(end = start+length-1)
```

```
> target_annotation
# A tibble: 340,928 x 4
   start length   end name
   <int>  <int> <dbl> <chr>
 1     1     14    14 GCTTTTTGCCATCC
 2     2     14    15 CTTTTTGCCATCCT
 3     3     14    16 TTTTTGCCATCCTG
 4     4     14    17 TTTTGCCATCCTGG
 5     5     14    18 TTTGCCATCCTGGG
 6     6     14    19 TTGCCATCCTGGGC
 7     7     14    20 TGCCATCCTGGGCG
 8     8     14    21 GCCATCCTGGGCGC
 9     9     14    22 CCATCCTGGGCGCT
10    10     14    23 CATCCTGGGCGCTA
# ... with 340,918 more rows
```

Fig. 1 The table `target_annotation`, as appearing in an R-console. This table contains positional information on the target regions, that is, start and end are the relative start and end position of the target region on the RNA target

For each length of target regions stored in the vector `oligo_lengths` a data frame with relative start positions and lengths are constructed by using `lapply()`, which applies a function to each element in a vector.

2. Extract the nucleobase sequence for each target region and store it in a column of `target_annotation` called "name":

```
target_regions = DNAStringSet(
  RNA_target[[1]],
  start=target_annotation$start,
  width=target_annotation$length)
names(target_regions) = as.character(target_regions)

target_annotation$name = names(target_regions)
```

The function `DNAStringSet()` as used here takes as input a DNA sequence and outputs substrings of this sequence with the provided start positions and lengths. Even though we are working on RNA sequences we use Biostrings data objects for DNA sequences for convenience. Therefore, sequences are represented with T (thymine) instead of U (uracil).

The table `target_annotation`, as appearing in an R-console, is shown in Fig. 1.

3.2 Identify Repeated Regions on the RNA Target

An improvement in potency has been observed for gapmers targeting repeated regions on an RNA target. The purpose of this code section is to count how many times a target region is occurring on the RNA target and add a column with this information to `target_annotation`.

1. Count how many times a nucleobase sequence occurs on the RNA target:

```
tr = target_annotation$name
replica = table(tr)
target_annotation$NoRepeats = as.vector(replica[tr])
```

The function `table()` returns a contingency table in an array format with unique names.

In Fig. 2, `target_annotation` is shown with the added column for the number of occurrences of a target region.

3.3 Evaluate Sequence Specificity

The purpose of this code section is to match target regions to all human pre-mRNAs and from this construct a data frame with information on target region specificity.

1. For each target region sequence, count the number of pre-mRNA transcripts with a perfect match to the sequence as well as the number of pre-mRNA transcripts with a single mismatch (*see* **Note 8**):

```
uni_tar = dplyr::select(target_annotation, name, length)
%>%
 unique() %>%
 split(.,.$length)

uni_tar = lapply(uni_tar, function(X){

  dict0 = PDict(X$name, max.mismatch = 0)
  dict1 = PDict(X$name, max.mismatch = 1)

  #perfect match count
  pm = vwhichPDict(
    pdict = dict0, subject = HS,
    max.mismatch = 0, min.mismatch=0)
  X$gene_hits_pm = tabulate(unlist(pm),nbins=nrow(X))

  #single mismatch count, without indels
  mm1 = vwhichPDict(
    pdict = dict1, subject = HS,
    max.mismatch = 1, min.mismatch=1)
   X$gene_hits_1mm  =  tabulate(unlist(mm1),nbins=nrow
(X))
  X
}) %>%
  bind_rows()
```

```
> target_annotation
# A tibble: 340,928 x 5
   start length   end name              NoRepeats
   <int>  <int> <dbl> <chr>                 <int>
 1     1     14    14 GCTTTTTGCCATCC            1
 2     2     14    15 CTTTTTGCCATCCT            1
 3     3     14    16 TTTTTGCCATCCTG            1
 4     4     14    17 TTTTGCCATCCTGG            1
 5     5     14    18 TTTGCCATCCTGGG            1
 6     6     14    19 TTGCCATCCTGGGC            1
 7     7     14    20 TGCCATCCTGGGCG            1
 8     8     14    21 GCCATCCTGGGCGC            1
 9     9     14    22 CCATCCTGGGCGCT            1
10    10     14    23 CATCCTGGGCGCTA            1
# ... with 340,918 more rows
```

Fig. 2 The table `target_annotation`, as appearing in an R-console. Compared to Fig. 1, information on the number of occurrences of a target region (`NoRepeats`) has been added

```
> uni_tar
# A tibble: 328,299 x 4
   name           length gene_hits_pm gene_hits_1mm
   <chr>           <int>        <int>         <int>
 1 GCTTTTTGCCATCC     14            5           355
 2 CTTTTTGCCATCCT     14           12           701
 3 TTTTTGCCATCCTG     14           25           774
 4 TTTTGCCATCCTGG     14           18           834
 5 TTTGCCATCCTGGG     14           11           607
 6 TTGCCATCCTGGGC     14           13           610
 7 TGCCATCCTGGGCG     14            5           311
 8 GCCATCCTGGGCGC     14            3           249
 9 CCATCCTGGGCGCT     14            4           271
10 CATCCTGGGCGCTA     14            4           109
# ... with 328,289 more rows
```

Fig. 3 Table with information on specificity named `uni_tar`

The columns "name" and "length" of the `target_annotation` data frame (*see* Fig. 2) are selected using `dplyr::select()` and the resulting data frame is split into a list of data frames depending on the "length" column. Then, `lapply()` is used on this list to match the target regions to the human genome by using the functions `PDict()`, which stores a dictionary of DNA patterns, and `vwhichPDict()`, which returns a vector with the number of matches for the dictionary. The output of `lapply()` is a list of data frames, which `bind_rows()` binds together by rows to construct the data frame `uni_tar` (*see* Fig. 3).

3.4 Estimate Transcript Accessibility for the RNA Target at Single-Nucleotide Resolution

In this code section the accessibility of each target region is evaluated by computing the probability that the RNA target is unfolded in the target region. A column with these probabilities is added to `target_annotation`.

1. Evaluate the accessibility of each target region on the RNA target:

```
accessibility = RNAplfold_R(RNA_target,
                            u.in = max(oligo_lengths))
%>%
  as_tibble() %>%
  mutate(end=1:l) %>%
  gather(length,accessibility, -end) %>%
  mutate(length=as.double(length))

target_annotation = left_join(target_annotation,
                              accessibility,
                              by=c('length','end'))
```

The `RNAplfold_R` function wrapper is applied to the RNA target sequence and pair probabilities are calculated for regions of length 1 to the maximum target region length. The output of `RNAplfoldR()` is transformed to a tibble object with columns for the end position, length, and computed accessibility of the target regions. The transformed output is then merged with `target_annotation` based on the "length" and "end" columns of both data frames using the `left_join()` function. The addition of the accessibility column to the `target_annotation` is shown in Fig. 4.

```
> target_annotation
# A tibble: 340,928 x 6
   start length   end name           NoRepeats accessibility
   <int>  <dbl> <dbl> <chr>              <int>         <dbl>
 1     1     14    14 GCTTTTTGCCATCC         1      0.00615
 2     2     14    15 CTTTTTGCCATCCT         1      0.00654
 3     3     14    16 TTTTTGCCATCCTG         1      0.00693
 4     4     14    17 TTTTGCCATCCTGG         1      0.000613
 5     5     14    18 TTTGCCATCCTGGG         1      0.000482
 6     6     14    19 TTGCCATCCTGGGC         1      0.000485
 7     7     14    20 TGCCATCCTGGGCG         1      0.000453
 8     8     14    21 GCCATCCTGGGCGC         1      0.000520
 9     9     14    22 CCATCCTGGGCGCT         1      0.00423
10    10     14    23 CATCCTGGGCGCTA         1      0.00174
# ... with 340,918 more rows
```

Fig. 4 The table `target_annotation`, as appearing in an R-console. Compared to Fig. 2, information on predicted accessibility of a target region (`accessibility`) has been added

3.5 High-Frequency Polymorphisms

To avoid designing gapmers that will not have a perfect match to the RNA target in certain patient populations due to polymorphisms, the highest frequency of any polymorphism within a target region is annotated to that target region.

1. From the relative start positions in `target_annotation` find the chromosomal position by using the information in the `chr_coord` data frame. Then, for each target region, note the frequency of the most frequent polymorphism found within that region:

```
if (chr_coord['strand'] == 1) {
  target_annotation$chr_start = chr_coord['start'] +
    target_annotation$start - 1
  target_annotation$chr_end = chr_coord['start'] +
    target_annotation$end - 1
} else {
  target_annotation$chr_start = chr_coord['end'] -
    target_annotation$end + 1
  target_annotation$chr_end = chr_coord['end'] -
    target_annotation$start + 1
}

PMmax = PMs %>%
  mutate(name = map(chr_start, function(X){
    filter(target_annotation,
           chr_start <= X,
           chr_end >= X)$name
  })) %>%
  unnest() %>%
  arrange(desc(PM_freq)) %>%
  filter(!duplicated(name))

target_annotation = left_join(
  target_annotation, PMmax,
  by = c("name", "chr_start"))
```

The function `map()` works like `lapply()` within a data frame, that is, it applies a function to values in a specified column. In the code above, `map()` extracts target regions from `target_annotation` that overlaps with a specified chromosomal position in a list. The tibble containing the polymorphisms is then reshaped and merged with `target_annotation`.

```
> PMmax
# A tibble: 139,560 x 3
   PM_freq chr_start name
     <dbl>     <int> <chr>
 1   0.482  35308276 AGTTCCTTTTCTCT
 2   0.482  35308276 GTTCCTTTTCTCTT
 3   0.482  35308276 TTCCTTTTCTCTTT
 4   0.482  35308276 TCCTTTTCTCTTTT
 5   0.482  35308276 CCTTTTCTCTTTTT
 6   0.482  35308276 CTTTTCTCTTTTTT
 7   0.482  35308276 TTTTCTCTTTTTTT
 8   0.482  35308276 TTTCTCTTTTTTTT
 9   0.482  35308276 TTCTCTTTTTTTTT
10   0.482  35308276 TCTCTTTTTTTTTT
# ... with 139,550 more rows
```

Fig. 5 The table with high-frequency polymorphisms (`PM_freq`), chromosomal position of the PM (`chr_start`) and sequence of target region

```
> target_annotation
# A tibble: 340,928 x 9
   start length   end name           NoRepeats accessibility chr_start  chr_end PM_freq
   <int>  <dbl> <dbl> <chr>              <int>         <dbl>     <dbl>    <dbl>   <dbl>
 1     1     14    14 GCTTTTTGCCATCC         1      0.00615   35299275 35299288      NA
 2     2     14    15 CTTTTTGCCATCCT         1      0.00654   35299276 35299289      NA
 3     3     14    16 TTTTTGCCATCCTG         1      0.00693   35299277 35299290      NA
 4     4     14    17 TTTTGCCATCCTGG         1      0.000613  35299278 35299291      NA
 5     5     14    18 TTTGCCATCCTGGG         1      0.000482  35299279 35299292      NA
 6     6     14    19 TTGCCATCCTGGGC         1      0.000485  35299280 35299293      NA
 7     7     14    20 TGCCATCCTGGGCG         1      0.000453  35299281 35299294      NA
 8     8     14    21 GCCATCCTGGGCGC         1      0.000520  35299282 35299295      NA
 9     9     14    22 CCATCCTGGGCGCT         1      0.00423   35299283 35299296      NA
10    10     14    23 CATCCTGGGCGCTA         1      0.00174   35299284 35299297      NA
# ... with 340,918 more rows
```

Fig. 6 The table `target_annotation`, as appearing in an R-console. Compared to Fig. 4, information on high-frequency polymorphisms for a target region (`PM_freq`) has been added

The table with high-frequency polymorphisms can be seen in Fig. 5, and in Fig. 6 is shown the `target_annotation` table with the column of high-frequency polymorphisms added.

3.6 Match RNA Target Regions to the Mouse Ortholog

If the gapmers are to be evaluated pharmacodynamically in mice, they need to have a perfect match in the pre-mRNA of the mouse ortholog of the RNA target. For some RNA targets a mouse ortholog might not exist or several orthologs may exist.

1. Identify which human target regions are conserved in the mouse ortholog pre-mRNA:

```
> uni_tar
# A tibble: 328,299 x 5
   name              length gene_hits_pm gene_hits_1mm conserved_in_mmusculus
   <chr>              <int>        <int>         <int> <lgl>
 1 GCTTTTTGCCATCC        14            5           355 FALSE
 2 CTTTTTGCCATCCT        14           12           701 FALSE
 3 TTTTTGCCATCCTG        14           25           774 FALSE
 4 TTTTGCCATCCTGG        14           18           834 FALSE
 5 TTTGCCATCCTGGG        14           11           607 FALSE
 6 TTGCCATCCTGGGC        14           13           610 FALSE
 7 TGCCATCCTGGGCG        14            5           311 FALSE
 8 GCCATCCTGGGCGC        14            3           249 FALSE
 9 CCATCCTGGGCGCT        14            4           271 FALSE
10 CATCCTGGGCGCTA        14            4           109 FALSE
# ... with 328,289 more rows
```

Fig. 7 The table `uni_tar`, as appearing in an R-console. Compared to Fig. 3, information on the conservation to mouse of a target region (`conserved_in_mmusculus`) has been added

```
lm = width(RNA_target_mouse)
MM_tab = lapply(oligo_lengths, function(i){
  tibble(st=1:(lm-i+1),w=i)}) %>%
  bind_rows()

RNAsitesMM = DNAStringSet(
  RNA_target_mouse[[1]],
  start=MM_tab$st,
  width=MM_tab$w)

uni_tar$conserved_in_mmusculus =
  uni_tar$name %in% RNAsitesMM
```

In Fig. 7, the data frame with the unique target regions (`uni_tar`) is shown after the addition of the column with conservation to mouse.

3.7 Occurrences of CGs Nucleobase Sequences, Duplex and Self-Folding

In this and the following code section, properties relating to the gapmer nucleobase sequence are calculated.

1. Count the occurrence of CG dinucleotides in gapmer nucleobase sequences:

```
uni_tar$CGs = ( uni_tar$length -
        nchar(gsub(’CG’,”,uni_tar$name)) )/2
```

2. Define by the reverse complement of the target sequences the nucleobase sequences of the gapmers (`oligo_seq` column):

```
> uni_tar
# A tibble: 328,299 x 9
   name       length gene_hits_pm gene_hits_1mm conserved_in_mmu…   CGs oligo_seq  sec_energy duplex_energy
   <chr>       <int>        <int>         <int> <lgl>              <dbl> <chr>           <dbl>         <dbl>
 1 GCTTTTT…       14            5           355 FALSE                  0 GGATGGCAA…          0          -3
 2 CTTTTTG…       14           12           701 FALSE                  0 AGGATGGCA…          0          -3.7
 3 TTTTTGC…       14           25           774 FALSE                  0 CAGGATGGC…          0          -7.7
 4 TTTTGCC…       14           18           834 FALSE                  0 CCAGGATGG…          0          -8.4
 5 TTTGCCA…       14           11           607 FALSE                  0 CCCAGGATG…       -0.2          -7.1
 6 TTGCCAT…       14           13           610 FALSE                  0 GCCCAGGAT…       -3.8          -7.7
 7 TGCCATC…       14            5           311 FALSE                  1 CGCCCAGGA…       -3.6          -8.2
 8 GCCATCC…       14            3           249 FALSE                  1 GCGCCCAGG…       -2.4          -7.1
 9 CCATCCT…       14            4           271 FALSE                  1 AGCGCCCAG…          0          -6.3
10 CATCCTG…       14            4           109 FALSE                  1 TAGCGCCCA…          0          -2.4
# ... with 328,289 more rows
```

Fig. 8 The table `uni_tar`, as appearing in an R-console. Compared to Fig. 6, information on CG-count and duplex- and self-folding energies has been added

```
nucleobase_seq =
unique(reverseComplement(target_regions))
uni_tar$oligo_seq =
as.character(nucleobase_seq[uni_tar$name])
```

3. Estimate the minimum free energies for self-folding and duplex formation of the gapmers:

```
uni_tar$sec_energy = RNAselffold_R(uni_tar$oligo_seq)
uni_tar$duplex_energy = RNAduplex_R(uni_tar$oligo_seq)
```

4. The addition of the CG-count and the duplex- and self-folding energies to the `uni_tar` table is done by executing the code above and the resulting table is shown in Fig. 8.

3.8 Selecting Nucleobase Sequences for Gapmer Design

In the R-environment there are now two data frames: `target_annotation` (*see* Fig. 6) and `uni_tar` (*see* Fig. 8). The first contains columns with positional information for the target regions, that is, relative start and stop positions on the RNA target and chromosomal positional information. It also contains information on high frequency polymorphisms, number of occurrences of a target region in the RNA target and pair probabilities for the accessibility of target regions. The latter contains columns with target region specificity, that is, the number of human pre-mRNAs with a perfect match or a single mismatch to the target region. It also contains information on the gapmer nucleobase sequence properties, that is, energies for duplex formation, self-folding, and the number of occurrences of CGs.

1. Merge the two data frames `target_annotation` and `uni_tar` based on the column with target region sequences and length:

```
target_regions = left_join(
  target_annotation,
  uni_tar,
  by=c('name','length'))
```

2. Select sequences according to the following criteria (*see* **Note 9**).
   - Select sequences that match perfectly only to the intended RNA target. Do not allow target regions with a single mismatch in more than 50 transcripts.
   - For pharmacodynamic evaluation of target engagement in mouse, select sequences with perfect matches in the mouse ortholog of the RNA target.
   - Discard target regions containing sites of known polymorphisms with minor allele frequencies >5%.
   - Remove highly inaccessible regions by only allowing regions with predicted accessibility $>10^{-6}$.

   Filter target regions using these criteria as follows:

```
target_region_select = filter(
  target_regions,
  gene_hits_pm ==1,
  gene_hits_1mm <= 50,
  accessibility > 1E-6,
  PM_freq < 0.05 | is.na(PM_freq),
  conserved_in_mmusculus )
```

3. Select regions across the RNA target by dividing the start positions of the identified target regions into *K* clusters using a *K*-medoids distance-based clustering algorithm, and select one target region from each cluster as follows (*see* **Note 10**):

```
library(cluster)
K = 10
start_pos = sort(unique(target_region_select$start))

cluster_tab = tibble(
  start = start_pos,
  cluster = clara(x = start_pos, k = K,
                  metric = 'euclidean',
                 pamLike = T, samples=100)$clustering)

nucleobase_select = left_join(target_region_select,
                              cluster_tab, by='start') %>
%
  group_by(cluster) %>%
  sample_n(1) %>%
  ungroup()
```

Table 1 shows $K = 10$ target regions selected for *TOM1* in the manner described above (*see* **Note 11**).

This concludes the workflow for identifying target regions suitable for gapmers.

Table 1
Target regions selected for TOM1

Nucleobase sequence	Start position (nt)	Length (nt)	Single mismatch count	log10 accessibility	Polymorphism frequency	Duplex formation (kcal/mol)	Self-folding (kcal/mol)
GAAGTATTTCTTGCCCAAG	2809	19	1	−5.04	NA	−6.3	0.0
GATGTAACTAACTATA	9533	16	24	−2.18	NA	−1.4	0.0
GAGGGCCCAGTCCTCG	18631	16	13	−3.87	NA	−11.9	−8.1
ACAGCATGTCCAGGTCAG	24316	18	5	−2.57	NA	−12.2	0.0
CTCACTGCGCAGCTTC	28002	16	27	−4.28	NA	−1.2	0.0
CTACCGTTCATGGCGCAG	31193	18	0	−3.86	NA	−8.9	−0.5
AAACCTACAAGACAGAAAA	33692	19	9	−1.62	NA	−10.0	0.0
CGTTGGTCAGCCAGTGAGC	35150	19	0	−4.88	NA	−8.9	−2.7
AGGCAAACAGCATGTC	47915	16	40	−1.90	NA	−15.8	−0.6
GATACAAAAGGCACCTCT	48660	18	0	−3.28	NA	−20.5	0.0

4 Notes

1. For reproducibility the versioning of R and the applied R-packages are listed below:
   - R version 3.5.1.
   - BSgenome.Hsapiens.NCBI.GRCh38_1.3.1000.
   - GenomicFeatures_1.32.2.
   - Biostrings_2.48.0.
   - biomaRt_2.36.1.
   - AnnotationDbi_1.42.1.
   - tidyverse_1.2.1.
   - cluster_2.0.7-1.
2. The R-script `biocLite.R` installs core Bioconductor packages. Additional Bioconductor packages can then be installed by use of the function `biocLite()`.
3. Positional information can be extracted from a GRanges object by applying the accessor functions `seqnames()`, `start()`, `end()`, and `strand()` to retrieve information on chromosome, genomic start position, genomic end position and chromosome strand, respectively.
4. The function `useMart()` connects to the selected BioMart database and dataset, here mouse and human gene sequences from Ensembl. By using `getBM()` with the desired filters and values, lists of attributes can be retrieved through this connection. The attributes retrieved here are first the mouse homolog (s) of the RNA target, which are stored in `ortho_ENS`, and then the pre-mRNA sequence(s) of the mouse homolog(s), which are stored in `RNA_target_mouse`.
5. The R-functions defined in this section can be easily modified to call other structure prediction tools as long as they can be run from the terminal.
6. For all R-functions where we call algorithms that are run from the terminal we assume a unix-like environment. Specifically, for the `RNAplfold_R` function the pipe connection opened by the `cat` command is dependent on the operating system.
7. The `RNAdupex_R` and `RNAselffold_R` functions both use the `system` command which is dependent on the operating system. Here we assume a unix-like environment.
8. Note that matching of sequences using the R-function `vwhichPDict()` currently not allows for insertions and deletions (indels) even though there is an input parameter named `with.indels` which can be set to TRUE or FALSE. Future versions of the Biostrings package may address this.

9. We have found the criteria listed to be good starting points for short-listing of preferred target regions. They can of course be adjusted depending on specific project aims and resources available.
10. For target regions that pass the criteria, the final selection of *K* regions can also be done simply at random.
11. For each nucleobase sequence in Table 1, a standard LNA/DNA design could be to modify each flank with three LNAs. However, this is not necessarily the optimal design. Alternatively, the LNA/DNA design pattern that best achieves a certain predetermined binding affinity could be predicted, as described previously [14].

Acknowledgments

We thank Matteo Cassotti, Lukasz Kielpinski, and Sindri Traustason for helpful discussions during preparation of the manuscript.

References

1. Hughes JP, Rees S, Kalindjian SB, Philpott KL (2011) Principles of early drug discovery. Br J Pharmacol 162:1239–1249
2. Muller PY, Milton MN (2012) The determination and interpretation of the therapeutic index in drug development. Nat Rev Drug Discov 11:751–761
3. Huggins DJ, Sherman W, Tidor B (2012) Rational approaches to improving selectivity in drug design. J Med Chem 55:1424–1444
4. Hagedorn PH, Hansen BR, Koch T, Lindow M (2017) Managing the sequence-specificity of antisense oligonucleotides in drug discovery. Nucleic Acids Res 45:2262–2282
5. Hagedorn PH, Pontoppidan M, Bisgaard TS et al (2018) Identifying and avoiding off-target effects of RNase H-dependent antisense oligonucleotides in mice. Nucleic Acids Res 46:5366–5380
6. Bennett CF, Swayze EE (2010) RNA targeting therapeutics: molecular mechanisms of antisense oligonucleotides as a therapeutic platform. Annu Rev Pharmacol Toxicol 50:259–293
7. Wahlestedt C, Salmi P, Good L et al (2000) Potent and nontoxic antisense oligonucleotides containing locked nucleic acids. PNAS 97:5633–5638
8. Lützelberger M, Kjems J (2006) Strategies to identify potential therapeutic target sites in RNA. In: RNA towards medicine. Springer, Berlin, Heidelberg, pp 243–259
9. Watson JD, Crick FH (1953) Molecular structure of nucleic acids; a structure for deoxyribose nucleic acid. Nature 171:737–738
10. Hagedorn PH, Persson R, Funder ED et al (2018) Locked nucleic acid: modality, diversity, and drug discovery. Drug Discov Today 23:101–114
11. Freier SM, Watt AT (2007) Basic principles of antisense drug discovery. In: Antisense drug technology principles. Springer, Berlin, Heidelberg, pp 117–141
12. Laxton C, Brady K, Moschos S et al (2011) Selection, optimization, and pharmacokinetic properties of a novel, potent antiviral locked nucleic acid-based antisense oligomer targeting hepatitis C virus internal ribosome entry site. Antimicrob Agents Chemother 55:3105–3114
13. SantaLucia J (1998) A unified view of polymer, dumbbell, and oligonucleotide DNA nearest-neighbor thermodynamics. PNAS 95:1460–1465
14. Pedersen L, Hagedorn PH, Lindholm MW, Lindow M (2014) A kinetic model explains why shorter and less affine enzyme-recruiting oligonucleotides can be more potent. Mol Ther Nucleic Acids 3:e149
15. Tafer H, Ameres SL, Obernosterer G et al (2008) The impact of target site accessibility

on the design of effective siRNAs. Nat Biotechnol 26:578–583

16. Matveeva OV, Mathews DH, Tsodikov AD et al (2003) Thermodynamic criteria for high hit rate antisense oligonucleotide design. Nucleic Acids Res 31:4989–4994
17. Lorenz R, Bernhart SH, Höner Zu Siederdissen C et al (2011) ViennaRNA Package 2.0. Algorithms Mol Biol 6:26
18. Kielpinski LJ, Hagedorn PH, Lindow M, Vinther J (2017) RNase H sequence preferences influence antisense oligonucleotide efficiency. Nucleic Acids Res 45:12932–12944
19. Watanabe DTA, Geary RS, Levin AA (2006) Plasma protein binding of an antisense oligonucleotide targeting human ICAM-1 (ISIS 2302). Oligonucleotides 16:169–180
20. Crooke ST, Wang S, Vickers TA et al (2017) Cellular uptake and trafficking of antisense oligonucleotides. Nat Biotechnol 35:230–237
21. Hung G, Xiao X, Peralta R et al (2013) Characterization of target mRNA reduction through in situ RNA hybridization in multiple organ systems following systemic antisense treatment in animals. Nucleic Acid Ther 23:369–378
22. Liang X-H, Sun H, Shen W, Crooke ST (2015) Identification and characterization of intracellular proteins that bind oligonucleotides with phosphorothioate linkages. Nucleic Acids Res 43:2927–2945
23. Denayer T, Stöhr T, Van Roy M (2014) Animal models in translational medicine: validation and prediction. Eur J Mol Clin Med 2:5
24. Vickers TA, Freier SM, Bui H-H et al (2014) Targeting of repeated sequences unique to a gene results in significant increases in antisense oligonucleotide potency. PLoS One 9: e110615–e110612
25. Zerbino DR, Achuthan P, Akanni W et al (2018) Ensembl 2018. Nucleic Acids Res 46: D754–D761
26. Krieg AM (2006) Therapeutic potential of toll-like receptor 9 activation. Nat Rev Drug Discov 5:471–484
27. Burdick AD, Sciabola S, Mantena SR et al (2014) Sequence motifs associated with hepatotoxicity of locked nucleic acid--modified antisense oligonucleotides. Nucleic Acids Res 42:4882–4891
28. Hagedorn PH, Yakimov V, Ottosen S et al (2013) Hepatotoxic potential of therapeutic oligonucleotides can be predicted from their sequence and modification pattern. Nucleic Acid Ther 23:302–310
29. Mitsuhashi M (1997) Strategy for designing specific antisense oligonucleotide sequences. J Gastroenterol 32:282–287
30. Schiavone N, Donnini M, Nicolin A, Capaccioli S (2004) Antisense oligonucleotide drug design. Curr Pharm Des 10:769–784
31. Chan JHP, Lim S, Wong WSF (2006) Antisense oligonucleotides: from design to therapeutic application. Clin Exp Pharmacol Physiol 33:533–540
32. Chalk AM, Sonnhammer ELL (2002) Computational antisense oligo prediction with a neural network model. Bioinformatics 18:1567–1575
33. Camps-Valls G, Chalk AM, Serrano-López AJ et al (2004) Profiled support vector machines for antisense oligonucleotide efficacy prediction. BMC Bioinformatics 5:135
34. Fawcett T (2006) An introduction to ROC analysis. Pattern Recogn Lett 27:861–874
35. Stanton R, Sciabola S, Salatto C et al (2012) Chemical modification study of antisense gapmers. Nucleic Acid Ther 22:344–359
36. R Core Team (2017) R: a language and environment for statistical computing, Vienna
37. Wickham H (2017) Tidyverse: easily install and load the "Tidyverse." R package
38. Maechler M, Rousseeuw P, Struyf A, et al (2017) Cluster: cluster analysis basics and extensions. R package
39. Lawrence M, Huber W, Pagès H et al (2013) Software for computing and annotating genomic ranges. PLoS Comput Biol 9:e1003118
40. Durinck S, Spellman PT, Birney E, Huber W (2009) Mapping identifiers for the integration of genomic datasets with the R/bioconductor package biomaRt. Nat Protoc 4:1184–1191
41. Pagès H, Carlson M, Falcon S, Li N (2017) AnnotationDbi: annotation database interface. R package

Chapter 17

RACE-SEQ and Population-Wide Polymorphism Susceptibility Testing for Endonucleolytically Active, RNA-Targeting Therapeutics

Louise Usher, Pantazis I. Theotokis, and Sterghios A. Moschos

Abstract

High-throughput sequencing of the products of 5′ RNA ligase-mediated rapid amplification of cDNA ends (5′ RLM-RACE) reactions (RACE-SEQ) enables the mapping and digital enumeration of expected and novel 5′ ends in RNA molecules. The resulting data are essential in documenting the mechanism of action and precision of endonucleolytically active, RNA-targeting drugs such as RNase H-active antisense or small interfering RNA. When applied to error-prone replication systems such as RNA viruses or in vitro RNA replicon systems, the method can additionally report the relative susceptibility of known and unknown polymorphisms to a prospective sequence-specific drug, making it a powerful tool in patient selection and stratification as well as resistance prediction.

We describe the preparation of sequencing libraries for ultra-high depth 5′ RLM-RACE analysis on two popular second-generation high-throughput sequencing platforms (Illumina, Ion Torrent) and supply a detailed bioinformatics analysis pipeline for target site activity definition and enumeration. We further illustrate how the pipeline can be simply modified to generate polymorphism-specific drug susceptibility data from in vitro replicon experiments (RACE-SEQ-MM), in a patient-free manner, to cover both known and unknown target site variants in the population.

Key words RACE, 5′ RLM-RACE, RACE-SEQ, RACE-SEQ-MM, RNAi, siRNA, Antisense, Mechanism of action, Pipeline

1 Introduction

It is now well accepted that one of the critical requirements for realizing the translational potential of molecular therapeutics is the availability of conclusive evidence of an on-target mechanism of action [1]. Experimental data must therefore evidence effective target engagement and, where an enzymatic function is involved, the appropriate reaction products [2]. For sequence-specific, endonucleolytically active, RNA-targeting molecular therapeutics such as RNase H-active antisense and small interfering RNA (siRNA) mediators of RNA interference (RNAi), these reaction products are

Olof Gissberg et al. (eds.), *Oligonucleotide-Based Therapies: Methods and Protocols*, Methods in Molecular Biology, vol. 2036, https://doi.org/10.1007/978-1-4939-9670-4_17,

the novel 5′ ends in the targeted RNA, at the anticipated site of action [3].

Traditionally, 5′ RNA ligase-mediated rapid amplification of cDNA ends (5′ RLM-RACE) reactions were used to document such novel 5′ ends. Briefly, this involved the ligation of a known, synthetic RNA adapter to free 5′ RNA ends, production of cDNA using gene-specific reverse transcription primers (GSP), and the generation of PCR/nested PCR amplicons using primers specific to the ligated RNA adapter (upstream) and the gene specific primer (downstream) surrounding the drug active site. The resulting amplicon would then be sized by gel electrophoresis, excised, purified, and Sanger-sequenced to determine the drug site of action as the point at which the known RNA adapter sequence would stop and the targeted RNA sequence would start (Fig. 1). However, this qualitative method routinely generated unexpected electrophoresis gel bands, and/or minor Sanger sequencing traces; these were typically overlooked as non-specific amplification artifacts or contaminants, respectively. Using high throughput, second generation sequencing on such 5′ RLM-RACE products (RACE-SEQ) revealed that the minor Sanger sequencing traces were due to the imprecise Slicer activity of siRNA-induced silencing complexes (siRISC) [4]. Furthermore, as additional data emerged on the method from multiple laboratories, it became clear that the extent of information returned from this analytical approach was a

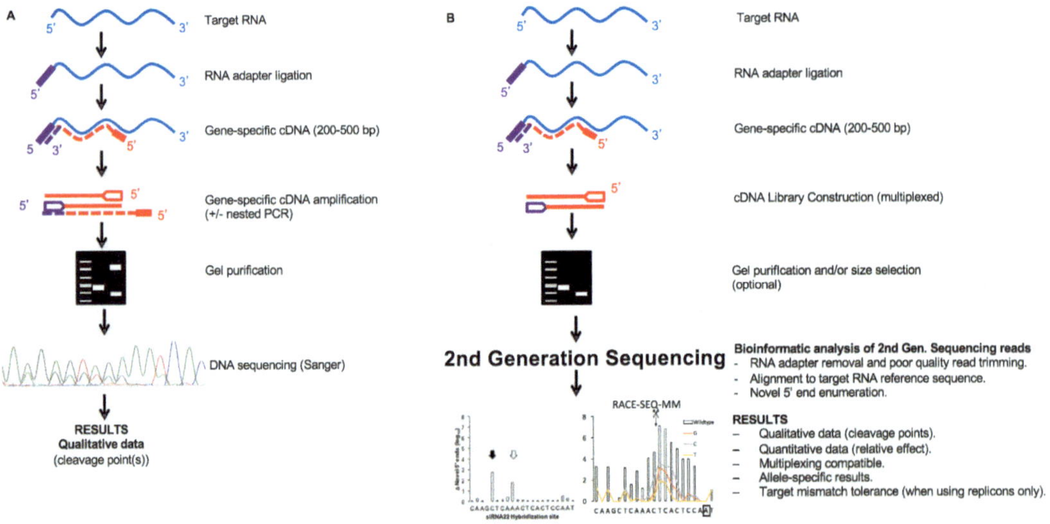

Fig. 1 Comparative features of 5′ RLM-RACE and RACE-SEQ, or RACE-SEQ-MM. The gold-standard method for defining novel 5′ ends in target RNAs is a manual, labor-intensive, qualitative approach that can deal with single samples at a time, returning sometimes inconclusive data (**a**) such as mixed Sanger traces. RACE-SEQ on the other hand (**b**) can be optimized to parallel process multiple samples generating a wealth of quantitative and qualitative data through a series of bioinformatic processing steps, including the anticipated impact of unknown target polymorphisms on drug efficacy (RACE-SEQ-MM)

function of the biology of the experimental setup, and the data analysis pipeline implemented. Thus, parameters such as the mutation rate of the RNA target (tissue RNA [5–7], endogenous targets in cell culture [8], viral RNA or replicon RNA in cell culture [4, 9, 10]) and depth of sequencing and breadth of sequencing [4] orchestrate the observed outcomes, including predictive pharmacogenomic assessment of drug efficacy against targets mismatched to the drug (RACE-SEQ-MM [9]).

The RACE-SEQ method has been applied on the Illumina and Ion Torrent platforms, two of the most popular second generation sequencing systems available to, or accessible by most laboratories. Despite their radically different chemistries and physics, RACE-SEQ workflows on both platforms can be summarized into three steps: 5′ RLM RACE-based sequencing library preparation, sequencing, and data analysis. In this chapter we focus on the library preparation (RNA adapter ligation, reverse transcription, sequencing amplicon generation) and data interpretation aspects, and highlight opportunities to reduce process complexity and cost where possible. For example, the following protocol covers RACE-SEQ or RACE-SEQ-MM library preparation without sample multiplexing, or sequencing adapter-tagging at the PCR/nested PCR step, approaches that can reduce the number of handling steps. Likewise, the data analysis components indicate how datasets can be processed either for cleavage point characterization (RACE-SEQ) or polymorphism tolerance testing (RACE-SEQ-MM).

2 Materials

Standard good laboratory practice procedures for RNA work apply throughout these methods, that is, RNA quality between $OD_{260/280}$ 1.8–2.1 or Agilent Bioanalyzer RNA integrity number (RIN) >6.0, use of certified RNase-free barrier tips and plastic ware (including during sequencing library preparation steps), use of precision (electronic by preference) pipettors, pretreatment of any in-house containers with 0.1% v/v diethylpyrocarbonate (DEPC), and workspace/glove treatment with RNase ZAP™ or equivalent.

2.1 Preparation of 5′ RLM RACE-Based Sequencing Amplicons

A wide variety of 5′ RLM RACE kits are available from a number of commercial reagent suppliers, including Merck (previously known as Sigma-Aldrich), Thermo Fisher Scientific (Life Technologies, Invitrogen), and Clontech, among others. The kits may cover all steps up to and including library purification allowing them to be ready for (Sanger) sequencing. The reader is invited to use any of these (RACE-SEQ was independently developed by two separate groups using the Invitrogen GeneRacer kit [4, 5]) provided attention is paid to key parameters as detailed in the steps below.

Alternatively, the required kit components such as RNA adapter oligonucleotides, primers, enzymes, buffers, and purification components can be sourced independently (e.g., Integrated DNA Technologies, Eurogentec, Guangzhou Ribobio Company, and New England Biolabs) for a fraction of the cost.

2.1.1 RNA Adapter Ligation

1. Total RNA in excess of 0.4 μg from a biological experiment (in a maximum volume of 12.5 μl for a 20 μl adapter ligation reaction).
2. Nuclease-free water (*see* **Note 1**).
3. 5′ RACE RNA adapter: 0.1 mM 5′ RACE RNA adapter *without* a 5′ phosphate (we routinely use for experiments in *Homo sapiens* 5′-GGA CAC UGA CAU GGA CUG AAG GAG UAG AAA-3′), desalted purity level, in nuclease-free water (*see* **Notes 2–7**). Store in aliquots at −80 °C.
4. T4 RNA ligase I, 10,000 units/ml (*see* **Note 8**).
5. 10× T4 RNA ligase I buffer: 500 mM Tris–HCl, 100 mM $MgCl_2$, 100 mM dithiothreitol, pH 7.5 at 25 °C.
6. RNase Inhibitor: 40,000 units/ml murine RNase Inhibitor (New England Biolabs). Store at −20 °C.
7. GlycoBlue: 15 mg/ml GlycoBlue coprecipitant, RNase and DNase free, (ThermoFisher Scientific, Loughborough, UK).
8. 10 mM adenosine 5′ triphosphate (ATP).
9. Phenol–chloroform: 5/1 ratio (v/v) Phenol, chloroform (molecular biology grade).
10. Absolute ethanol (EtOH) (molecular biology grade).
11. 70% v/v EtOH: v/v molecular biology grade EtOH in nuclease-free water.
12. 3 M Sodium acetate, pH 5.2 at 25 °C.
13. Nuclease-free PCR microcentrifuge tubes (typically 0.2 ml).
14. Nuclease-free 1.5 ml microcentrifuge tubes.
15. Thermal cycler.
16. Wet ice.
17. Dry ice (or accessible −80 °C freezer shelf).
18. Refrigerated microtube centrifuge.

2.1.2 Reverse Transcription

1. Gene-specific primer (GSP): Primer for reverse transcription, designed to anneal downstream from the anticipated drug cleavage point on the target RNA, stored at 0.1 mM stock concentration in nuclease-free water, at −20 °C (*see* **Notes 9–15**).
2. Moloney murine leukemia virus reverse transcriptase (Mo-MuLV RT): 200,000 units/ml (New England Biolabs).

3. 10× RT reaction buffer (New England Biolabs; *see* **Note 16**).
4. RNase Inhibitor: 40,000 units/ml murine RNase Inhibitor.
5. dNTP mix: 10 mM each of adenosine triphosphate, cytosine triphosphate, guanosine triphosphate, and thymidine triphosphate.
6. Nuclease-free PCR microcentrifuge tubes.
7. Nuclease-free water.
8. Thermal cycler.
9. Wet ice.

2.1.3 Sequencing Amplicon Generation, Size Selection, and Purification

PCR amplification offers several opportunities to streamline library preparation ahead of second generation sequencing. The approach to be taken may be influenced by the choice of sequencing platform, RACE-SEQ application, and/or sequencing kit selection (*see* **Notes 17–21**). The reader may also prefer to outsource second generation sequencing; performing library preparation and validation in house can substantially reduce outsourced sequencing costs.

1. GeneRacer Forward: A forward PCR primer corresponding to the 5′ RNA adapter, such as 5′-GGA CAC TGA CAT GGA CTG AAG GAG TA-3′, stored at 0.1 mM stock concentration in Tris-EDTA or nuclease-free water (*see* **Note 22**).
2. The GSP used during reverse transcription (*see* Subheading 2.1.2, **item 1**), or a nested GSP primer (*see* **Note 23**).
3. Q5 Hot Start High Fidelity 2× Master Mix (New England Biolabs; *see* **Note 24**).
4. AxyPrep beads: AxyPrep Mag Paramagnetic PCR reaction cleanup beads (Appleton Woods Ltd., Birmingham, UK).
5. AMPure XP beads: Agencourt AMPure XP beads. (Beckman Coulter, High Wycombe, UK; *see* **Note 25**.)
6. Neodymium magnet.
7. Column-based nucleic acid gel extraction kit (e.g., New England Biolabs Monarch DNA Gel Extraction Kit).
8. Nuclease-free PCR microcentrifuge tubes (0.2 ml).
9. Nuclease-free 1.5 ml microcentrifuge tubes.
10. Nuclease-free water.
11. 70% ethanol (molecular biology grade) in nuclease-free water.
12. Agarose, low melting point.
13. Gel electrophoresis equipment.
14. 100 bp DNA ladder.
15. DNA loading dye: 6× Orange DNA loading Dye.
16. DNA staining dye (e.g., ThermoFisher SYBR Safe).

17. 1× Tris–borate–EDTA (TBE) buffer: 89 mM Tris–borate, 2 mM EDTA, pH 8.3 at 25 °C.
18. Tris-EDTA (TE) buffer: 10 mM Tris–HCl pH 8.0 at 25 °C, 0.1 mM EDTA.
19. Thermal cycler.
20. Isopropanol.
21. UV transilluminator compatible with gel band excision.
22. Sterile scalpel.
23. Wet ice.
24. High sensitivity spectrophotometric nucleic acid quantification system (ThermoFisher NanoDrop or QuBit).

2.2 Bioinformatics

You will need to use a Linux operating system for the RACE-SEQ-lite script to run the necessary command line packages. If you are using a Bio-Linux distribution (Bio-Linux 8), then you will have most of the packages preinstalled system-wide (*see* **Note 26**).

2.2.1 Software Packages

1. To trim the RACE adapter, the default package is Cutadapt (≥v. 1.2).
2. For the alignment of the reads to the reference sequence you will need Bowtie (v. 1.0.0) for reads generated with Illumina sequencers (NextSeq, MiSeq, NovaSeq, HiSeq, etc.; *see* **Note 27**).
3. A reference sequence of your target transcript in fasta format (*see* **Note 28**).
4. You will need the Samtools (≥v. 1.3.1) and Bedtools (≥v. 2.17.0) software packages installed.
5. To run the RACE-SEQ-lite script you will need to have a version of R (≥v. 3.4) installed on your system. All the necessary R packages will get installed and loaded automatically.
6. All command line packages need to be installed system-wide.

3 Methods

3.1 Preparation of 5′ RLM RACE-Based Sequencing Amplicons

3.1.1 RNA Adapter Ligation

1. Working on wet ice, prepare the adapter ligation reaction by adding <12.5 μl of total RNA extract (>0.4 μg; volume can be made up to 12.5 μl with nuclease-free water) to 2 μl of RNA adapter (0.1 mM) in a nuclease-free thermal cycling tube (tube 1; *see* **Note 29**).
2. Heat tube 1 in a thermal cycler to 65 °C for 5 min and immediately transfer the tube 1 to wet ice. Cool on wet ice for 2 min.

3. Working on wet ice, in a separate nuclease free tube (tube 2) prepare the RNA ligase mix, consisting of 2 μl of 10× T4 RNA ligase I buffer, 2 μl of 10 mM ATP, 0.5 μl of RNase Inhibitor, and 1 μl of T4 RNA ligase I (*see* **Note 30**).
4. Pipette mix tube 2 gently, and briefly centrifuge for 10 s at 10,000 × *g* (*see* **Note 31**).
5. Working on wet ice, transfer 5.5 μl of the ligase mix (tube 2) to the annealed RNA (tube 1); discard tube 2.
6. Using a thermal cycler, perform RNA adapter ligation in tube 1 at 37 °C for 1 h, with the heated lid switched off (*see* **Note 32**).
7. Bring the RNA adapter ligation reaction volume in tube 1 up to 0.1 ml using nuclease-free water.
8. Add 0.1 ml phenol-chloroform to the RNA adapter ligation reaction (tube 1).
9. Vortex the mix at full speed for 30 s.
10. Centrifuge at 12,000 × *g* for 5 min at room temperature.
11. *Carefully* remove tube 1 from microcentrifuge *without* disturbing the oil-water interphase (*see* **Note 33**).
12. *Carefully* transfer the upper aqueous phase (~0.1 ml) into a new 1.5 ml nuclease-free microcentrifuge tube (tube 3) using nuclease-free barrier tips. Record the volume transferred.
13. Add to tube 3 the following materials in the specified order: 1.5 μl GlycoBlue, 10 μl of 3 M sodium acetate, and 2× volumes absolute EtOH relative to the amount transferred in **step 12** (*see* **Note 34**).
14. Vortex tube 3 for 30 s.
15. To precipitate the RNA, incubate tube 3 on dry ice for 30 min (*see* **Note 35**).
16. Centrifuge tube 3 at 16,000 × *g* for 20 min at 4 °C.
17. *Carefully* remove tube 3 from the centrifuge, and aspire the supernatant without disturbing the pellet: discard the supernatant.
18. Wash the pellet by adding 0.5 ml of 70% v/v EtOH to tube 3. Mix by inversion ×3.
19. Vortex tube 3 for 10 s.
20. Centrifuge tube 3 at 16,000 × *g* for 2 min at 4 °C and remove the supernatant as per **step 17**.
21. Centrifuge tube 3 for a further 10 s to collect and remove residual supernatant EtOH as per **step 17**.
22. Air dry pellets for up to 5 min.

23. Resuspend the adapter-ligated RNA pellet in 11–20 μl of RNase-free water and mix well by pipetting.
24. Keep on wet ice or store at −20 °C (up to 2 weeks) or −80 °C (long term).

3.1.2 Reverse Transcription

1. Transfer 11 μl of adapter ligated RNA produced in the previous section into a nuclease-free PCR microcentrifuge tube (tube 4; *see* **Note 36**).
2. To the 11 μl of adapter ligated RNA (tube 4), add 1 μl of GSP diluted to a 1 μM working concentration using nuclease-free water, and 1 μl of dNTPs (10 mM each; *see* **Note 37**).
3. Transfer tube 4 onto a thermal cycler and heat for 5 min at 65 °C to remove secondary RNA structure. Immediately transfer tube 4 onto wet ice for 2 min.
4. In a separate nuclease-free tube (tube 5), create a reverse transcription master mix consisting of 2 μl 10× Mo-MuLV RT reaction buffer, 0.2 μl RNase Inhibitor, 1 μl of Mo-MuLV RT enzyme, and 5.8 μl of nuclease-free water (9 μl final volume; *see* **Note 38**).
5. Transfer the 9 μl contents of the reverse transcription master mix (tube 5) to the adapter-ligated RNA (tube 4) to give a total volume of 20 μl and keep it on wet ice; discard tube 5.
6. Transfer reverse transcription mix (tube 4) onto a thermal cycler and perform reverse transcription at 55 °C for 30 min followed by enzyme inactivation at 70 °C for 15 min.
7. Store resulting cDNA at −20 °C (2 weeks), −80 °C (indefinitely), or proceed to sequencing amplicon generation.

3.1.3 Sequencing Amplicon Generation, Size Selection, and Purification

1. Create a PCR reaction in a nuclease-free PCR microcentrifuge tube (tube 6) consisting of the following materials: For a 40 μl reaction, add 20 μl Q5 Hot Start High-fidelity 2× Master Mix, 2 μl of 10 μM GeneRacerF1 primer, 2 μl of 10 μM GSP, 4 μl of cDNA template from tube 4 (cDNA volume should be up to 10% v/v of the PCR reaction volume) and 12 μl of nuclease-free water (*see* **Note 39**).
2. Transfer the PCR mix (tube 6) onto a thermal cycler and perform PCR as follows: 98 °C for 30 s; 35 amplification cycles (95 °C for 15 s, 60 °C for 10 s, and 72 °C for 15 s), 72 °C for 2 min, and 4 °C hold (*see* **Notes 40** and **41**).
3. Prepare a 2% w/v low melting point agarose gel in TBE buffer and supplement with appropriate DNA staining dye (e.g., 2 μl of SYBR Safe per 50 ml of gel; *see* **Notes 42** and **43**).
4. Use an agarose gel well comb appropriate for your number of samples and gel size, and allow gel to set fully.

5. Dilute 5–20 μl of PCR product 1:6 with 6× Orange loading Dye.
6. Load the dye-diluted PCR product onto the agarose gel alongside an appropriate DNA ladder.
7. Run at 100 V for 40–60 min or until the dye front reaches the edge of the gel (*see* **Note 44**).
8. Visualize bands under a blue light transilluminator, and excise target bands using a sterile scalpel into nuclease-free 1.5 ml microcentrifuge tubes; do not use UV transilluminators if the excised DNA band is to be extracted and used for sequencing.
9. Purify the DNA from the agarose using a gel extraction kit; **steps 9–13** describe the steps relevant to the New England Biolabs Monarch DNA Gel Extraction kit. Place gel in 4× volumes of gel dissolving buffer and incubate at 50 °C for 5–10 min.
10. Transfer entire volume onto the Monarch DNA cleanup column in batches of 0.8 ml.
11. Centrifuge column at 13,000 × *g* for 1 min and discard flow through (repeat **steps 10** and **11** to process entire volume).
12. Wash column 2× with 0.2 ml DNA wash buffer by centrifuging at 13,000 × *g* for 1 min, discarding the flow through.
13. Elute in 20 μl NEB elution buffer, TE buffer, or nuclease free water.
14. To further purify and concentrate DNA if necessary, for example, for the removal of primer dimers, for >100 bp amplicons continue at **step 15**, for <100 bp amplicons go to **step 28**, or proceed directly to **step 38**.
15. Add 1.6× volumes (32 μl) of room temperature AMPure XP beads.
16. Mix by pipetting at least 5×.
17. Incubate on bench for 8 min.
18. Place on neodymium magnet (or rack) for 3 min. The AMPure XP beads should form a visible pellet collect close to the magnet.
19. Remove supernatant by pipetting, taking care not to disturb the pellet.
20. Wash the AMPure XP beads 2× with 0.3 ml of 70% v/v EtOH without disturbing the pellet.
21. Remove residual ethanol by pipetting.
22. Air-dry for 3–5 min.
23. Resuspend in 25 μl of TE by pipetting.
24. Vortex at full speed for 10 s.

25. Centrifuge at 300 × *g* for 5 s.
26. Place on neodymium magnet for 2 min.
27. Collect cleaned PCR product (~23 μl) into a new nuclease-free tube and proceed to **step 38**.
28. Prepare a mix of 0.07 ml isopropanol and 0.18 ml AxyPrep beads.
29. Transfer 25 μl of the AxyPrep bead-isopropanol beads to 10 μl of PCR product.
30. Mix by pipetting 5×.
31. Incubate at room temperature for 5 min.
32. Transfer tubes to neodymium magnet (or rack) for 3 min.
33. Remove supernatant by pipetting without disturbing the AxyPrep bead pellet proximal to the magnet.
34. Wash 2× with 0.2 ml 70% EtOH without disturbing the pellet.
35. Remove residual EtOH by 300 × *g* 5 s centrifugation and pipetting.
36. Air dry the pellet for <5 min.
37. Resuspend the pellet in 40 μl of TE buffer, place on the magnet for 2 min and collect the cleaned PCR product.
38. Quantify using high sensitivity spectrophotometric approach.
39. Proceed to library preparation in accordance to the sequencing library kit protocol suited to amplicon size and sequencing platform of choice.
40. Retrieve FASTQ data at sequencing run end for bioinformatic analysis.

3.2 Bioinformatic Software Installation

1. Launch your Linux-based bioinformatics environment (*see* **Note 26**).
2. Check if you have python installed by typing.

```
python --version OR
python3 --version
```

3. Once you know you have either python or python3 working, download and install python-pip from the command line using apt-get.

```
sudo apt-get install python-pip
```

4. Once you have python-pip installed, download and install the latest Cutadapt version using the pip trusted repository.

```
sudo pip install cutadapt
```

For more information and troubleshooting please read the Cutadapt documentation (*see* **Note 45**).

5. Install Bowtie, Samtools and Bedtools from the command line using apt-get. If you are working on a Bio-Linux machine you have Bowtie, Samtools and Bedtools already preinstalled. Otherwise use the following command to download the latest versions.

```
sudo apt-get install bowtie samtools bedtools
```

6. Download and install the latest version of the R environment system-wide using the command.

```
sudo apt-get install r-base
```

7. For Ion Torrent-generated data, use the Tmap aligner for optimal alignment results (*see* **Note 46**).

3.3 Data Preprocessing

Depending on the sequencing platform (e.g., Illumina, IonTorrent) and whether it has been carried out in-house or externally you will need to follow a slightly different data preprocess step.

1. Concatenate the files. If you are using IonTorrent you will have a fastq file for every sample with single-end reads. If you are using an Illumina sequencer you will have paired end reads in two different files. For pair end reads concatenate the files using the cat command to perform a duplex-like sequencing dataset.

```
cat your_reads1.fastq your_reads2.fastq > your_-
reads.fastq
```

2. Trim the adaptor sequence. During the initial adapter trimming stage, cutadapt filters for the reads that contain the exact adapter sequence on the 5-prime end of the reads. It then trims the RACE adapter sequence from these reads and outputs only the processed sequence. Any reads that do not contain the exact adapter sequence on their 5-prime end will be discarded (*see* **Notes 47–52**).

3. Check if your reference file has only one header using the following command, which should return "1" if true (*see* **Note 28**).

```
grep '^>' your_reference.fasta | wc -l
```

4. Download the RACE-SEQ-lite script from the GitHub repository (*see* **Note 53**) and place it in your working directory along with your reference fasta file and only one sample fastq file that you want to process.

3.4 Run the RACE-SEQ Pipeline

1. Run the RACEseqMM.r script using the Rscript command and the *--help* option to bring up a short description and the help page (Table 1).

```
Rscript RACE-SEQ.r -h
```

2. While you run the script, it automatically identifies and imports the reference file in fasta format and the reads file in fastq format as standard inputs. If there is more than one fasta or fastq file in your working directory the script will exit with an error.

Table 1
Command line options for the RACE-SEQ R script

Options	Description
-s, --start	Input the first nucleotide genomic location
-e, --end	Input the last nucleotide genomic location
-a, --adapter	Input the RACE adapter sequence [default: NO]
-m, --mismatch	Input number of mismatches during alignment [default: 0]
-p, --plot	Print output graph [default: NO]
-t, --tmap	Use the tmap aligner instead of bowtie [default: NO]
--notsv	Do not print output TSV file [default: YES]
-i, --iterate	Create the alternative references to cover all the possible SNPs of the reference between the genomics locations specified by *-s* and *-e* and then perform global alignment and generate graph [default: YES]
-h, --help	Print this help page

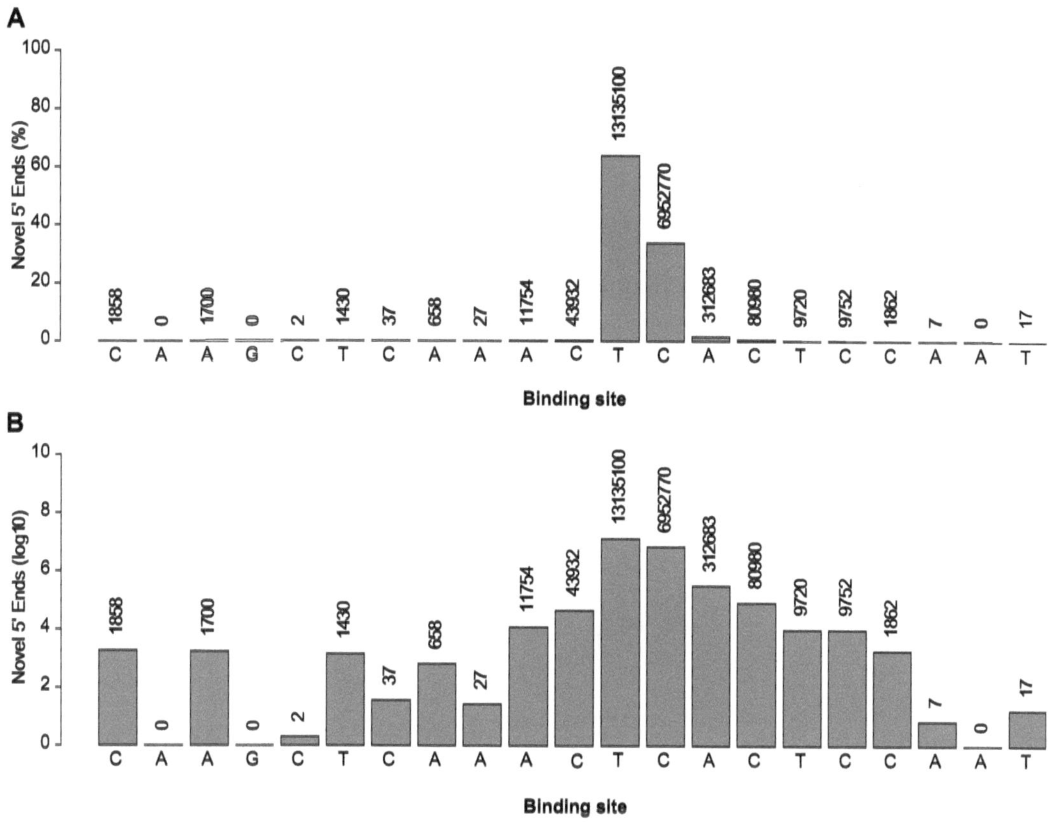

Fig. 2 An example of the graph generated using the -p option while running RACE-SEQ. The two graphs representing the novel 5′ cleavage incidents recorded on the same dataset between the specified genomic locations, in a linear (**a**) and a logarithmic (**b**) scale. Absolute counts of novel 5′ ends at each position are also returned above each bar. The logarithmic scale unveils important details about the cleavage products that otherwise would have been overlooked due to the huge number of reads generated during RACE-SEQ. Users are strongly advised to favor logarithmic data representation in line with data normal distribution principles.

3. The minimum parameters you need to set for the script to run are the --*start* and --*end* options, which will set the genomic locations for the default .tsv (tab separated values) output file. The following example command will perform alignment using Bowtie with 0 mismatches and output a .tsv formatted table with the number of the cleavage incidents in the span of the genomic region specified, in a linear scale (%) and in a logarithmic scale (log10; *see* **Note 54**). To generate plots of the enumerated cleavage points in the region of interest, an example of which is shown in Fig. 2, use the --*p* option.

```
Rscript RACEseqMM.r -s 9478 -e 9498
```

4. Using the following command, the script will use the Tmap aligner instead of the default Bowtie with 0 mismatches during alignment. Then it will output a graph of the region of interest but no table with values, on account of the *--notsv* switch.

```
Rscript RACEseqMM.r -s 9478 -e 9498 -t -p --notsv
```

5. The following example command will perform the RACE adapter trimming on the 5′ end of the reads using the specific nucleotide sequence provided with 0 mismatches in the trimming process. Then it will perform alignment with the reference sequence using the default Bowtie aligner and allow for 2 mismatches during alignment. Then it will output a graph plotted between the specified genomic locations but not a .tsv table (*see* **Notes 51**, **52**, and **55**).

```
Rscript RACEseqMM.r -s 9478 -e 9498 -a GGACACTGACATG-
GACTGAAGGAGTAGAAA -m 2 - p --notsv
```

4 Notes

1. Either manufactured in-house using >18 MOhm water treated with 0.1% diethylpyrocarbonate (DEPC) overnight and autoclaved to degrade DEPC or commercially procured.
2. The RACE-SEQ method was originally developed using the Life Technologies Generacer 5′ RLM-RACE Kit, which was designed to analyze full-length coding RNAs with intact 5′ caps. Thus, in the first step of 5′ RLM RACE, a phosphatase is used to remove 5′ phosphates from mRNA fragments (such as those generated by endonucleotically active antisense and Slicer-active RNAi drugs) and non-mRNA transcripts. In the second step, a pyrophosphatase is used to remove 5′ caps from full-length, capped mRNAs, leaving them as the only RNA species in a sample with a 5′ phosphate group. The third step involves the ligation of a synthetic RNA adapter of known sequence to these free 5′ phosphorylated ends using an RNA ligase. In RACE-SEQ the molecular species of interest are truncated RNAs, making the phosphatase step redundant, as a minimum. The redundancy of the pyrophosphatase step is a function of experimental design (e.g., drug cleavage site distance from the canonical 5′ end of the target, presence of 5′ cap structure(s), and need for relative quantification of intact/cleaved species).

3. Kit-derived or custom RNA adapters must be confirmed to be absent from the host genome by BLASTn before use to avoid spurious amplicon artifacts.
4. RNA adapter length can be adjusted at either the 5′ or 3′ end to conform with amplicon size needs. For example, the RNA adapter described herein is a shortened version of the RNA Adapter originally described in the Invitrogen GeneRacer kit: 5′-CGA CUG GAG CAC GAG GAC ACU GAC AUG GAC UGA AGG AGU AGA AA-3′.
5. Review the RNA ligase documentation for any specific enzymatic preferences regarding end nucleotide composition on any custom RNA adapters.
6. When purchasing custom synthesized RNA adapters, ensure that these are not 5′ phosphorylated so that adapter concatamerization is avoided during the RNA adapter ligation step.
7. Custom-manufactured RNA adapters supplied at standard desalted purity (lowest manufacturing cost) are adequate for 5′ RLM-RACE.
8. In our experience, and knowledge from other fields of NGS such as metagenomics, the enzymes used, from RNA extraction onto NGS library preparation may contribute contaminating reads to sequencing data. This happens largely because nucleic acids in the enzyme production systems are carried over into the final enzyme formulations used in RNA sample processing and NGS library preparation. A biological control sample consisting of cells/tissue not subjected to endonucleolytic drug activity is strongly advised to ascertain background levels of sequence contamination in addition to aligner-based data curation. Equally, it is strongly advised to maintain enzyme supplier and batch/lot consistency within experiments to minimize data variability between samples.
9. Guidance for the identification of GSP binding sites is available in the manuals of 5′ RLM RACE kits from ThermoFisher, Clontech, Roche, and Merck. In our experience, use of standard nearest neighbor-based primer design software such as PrimerQuest, Primer 3, and VisualOMP are fit for purpose with additional attention placed on primer length (22–28 nt), relatively high GC content (50–70%) for high melting temperature-based selectivity, and a maximum of two 3′ terminal guanines or cytosines. Standard PCR primer exclusion criteria such as primer dimer and hairpin formation apply. It is recommended that the GSP melting temperature is similar to the RNA Adapter-specific forward primer.
10. Critical to experimental success is the size of the 5′ RLM RACE sequencing library amplicon to be generated by PCR or nested PCR from the RNA adapter-tagged, GSP reverse-transcribed

cDNA. The amplicon must be compatible with the second generation sequencing platform operating parameters. Both Illumina and Ion Torrent are well suited to small (<400 bp) DNA library sequencing, although practical limitations usually restrict library sizes to <300 bp, which is usually adequate for appropriate GSP binding site identification.

11. Both technologies can perform bidirectional sequence reading which markedly improves the reliability of resulting reads [10, 11], although only Illumina can perform true paired end sequencing on libraries exceeding nominal read length limitations (i.e., >300 bp). This is because of the physical limitations of Ion Torrent sequencing methods (bead-based emulsion extension reactions that do not physically accommodate libraries >400 bp), which do not apply on Illumina.
12. In the unlikely scenario that a suitable GSP site cannot be defined within the typical library size limits of Illumina, paired end read fidelity can be sacrificed to generate longer cDNAs; crucially, this does not impact on read quality over the definition of the novel 5′ ends as these universally fall within the high-quality read length region of the platform. Alternatively, third generation sequencing platforms can be used such as Oxford Nanopore or Pacific Biosciences. However, the end user must note the currently poor accuracy of Oxford Nanopore compared to Illumina and Ion Torrent, and the relatively high cost per base of Pacific Biosciences for a given read depth, which would limit use to restriction site definition but render mismatched target cleavage tolerance (RACE-SEQ-MM) pharmacogenomics unreliable.
13. For A/T rich target sequences, the use of high melting temperature nucleoside modifications such as locked nucleic acid (LNA) can reduce GSP length to <28 nt. When using LNA ensure these are located at the 5′ end of the GSP binding site, with at least one non-LNA spacer nucleotide between modifications.
14. LNA-modified GSPs are not suitable for RACE-SEQ-MM as these will introduce specificity bias toward the "locked" nucleotides in the target sequence queried.
15. Standard desalted primers are adequate for all steps; typically stored at 0.1 mM in TE and diluted to working concentrations in nuclease-free water.
16. Alternatively, the ThermoFisher Scientific Superscript III reverse transcriptase can be used to comparable outcomes; the reaction would need to be supplemented with RNase Inhibitor to a final concentration of 4000 units/ml, and 5 μM final concentration of DTT.

17. The extent of amplicon processing following this step is a function of the sequencing platform and kit to be used; here we provide the minimum necessary processing for maximal usable read return after sequencing.
18. The Ion Torrent PGM and Illumina MiSeq can only analyze 1–2 samples by RACE-SEQ (one million read minimum requirement). Large output sequencers (e.g., Illumina HiSeq, NovaSeq; Ion Torrent Proton) permit sample multiplexing through library barcoding, but only for RACE-SEQ; RACE-SEQ-MM requires 100 million reads as a minimum. Barcoded RACE-SEQ-MM is currently possible only on the Illumina NovaSEQ platform.
19. For downstream second generation sequencing, kits tailored to the Illumina and Ion Torrent platforms can be purchased from the instrument manufacturers or reliable third party suppliers such as New England Biolabs, Roche (KAPA Biosystems), BIOO Scientific, Labgene Scientific S.A., and Bioline. These kits usually come with comprehensive instructions relevant to each platform, and are sold in versions for specific applications such as RNA-SEQ, genomic DNA sequencing, amplicon sequencing etc. The reader is advised to carefully review the sequencing kit protocol and sequencing adapter approach used per platform/kit supplier to select an appropriate solution for their experimental setup.
20. In our experience, standard library kits for sequencing DNA amplicons results in less troubleshooting around library preparation and validation.
21. All platforms have unique chemistry specifications with regards to sequencing adapter ligation to the sequencing library. The user can eliminate the need for such additional ligation steps by 5′ tagging the GSP/RNA Adapter primer, or the nested PCR primers if nested PCR is used, with the relevant sequencing adapter nucleotides (and nucleotide barcodes, when multiplexing). For more information regarding these sequences please consult the user manuals of your sequencing platform. If applying such extensions to your primers it is necessary to reconfirm lack of primer dimers/hairpins for the extended primer sequence, and to evaluate reaction cleanup protocols for nucleic acid size limits based on the new sequencing library length.
22. A nested PCR primer, or shorter PCR primer can also be used; in the case of the 5′ RLM RACE RNA adapter proposed, the nested PCR primer can be 5′-GGA CAC TGA CAT GGA CTG AAG G-3′. When performing RACE-SEQ-MM, data fidelity can be improved by modifying primers according to Kennedy et al. [11] for bidirectional sequencing; this does not apply for

Illumina paired end sequencing, unless the library size is within the read length limits of the platform/sequencing kit used. Comparable fidelity can be achieved through RNA adapter sequence filtering at 100% identity in paired end sequencing.

23. The user may also reduce the need for 5′ RLM RACE amplicon ligation to sequencing adapters and barcodes by 5′ modifying the forward primer or nester PCR primer with sequences appropriate to the sequencing platform to be used.
24. A high-fidelity polymerase is essential for next generation sequencing, and particularly so for RACE-SEQ-MM; it is advised to use best-in-class enzymes in these experiments and regularly review supplier offerings.
25. For efficient size selection of <100 bp amplicons use AxyPrep beads. For >100 bp amplicons use AMPure XP beads.
26. We strongly recommend you opt for a Bio-Linux distribution as a bioinformatics operating system environment for this work, as it will save you a substantial amount of time on installing, setting up and troubleshooting your machine and your environment. If you use another Linux distribution, install the required software packages system-wide; you will need to have administrator privileges on your Linux system. Administrator privileges are necessary if you want to download and install new packages in your system or edit and get access to protected files created by other users. If you are setting up a new workstation with a Linux based operating system involving a virtual operating system hosted within a Windows or MacOS environment, we again strongly recommend that you opt for a Bio-Linux distribution, as the same benefits apply here as well; make sure that data storage is handled in the host operating system to optimize disk drive allocation to the Virtual Machine.
27. Tmap (≥v. 3.4.1) is the preferred aligner for reads generated with an Ion Torrent sequencer (e.g., PGM, PROTON). If the sequencing has been performed using Illumina technology, then the Tmap aligner does not need to be installed as in that case the aligner of preference is Bowtie.
28. Ensure there is only one header written in the fasta file. Edit the fasta file in a text editor to remove unnecessary text and additional headers/sequences if present.
29. The reaction can be scaled down to 10 μl with no impact to data, but do not reduce RNA mass in the reaction. This step is not suited to multiplexing but is suited to parallel sample processing to increase throughput. When performing the reaction on multiple samples in parallel, equilibrate RNA concentration across samples by adjusting RNA sample volume with

nuclease-free water to match the lowest concentration in your sample set.

30. A master mix can be generated to perform multiple sample reactions in parallel, by scaling components appropriately; if doing so, always adjust volumes up by 15% to avoid any liquid loss due to evaporation and use separate tips for each dispensing step.
31. 4 °C centrifugation is not necessary, but preferred.
32. A 4 °C final hold step is useful for maintaining sample integrity.
33. Centrifugation separates aqueous from solvent phase, with the RNA in the aqueous phase. If the interface is disturbed, simply repeat the centrifugation step.
34. That is, if 0.1 ml was transferred at **step 12**, add 0.2 ml of 100% v/v EtOH.
35. If no dry ice is available, place tubes directly onto the shelf of a −80 °C freezer.
36. A brief centrifugation step of tube 3 at 10,000 × *g* for 1 min at 4 °C ahead of the transfer is advised to ensure maximal material collection and transfer.
37. This step is not suited to the preparation and use of master mixes due to the substantial cross-contamination risk: Single pipetting step dispensing and use of fresh tips per dispensation is strongly advised.
38. A master mix can be generated to perform multiple sample reactions in parallel, by scaling components appropriately; if doing so, always adjust volumes up by 15% to avoid any liquid loss due to evaporation, and use separate tips for dispensing. If using ThermoFisher's SuperScript III reverse transcriptase prepare a master mix consisting of 4 μl 5× First strand buffer, 1 μl of 0.1 mM DTT, 0.2 μl RNase Inhibitor, 1 μl of SuperScript III reverse transcriptase enzyme, and 0.8 μl of nuclease-free water (7 μl final volume).
39. The reaction volume can be scaled down for economy provided the product is forward compatible with the required library handling steps applicable to your sequencing platform of choice. It is recommended that you briefly centrifuge tube 4 at 10,000 × *g* at 4 °C for 1 min prior to use.
40. A touchdown protocol can be used in the case of non-specific amplification, or due to low primer melting temperatures compared to 5′ RLM RACE kit provider recommendations due to, for example, high A/T content on the target of interest. A reliable starting touchdown cycling protocol involves 98 °C for 30 s; 20 cycles of (a) 95 °C for 15 s, (b) 70 °C for 10 s reduced by 0.5 °C per cycle, and (c) 72 °C for 15 s; 20 cycles of

(a) 95 °C for 15 s, (b) 60 °C for 10 s, and (c) 72 °C for 15 s; 72 °C for 2 min; 4 °C hold.

41. If performing nested PCR, scale down the first reaction to 15 μl and use the New England Biolabs Rapid PCR Cleanup Enzyme Set to degrade residual primers and dephosphorylate dNTPs (per 5 μl of first PCR amplicon add 1 μl of exonuclease I and 1 μl of shrimp alkaline phosphatase included in this kit; using a thermal cycler, heat to 37 °C for 5 min and inactivate enzymes at 80 °C for 10 min). After cleanup of the first reaction, transfer 4 μl to a new nuclease free PCR microcentrifuge tube supplemented with materials as per **steps 1** and **2** in this protocol to 40 μl total volume (use nested PCR primers instead of GeneRacer Forward and GSP), and use the same cycling conditions (assumes nested PCR primer melting temperatures of comparable (±2.0 °C melting temperature).
42. Adjust agarose content to required concentration for anticipated amplicon size.
43. Agarose gel electrophoresis allows for PCR analysis and gel extraction-based size selection and cleanup. Alternatives to agarose electrophoresis include the PerkinElmer Labchip XT platform (set extraction window to ±10% amplicon size and proceed to cleanup product by ethanol precipitation or PCR cleanup columns) or the ThermoFisher Size Select E-gel system.
44. Adjust voltage to low melting point agarose tolerance levels in line with low melting point agarose supplier recommendations to avoid gel melting in the tank.
45. Https://cutadapt.readthedocs.io/.
46. To download and install system-wide the latest version of the Tmap aligner as a separate command line package please follow the instructions on their official repository on GitHub (https://github.com/iontorrent/TS/tree/master/Analysis/TMAP).
47. The nucleic acid precipitation and purification steps during 5′ RLM RACE have been proven in our experience, necessary, albeit insufficient for adequate depletion of excess adapter. This results in RNA adapter carryover into the sequencing adapter ligation step.
48. Size selection approaches that fail to remove small amplicons such as gel excision, bead-based size selection, etc. can significantly reduce data due to adapter ligation amplification. The efficiency of this process depends on the size difference between the adapter ligation by-products and the 5′ RLM-RACE amplicon. It is therefore important to aim for a library size that allows for efficiency when a bead cleanup step is

implemented in removing adapter and primer dimers. In our hands, aiming for amplicons in excess of 150 bp allow for efficient separation using appropriate cutoff range paramagnetic beads. Any remaining contaminating adapter sequences can be easily eliminated from the dataset computationally.

49. Running the Cutadapt trimming software on your fastq dataset independently and using the verbose option will give you a very detailed initial summary statistics report. Based on that report you can further adjust Cutadapt's huge array of options to filter, quality control and process the raw sequencing reads based on various parameters to reflect your experiment.

50. Based on the sequencing technology used the length of the sequencing reads may vary, thus set the minimum and maximum length threshold at a specific cutoff level with the *-m* and -M parameters respectively, as an initial filtering step based on your experiment design. In conjunction with the cut-off length parameters you can choose the *--too-short-output = FILE* and *--too-long-output = FILE* options to output the filtered reads individually for further investigation and troubleshooting. Another useful filtering parameter is the *--untrimmed-output = FILE* which will output all the reads that do not contain the RACE adapter and can be used in combination with --discard-untrimmed.

51. Looking in the filtered reads output files can give you valuable insights to the sequenced reads and will help you troubleshoot any mistakes that might have occurred during the RACE adapter hybridization, library preparation, or PCR steps. To achieve these initial filtering steps, it is advised to run the Cutadapt trimming step prior to running your dataset through the RACE-SEQ(−MM) pipeline.

52. The RACE-SEQ pipeline has been built with the option to skip the initial adapter trimming step which has been preconfigured to run with the minimum default options. After manually generating an optimally filtered and quality controlled trimmed dataset based on your experiment specifications you can simply run it through the RACE-SEQ pipeline. This way you will generate the final outputs optimally, saving on alignment steps, which is arguably the most computationally intensive procedure.

53. https://github.com/pantastheo/RACE-SEQ-lite.

54. Bowtie v. 2.0.0 or later is not suited to RACE-SEQ due to its mismatch-tolerating read alignment methodology around alignment seed length [9].

55. Most importantly, the RACE-Seq-MM pipeline introduces the *--iterate* option. Using this option, the script will generate an index from the reference sequence with all the possible

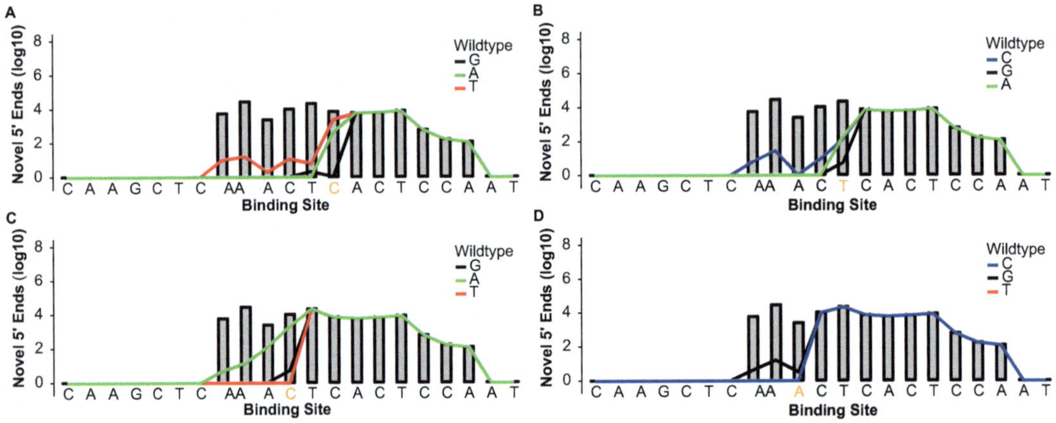

Fig. 3 A combined graph generated using the *--iterate* parameter to generate RACE-SEQ-MM data. The bar plot depicts the cleavage incidents generated on the wild-type reference genome of a replicon targeted by a short interfering RNA. The three line plots are generated by substituting the nucleotide in the specified position on the drug target site reference genome (marked as a gold nucleotide on the *X* axis) with each of the 3 alternative ones, and aligning against the "mutated" reference sequence; these lines represent novel 5′ ends identified on replicon quasi-species genomes. This analytical approach is valid only when applied on highly mutable target RNAs, such as viral RNAs or in vitro replicon RNA virus systems encoding the target site of interest, and strongly depends on high read quality

nucleotide combinations spanning the region of interest, based on your input parameters. Then it will generate and write all the possible sequences containing the single nucleotide variations in the region of interest. Following that, it will try to perform alignment using bowtie and utilizing all the new sequences as reference iteratively, meaning the whole script will be run three time multiplied by the length of the region of interest, plus the wild-type sequence (e.g., $(3 \times 21) + 1 = 64$). The output graph generated is a combination plot with the cleavage incident generated by the wild-type reference sequence as a histogram superimposed by line plots of the single variations per nucleotide for every genomic position (Fig. 3).

References

1. Morgan P, Brown DG, Lennard S, Anderton MJ, Barrett JC, Eriksson U, Fidock M, Hamrén B, Johnson A, March RE et al (2018) Impact of a five-dimensional framework on R&D productivity at AstraZeneca. Nat Rev Drug Discov 17:167–181
2. Cook D, Brown D, Alexander R, March R, Morgan P, Satterthwaite G, Pangalos MN (2014) Lessons learned from the fate of AstraZeneca's drug pipeline: a five-dimensional framework. Nat Rev Drug Discov 13:419–431
3. Moschos SA, Usher L, Lindsay MA (2017) Clinical potential of oligonucleotide-based therapeutics in the respiratory system. Pharmacol Ther 169:83–103. https://doi.org/10.1016/j.pharmthera.2016.10.009
4. Denise H, S a M, Sidders B, Burden F, Perkins H, Carter N, Stroud T, Kennedy M, Fancy S-A, Lapthorn C et al (2014) Deep sequencing insights in therapeutic shRNA processing and siRNA target cleavage precision. Mol Ther Nucleic Acids 3:e145

5. Tabernero J, Shapiro GI, LoRusso PM, Cervantes A, Schwartz GK, Weiss GJ, Paz-Ares L, Cho DC, Infante JR, Alsina M et al (2013) First-in-humans trial of an RNA interference therapeutic targeting VEGF and KSP in cancer patients with liver involvement. Cancer Discov 3:406–417
6. Barve M, Wang Z, Kumar P, Jay CM, Luo X, Bedell C, Mennel RG, Wallraven G, Brunicardi FC, Senzer N et al (2015) Phase 1 trial of Bi-shRNA STMN1 BIV in refractory cancer. Mol Ther 23:1123–1130
7. Dudek H, Wong DH, Arvan R, Shah A, Wortham K, Ying B, Diwanji R, Zhou W, Holmes B, Yang H et al (2014) Knockdown of β-catenin with dicer-substrate siRNAs reduces liver tumor burden in vivo. Mol Ther 22:92–101
8. Ganesh S, Koser ML, Cyr WA, Chopda GR, Tao J, Shui X, Ying B, Chen D, Pandya P, Chipumuro E et al (2016) Direct pharmacological inhibition of β-catenin by RNA interference in tumors of diverse origin. Mol Cancer Ther 15:2143–2154
9. Theotokis PI, Usher L, Kortschak CK, Schwalbe E, Moschos SA (2017) Profiling the mismatch tolerance of argonaute 2 through deep sequencing of sliced polymorphic viral RNAs. Mol Ther Nucleic Acids 9:22–33
10. Thys K, Verhasselt P, Reumers J, Verbist BMP, Maes B, Aerssens J (2015) Performance assessment of the Illumina massively parallel sequencing platform for deep sequencing analysis of viral minority variants. J Virol Methods 221:29–38
11. Kennedy SR, Schmitt MW, Fox EJ, Kohrn BF, Salk JJ, Ahn EH, Prindle MJ, Kuong KJ, Shen JC, Risques RA et al (2014) Detecting ultralow-frequency mutations by duplex sequencing. Nat Protoc 9:2586–2606

Chapter 18

Studying the Biotransformation of Phosphorothioate-Containing Oligonucleotide Drugs by LC-MS

Christophe Husser, Erich Koller, Andreas Brink, and Simone Schadt

Abstract

Across the pharmaceutical industry, there is increasing interest and need to investigate the biotransformation of oligonucleotide drugs. The method of choice is high-resolution mass spectrometry due to its unmet sensitivity and specificity.

Here, we describe a method developed and applied in our laboratory studying the biotransformation of phosphorothioate-containing oligonucleotide drugs. This method is based on capillary flow liquid chromatography with column switching coupled to high-resolution mass spectrometry.

Key words Oligonucleotide biotransformation, UPLC, Column switching, High resolution mass spectrometry, All ion fragmentation

1 Introduction

Across the pharmaceutical industry, there is increasing interest and need to investigate the biotransformation of oligonucleotide drugs. Similar to small molecule drugs, where biotransformation studies are a well-established part of the submission package, also for oligonucleotide drugs the biotransformation might have an impact on drug disposition, efficacy, and safety [1, 2]. Therefore, it is important to gain an understanding of differences between animal species used in toxicity testing and humans. Oligonucleotides are usually administered subcutaneously (SC). Oligonucleotides containing a phosphorothioate backbone are over 90% bound to plasma proteins which prevents fast excretion [3–5]. Plasma peak concentrations are typically reached within 2–4 h after SC administration [3, 5–7]. Once c_{max} is reached oligonucleotides have a very fast distribution phase where they get distributed into tissues and the plasma concentration is decreasing 2–3 log units within 2 h [5]. This fast distribution phase is followed by a long termination phase. The terminal half-life is up to several weeks [5]. Once distributed in tissues the oligonucleotides get released very slowly

Olof Gissberg et al. (eds.), *Oligonucleotide-Based Therapies: Methods and Protocols*, Methods in Molecular Biology, vol. 2036,
https://doi.org/10.1007/978-1-4939-9670-4_18,

from tissue. There seems to be an equilibrium between plasma concentration and tissue concentration [5, 6]. Locked-nucleic acid (LNA) modifications increase affinity to the target RNA, but they also protect the oligonucleotide from exonuclease degradation [8, 9]. As a consequence, oligonucleotide metabolite concentrations in plasma are typically very low, often below the limit of detection. Therefore, tissues have to be analyzed to obtain information on the biotransformation. This is practically only feasible in preclinical but not in clinical studies, leaving a gap that might potentially be filled with in vitro investigations. For in vitro to in vivo correlations and species differences, a good understanding of the target exposure to drug and metabolites is of key importance and appropriate analytical techniques are required to provide information on the identity of the metabolites formed.

Here, we describe a method for studying the in vitro and in vivo biotransformation of phosphorothioate-containing oligonucleotide drugs. This method is based on capillary flow liquid chromatography (LC) with column switching coupled to high-resolution mass spectrometry (MS).

2 Materials

Prepare all solutions using analytical or LC-MS grade reagents. Prepare and store all reagents at room temperature (unless indicated otherwise).

2.1 Cell Culture and Cell Lysis

1. Freshly isolated primary hepatocytes.
2. Complete medium: Williams Medium E, 10% fetal bovine serum, 100 U/mL penicillin, 0.1 mg/mL streptomycin.
3. Collagen-coated 24-well plates.
4. Lysis buffer: 4 M guanidine thiocyanate in 0.1 M Tris–HCl, pH 7.5, available commercially as ready-to-use tissue homogenization buffer for molecular biology (Panreac/AppliChem) (*see* **Note 1**).

2.2 Cell and Tissue Homogenization

1. Ultrasound homogenizer Sonorex (Bandelin).
2. Thermomixer (Eppendorf, Hamburg, Germany).
3. 1.5 mL Protein LoBind Tube, PCR clean.
4. Precellys tissue tubes CK28 (Bertin Technologies, France).
5. Precellys Evolution SUPER Homogenizer (Bertin Technologies, France).
6. Lysis buffer: *see* **item 4** in Subheading 2.1.

2.3 Solid-Phase Extraction (SPE)

1. OASIS HLB 1 cc SPE cartridges.
2. Vacuum manifold with manometer.
3. Vacuum centrifuge.
4. SPE washing solution: H_2O–HFIP–DIPEA (100:1:0.1, v/v/v). Add 40 mL H_2O to a 50 mL vial, add 40 μL DIPEA (*N,N*-Diisopropylethylamine 99.5% biotech grade), and add 400 μL HFIP (1,1,1,3,3,3-hexafluoro-2-2propanol).
5. SPE dilution solution: H_2O–HFIP–DIPEA (100:2:0.2, v/v/v). Add 40 mL H_2O to a 50 mL vial, add 80 μL DIPEA, and add 800 μL HFIP.
6. SPE elution solution: H_2O–acetonitrile–TEA (40:60:1, v/v/v). Add 4 mL H_2O to a 15 mL polypropylene conical tube (Falcon), add 6 mL acetonitrile, vortex, add 100 μL TEA (triethylamine puriss. p.a.), and vortex.
7. Reconstitution solution: H_2O–MeOH–HFIP–DIPEA (80:20:1:0.1, v/v/v). Add 8 mL H_2O to a 15 mL polypropylene conical tube. Add 2 mL MeOH, vortex, add 10 μL DIPEA, add 100 μL HFIP, and vortex (*see* **Note 2**).

2.4 HPLC-MS Analysis

1. A high-resolution LC-MS system with autosampler (*see* **Note 3**).
2. Trapping column: Xbridge BEH C4, 300 μm ID × 50 mm, 5 μm, 300 A.
3. Analytical column: Xbridge BEH C18, 300 μm ID × 50 mm, 5 μm, 130 A (Waters, Baden, Switzerland).
4. External 6-port Rheodyne™ MX Series II™ divert/inject valve.
5. HPLC mobile phase A: H_2O–MeOH–HFIP–DIPEA, 98:2:1:0.1. Add 480 mL H_2O to 500 mL in a PFA bottle. Add 20 mL MeOH, mix, add 500 μL DIPEA, mix, and add 5 mL HFIP.
6. HPLC mobile phase B: H_2O–MeOH–HFIP–DIPEA, 10:90:1:0.1. Add 50 mL H_2O to a 500 mL PFA bottle. Add 450 mL MeOH, mix, add 500 μL DIPEA, mix, and add 5 mL HFIP.
7. HPLC trapping column (Xbridge BEH C4, 300 μm ID × 50 mm, 5 μm, 300 A).
8. HPLC analytical column (Xbridge BEH C18, 300 μm ID × 50 mm, 5 μm, 130 A) (Waters, Baden, Switzerland) (*see* **Note 4**).

3 Methods

Carry out all procedures at room temperature, unless otherwise specified.

3.1 Cell Culture

1. Suspend freshly isolated primary hepatocytes in complete medium and seeded into collagen-coated 24-well plates at a density of 2×10^5 cells/well.
2. Culture hepatocytes at 37 °C in a 5% CO_2 atmosphere for about 3 h to allow for attachment to cell culture plates.
3. Add phosphorothioate-linked antisense oligonucleotide compound at 10 mM final concentration.
4. Culture hepatocytes at 37 °C in a 5% CO_2 atmosphere for about 3 h.
5. Remove the medium, and wash once with complete medium.
6. Culture hepatocytes in fresh complete medium at 37 °C in a 5% CO_2 atmosphere for 3 h, 21 h and 69 h.
7. Remove medium from cell culture wells and add 150 μL lysis buffer per well and freeze at −20 °C.

3.2 Cell and Tissue Homogenization

3.2.1 Cell-Lysate Homogenization

1. Thaw cell lysates and sonicate with ultrasound homogenizer for 5 min.
2. Add an aliquot of 100–300 μL to a 1.5 mL Protein LoBind Tube (*see* **Notes 5** and **6**).
3. Add 700–900 μL of SPE dilution buffer and incubate at room temperature for 2 h with 1200 rpm in the Thermomixer (*see* **Note 7**).

3.2.2 Tissue Homogenization

1. Add 300 μL Lysis Buffer (*see* **Note 8**) to 100 mg of tissue in Precellys CK28 tissue tubes.
2. Homogenize by spinning the CK28 tubes in the Precellys Evolution SUPER Homogenizer at 7800 rpm for 20 s, pause for 1 min, then mix again for 20 s at 7800 rpm.

3.3 Solid-Phase Extraction (SPE)

1. Place OASIS HLB 1 cc cartridges on the vacuum manifold and set vacuum to 5–10 inHg.
2. Precondition SPE cartridges by adding 1 mL acetonitrile, then switch on vacuum (*see* **Note 9**).
3. Add 1 mL of SPE washing buffer to the SPE cartridge and switch on vacuum.
4. Load samples by pipetting 1000 μL of the prepared cell extract or tissue homogenate onto the cartridge and switch on vacuum.

5. Wash by pipetting 1 mL of SPE washing buffer.
6. Elute with 400 μL SPE elution buffer.
7. Evaporate the eluate in a vacuum centrifuge at 45 °C at 10 mbar for 1–2 h to near but incomplete dryness (*see* **Note 10**).
8. Redissolve in 150–200 μL reconstitution solution by shaking for 20 min at 150 rpm in the Thermomixer.

3.4 HPLC-MS Analysis

The configuration of the online extraction, column-switching UltiMate UPLC system is shown in Fig. 1 (*see* **Note 3**). The trapping column is connected via a stainless-steel tee device with the analytical column. The column-switching between the trapping column and analytical column is performed by an external 6-port divert/inject valve at a column temperature of 50 °C (*see* **Note 11**).

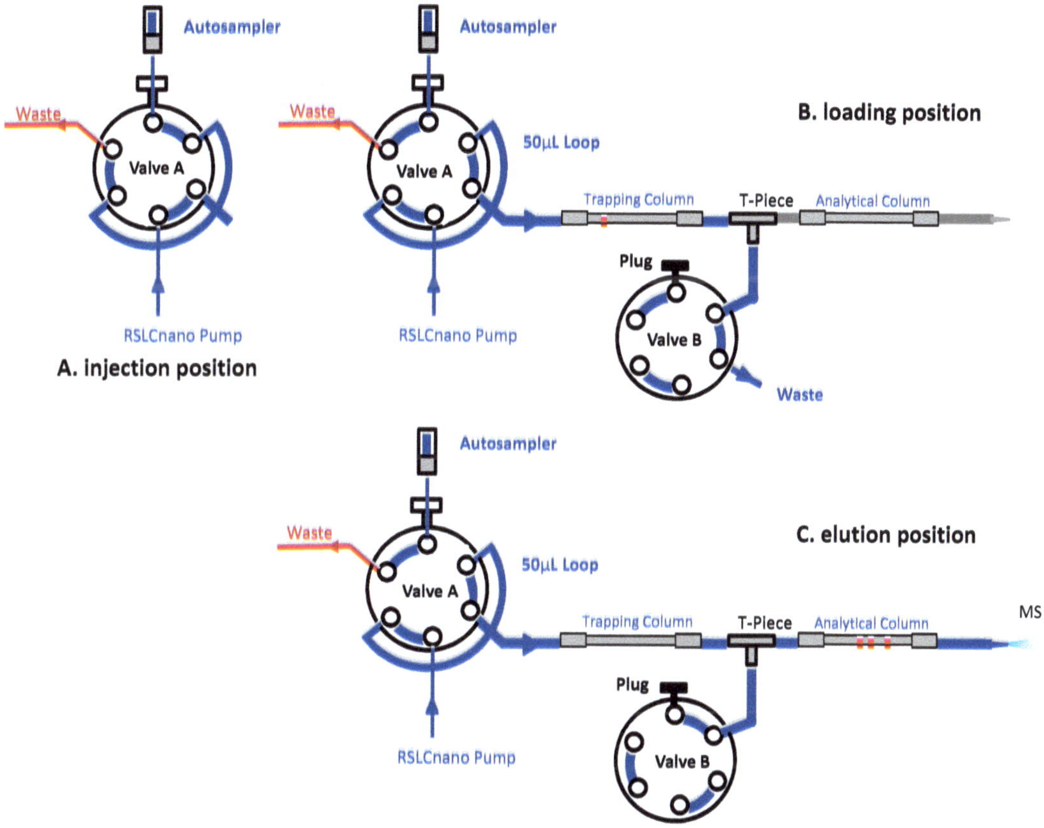

Fig. 1 Schematic configuration and valve positions of the LC-MS UltiMate column-switching system (**A**) injection position (valve A): Samples are injected via the auto sampler into the 50 μL loop. (**B**) loading position: Then valve A is switched and the sample is pumped by the RSLCnano Pump onto the trapping column. Because of the back pressure of the analytical column, the flow is directed from the T-piece into the waste. (**C**) elution position: Then, valve B is switched, and because of the back pressure of the plug, the flow is directed from the T-piece into the analytical column, and the oligonucleotides are eluted from the trapping column to the analytical column, and from the analytical column into the MS

Table 1
HPLC gradient

Time, min	Flow, μL/min	%B
0	20	2
8	20[a]	2
8.1	10	2
12	10	2
42	10	55
42.5	10	70
45	10	70
45.6	10	2
54.5	10	2
54.6	20	2
58	20	2

[a]First 8 min: loading of the trapping column

3.4.1 HPLC

1. Load 50 μL aliquots of the prepared sample onto the trapping column with a loading eluent consisting of 2% mobile phase B and 98% mobile phase A, delivered at a flow rate of 20 μL/min for 8.0 min and at a flow rate of 10 μL/min for further 2 min.
2. Switch the trapping column in line with the analytical column (Fig. 1). The HPLC conditions are listed in Table 1.
3. After 2 min using isocratic eluent B at 2% and at a flow rate of 10 μL/min, apply the gradient from 2% to 55% eluent B within 30.0 min.
4. Increase eluent B to 70% within 0.5 min and maintain for another 2.5 min.
5. Reequilibrate to start conditions 2% eluent B for 12 min (*see* **Note 12**).

3.4.2 MS Analysis

For MS analysis choose the following parameters on an Orbitrap Fusion instrument: negative ionization mode, sheath gas 10, auxiliary gas 0, sweep gas 0, ion transfer tube temperature 300 °C, spray voltage negative ion 2200 V, full scan mode 120,000, resolution, and scan range 550–1700. For data dependent higher energy collisional dissociation (HCD) fragmentation experiment: collision energy of 35% with detection in the ion trap at nominal mass resolution and a scan range of 150–2000, triggered on the most intense multiply charged ions in top speed mode. For all ion fragmentation (AIF) in HCD mode (*see* **Notes 13** and **14**): collision energy of 35%, resolution 30,000, isolation range 600–1800, and scan range 80–1200.

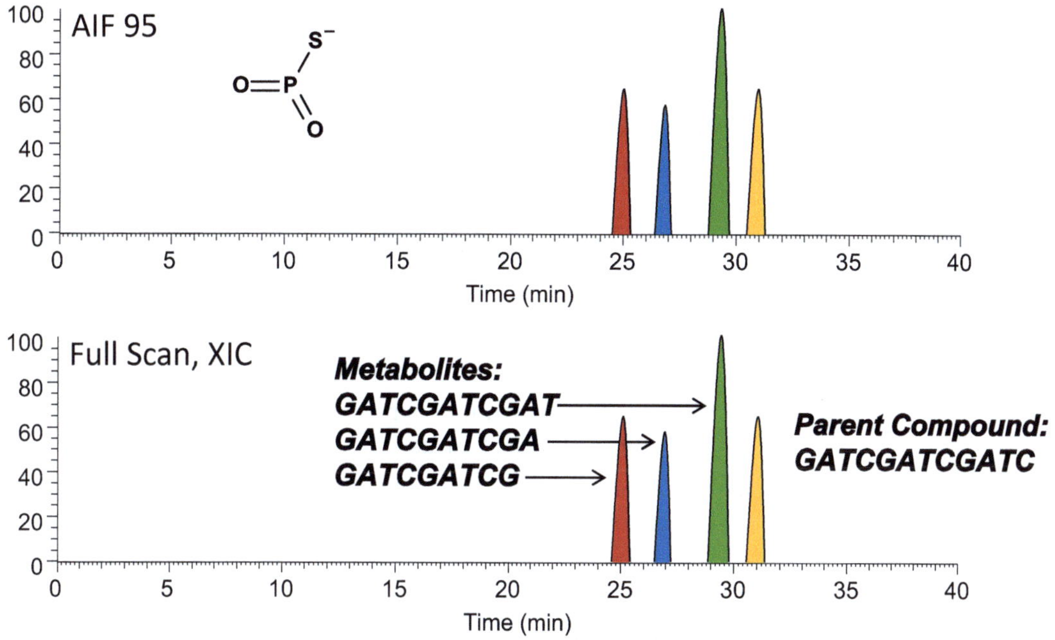

Fig. 2 Basic principle of the MS method combining all ion fragmentation (AIF) and full scan data. To find potential metabolites, the AIF trace is extracted for *m/z* 94.9362 which is a unique fragment of the phosphorothioate backbone (O_2PS^-). Peaks in the AIF trace extracted for *m/z* 94.9362 indicate elution of phosphorothioate containing oligonucleotides (top panel). In a second step, the full scan data at these retention times is investigated for *m/z* that can be assigned to potential oligonucleotide metabolites. The corresponding *m/z* values are displayed in an extracted ion chromatogram (XIC) (bottom panel)

3.5 Data Analysis

1. Extract *m/z* 94.9362, a unique fragment of the phosphorothioate backbone by collision-induced dissociation, in the AIF trace using Xcalibur or other MS software to identify peaks of possible metabolites [1] (*see* **Note 13**, Fig. 2).
2. Check MS spectrum of full scan data at the retention times of the peaks identified in the AIF trace by extracting *m/z* 94.9362. The mass spectra contain a series of peaks corresponding to different charge states of the oligonucleotides.
3. Deconvolute MS spectrum at the retention times of the peaks identified in the AIF trace with the Xtract software in Xcalibur to determine the exact mass of the metabolites (*see* **Note 14**).
4. Check MS^2 spectrum for characteristic fragments (*see* **Note 15**).

4 Notes

1. Guanidine thiocyanate may precipitate in 0.1 M Tris–HCl (pH 7.5). In this case, dissolve in a water bath at 30–40 °C. Instead of using the ready-to-use lysis buffer for molecular biology (Panreac/AppliChem), a lysis buffer can also be

prepared by adding 94.53 g guanidine thiocyanate to 200 mL 0.1 M Tris–HCl pH 7.5 buffer.

2. The MeOH content might need to be adjusted for different oligonucleotides depending on sequence and chemical backbone modifications.
3. A Binary Rapid Separation HPLC system (Thermo Scientific Dionex UltiMate NCP-3200RS) in combination with a Pal autosampler (CTC Analytics AG, Zwingen, Switzerland) and an Orbitrap Fusion Tribrid Mass Spectrometer (Thermo Scientific, Bremen, Germany) have been used in our laboratory. Other high-resolution LC-MS systems might be also used.
4. Similar columns from other vendors might also be used but have not been tested by us.
5. Tissue samples homogenates in H_2O are mixed 1:1 with lysis buffer for 10 min at 1200 rpm using a ThermoMixer.
6. If an internal standard is required, it can be added at this stage.
7. If another mixer is used, choose conditions where adequate shaking/mixing of the solution is ensured.
8. Alternatively, H_2O can also be used for lysis.
9. Always add the solvent before switching on vacuum. Reduce vacuum to the lowest possible setting.
10. It is important to avoid complete dryness, since this can result in solubility issues. In case complete dryness cannot be avoided, the reconstitution solution needs to be optimized for the compound and needs to contain a sufficiently high proportion of organic solvent.
11. Configuring the UPLC in column switching mode is important to enable loading of larger sample volumes to ensure increased sensitivity.
12. Keep the trapping column and the analytical column at 50 °C during the whole analysis sequence. Prior to the next injection, decouple the trapping column from the analytical column by switching the valves to loading position (Fig. 1).
13. We recommend drawing the structures and fragments of the oligonucleotide of interest in a chemistry drawing software, since fragments depend very much on the exact chemical structure. Examples can be found in the literature [1].
14. All ion fragmentation is an acquisition mode in which all precursor ions are fragmented without a preselection by the quadrupole. Fragmentation occurs in the higher energy collisional dissociation (HCD) cell, located at the far side of the C-trap.
15. In this case, MS^2 spectrum refers to fragmentation spectra from the data dependent HCD fragmentation experiment.

References

1. Husser C, Brink A, Zell M, Muller MB, Koller E, Schadt S (2017) Identification of GalNAc-conjugated antisense oligonucleotide metabolites using an untargeted and generic approach based on high resolution mass spectrometry. Anal Chem 89(12):6821–6826. https://doi.org/10.1021/acs.analchem.7b01244
2. Shemesh CS, Yu RZ, Gaus HJ, Greenlee S, Post N, Schmidt K, Migawa MT, Seth PP, Zanardi TA, Prakash TP, Swayze EE, Henry SP, Wang Y (2016) Elucidation of the biotransformation pathways of a Galnac3-conjugated antisense oligonucleotide in rats and monkeys. Mol Ther Nucleic Acids 5:e319. https://doi.org/10.1038/mtna.2016.31
3. Crooke ST (2008) Antisense drug technology: principles, strategies, and applications, 2nd edn. CRC Press, Boca Raton
4. Yu RZ, Kim TW, Hong A, Watanabe TA, Gaus HJ, Geary RS (2007) Cross-species pharmacokinetic comparison from mouse to man of a second-generation antisense oligonucleotide, ISIS 301012, targeting human apolipoprotein B-100. Drug Metab Dispos 35(3):460–468. https://doi.org/10.1124/dmd.106.012401
5. Geary RS, Norris D, Yu R, Bennett CF (2015) Pharmacokinetics, biodistribution and cell uptake of antisense oligonucleotides. Adv Drug Deliv Rev 87:46–51. https://doi.org/10.1016/j.addr.2015.01.008
6. Geary RS (2009) Antisense oligonucleotide pharmacokinetics and metabolism. Expert Opin Drug Metab Toxicol 5(4):381–391. https://doi.org/10.1517/17425250902877680
7. Yu RZ, Grundy JS, Geary RS (2013) Clinical pharmacokinetics of second generation antisense oligonucleotides. Expert Opin Drug Metab Toxicol 9(2):169–182. https://doi.org/10.1517/17425255.2013.737320
8. Juliano RL (2016) The delivery of therapeutic oligonucleotides. Nucleic Acids Res 44(14):6518–6548. https://doi.org/10.1093/nar/gkw236
9. Frieden M, Hansen HF, Koch T (2003) Nuclease stability of LNA oligonucleotides and LNA-DNA chimeras. Nucleosides Nucleotides Nucleic Acids 22(5-8):1041–1043. https://doi.org/10.1081/NCN-120022731

Chapter 19

ADME: Assessing Pharmacokinetic–Pharmacodynamic Parameters of Oligonucleotides

Rasmus Jansson-Löfmark, Christine Ahlström, and Peter Gennemark

Abstract

We describe tactics to assess pharmacokinetic (PK) and pharmacodynamic (PD) parameters of oligonucleotides. The chapter includes recommendations on the design of single-dose preclinical PK studies, preclinical PKPD studies, and toxicological studies, and on best practice for scaling PK and PD parameters from animal to human. We focus on single-stranded oligonucleotides, but relevant differences to double-stranded RNAs are also addressed.

Key words Pharmacokinetics, Pharmacodynamics, Oligonucleotides, Translation, Human dose prediction

1 Introduction

RNA-based drugs either upregulate or downregulate the level of a certain messenger RNA (mRNA), leading to increased or decreased expression of the corresponding protein [1–3]. Oligonucleotide therapies can be divided into single-stranded oligonucleotides (e.g., anti-microRNAs (anti-miRs), antisense oligonucleotides (ASOs), and aptamers), double-stranded RNA (e.g., short interfering RNA (siRNA), and miR-mimics), and synthetic mRNA [1, 3].

The pharmacokinetics (PK) of oligonucleotides differs from that of typical small-molecule drugs. First, the PK within each class of oligonucleotides is largely determined by the nucleotide backbone and independent of the nucleotide sequence. One can, therefore, get relatively good understanding of the PK from previous studies of drugs in the class. A prerequisite is that the previous studies have used the same nucleotide backbone of the drug, as well as the same administration route and drug formulation. The sequence independence also implies that scaling between species can become more straightforward compared to small-molecule drugs, provided there are sufficiently rich historical data available for the class. Second, the terminal half-life of oligonucleotides is

Olof Gissberg et al. (eds.), *Oligonucleotide-Based Therapies: Methods and Protocols*, Methods in Molecular Biology, vol. 2036, https://doi.org/10.1007/978-1-4939-9670-4_19,

typically longer than that of small-molecule drugs. This influences the design of in vivo studies. For example, sampling may be required over extended time periods, and drug accumulation may have to be considered in repeated-dosing studies. Finally, oral bioavailability is very low for oligonucleotides, making oral administration infeasible, at least in the absence of permeability enhancers.

On the pharmacodynamic (PD) side, it is generally known that the use of target-engagement data in drug discovery and development is associated with high success rate of candidate drugs [4–6]. For oligonucleotides, the target-engagement biomarker, that is, the mRNA, can be measured both in plasma and in tissue. This is an advantage compared to small-molecule drugs, for which a significant effort might be required to identify and measure the target-engagement biomarker. Furthermore, if the encoded mRNA is circulating in blood, the target-engagement biomarker can be measured over time in clinical trials. Such rich time-course data are useful to infer unobserved parameters such as the drug biophase half-life [7]. Finally, having access to a tissue target-engagement biomarker in the drug-discovery phase facilitates development and analysis of both in vitro and in vivo potency screens.

This chapter focuses on PKPD considerations for oligonucleotides. The scope is restricted in the following ways:

- We focus on single-stranded oligonucleotides, but relevant differences to double-stranded RNAs are also addressed. Synthetic mRNAs are pharmacologically different from other oligonucleotides and limited clinical data are available. This modality is therefore introduced but omitted from our main analysis.
- We do not cover recommendations on planning and analyzing drug-drug interaction studies. Assessment of potential drug-drug interactions is a requirement for regulatory filing, although no drug-drug interactions have been observed between small-molecule drugs and oligonucleotides in clinical studies. There are, however, some in vitro observations of such interactions [1]. Given the lack of clinical findings, it is common to back-load any in vitro studies until end of Phase 1.

We start by introducing relevant PK and PD parameters, and bioanalytical techniques used to measure oligonucleotides. The following main section addresses tactics and recommendations on the design and analysis of in vivo studies. Specifically, we have identified a couple of general questions that, in our experience, come up recurrently in the discovery phase of oligonucleotides (e.g., "How to design a single-dose preclinical PK study?"). The main section presents those questions and our answers to them. The chapter ends with concluding remarks.

This chapter is aimed for an audience with basic understanding of small-molecule PK, generation and interpretation of in vivo data, and of bioanalysis. Readers that are experienced in PK and PD analysis may skip parts of the "Background concepts" section.

2 Background Concepts

2.1 Pharmacokinetic Properties of Oligonucleotides

This section describes the distribution and elimination properties of the main types of oligonucleotides: single-stranded oligonucleotides, double-stranded RNAs, and synthetic messenger RNAs.

A single-stranded oligonucleotide normally consists of 12–20 base pairs with a total molecular weight of 6–9 kDa. It is highly soluble and generally polyanionic. The drug is mainly distributed to the liver and to certain segments of the kidney, and to a lower extent to other tissues and cells. The main route of elimination is via intracellular endonucleases and exonucleases in tissues [1]. They are also excreted renally; primarily the fraction of the oligonucleotides that is not bound to plasma proteins. Single-stranded oligonucleotides are commonly delivered intravenously, subcutaneously or intrathecally. Oral bioavailability is very low due to high molecular weight and very low transcellular permeability. Bioavailability can be increased by coadministering the drug with permeability enhancers that increase paracellular leakage [8]. Depending on the target tissue and the drug's PKPD properties, a single-stranded oligonucleotide might require a targeting ligand (i.e., GalNac-conjugate) to achieve its therapeutically relevant target exposure [2].

A double-stranded RNA consists of 20–25 base pairs, with a total molecular weight of 14–18 kDa. Physical-chemistry, distribution and excretion properties are similar to those of single-stranded oligonucleotides: high distribution to liver and to certain segments of the kidney, and elimination primarily via intracellular endonucleases and exonucleases in tissues [9]. Double-stranded RNAs are also excreted renally; primarily the fraction of the oligonucleotide that is not bound to plasma proteins. The intact siRNA does not elicit the main pharmacological action. Instead, it is the cleaved-off antisense strand that is pharmacologically active (i.e., similar to an active metabolite for a small-molecule drug) [2]. Double-stranded RNAs are commonly delivered intravenously or subcutaneously.

A synthetic mRNA or modified RNA has a molecular weight of 200–400 kDa and is highly soluble and polyanionic. It has limited tissue distribution, unless administered via a delivery system. If administered as a lipid nanoparticle (LNP) formulation, it distributes primarily to liver and spleen. However, tissue distribution can be altered by choice of formulation [10]. Modified RNAs bind to the ribosomes, where they use the endogenous protein synthesis machinery to synthesize the protein of the encoded mRNA sequence. Hence, they have a vastly different pharmacological feature compared to single and double stranded RNAs [11]. From a PKPD perspective, both the PK of the modified RNA and the synthesized protein need to be monitored. In summary, modified RNAs differ in mode of action and molecular weight compared to siRNAs and ASOs. The PKPD properties and translation to human can hence not be expected to be similar.

The use of in vitro data for PK characterization of oligonucleotides is relatively rare. The main in vitro parameter that is used is plasma protein binding (PPB) [12]. PPB of oligonucleotides influences tissue distribution and the fraction excreted via the kidneys. ASOs (with the commonly used phosphorothioate modification of the backbone) bind extensively to plasma proteins, mostly to albumin and to lower extent to alpha-macroglobulin. Binding is commonly linear with regard to concentration, unless excessively high plasma concentrations are achieved. PPB is reported to be similar across species, except that binding in mice could be lower [13, 14]. Unformulated and unmodified siRNA may have a lower level of PPB compared to ASOs, something that may lead to a higher fraction excreted via kidneys [15]. Although in vitro methods are not extensively used for oligonucleotides, we note some studies assessing metabolic pathways, the role of nucleases and transporter interactions [16–18].

2.2 Bioanalytical Techniques

Here we provide a brief overview of bioanalysis of oligonucleotides (*see* for example [19] for a comprehensive review).

Bioanalytical techniques for absolute quantification of oligonucleotides in biological matrices (i.e., plasma and tissue) can be broadly classified into hybridization-based assays and chromatographic assays. Hybridization-based assays commonly use probe oligonucleotides to hybridize the target oligonucleotides through a specific Watson-Crick base-pair mechanism. The formed hybridized complex is then quantified by techniques such as hybridization enzyme-linked immunosorbent assay (ELISA), quantitative polymerase chain reaction (qPCR), in situ hybridization, northern blot, microarray or next generation sequencing. Chromatographic-based assays commonly involve liquid chromatography (LC) separation followed by direct detection of target oligonucleotides using UV, fluorescence or mass spectrometry (MS). In general, chromatographic assays are more specific but less sensitive compared to hybridization-based assays. The sensitivity of a particular bioanalytical method also depends on the analyte characteristics, such as structure and length of the oligonucleotide.

LC-MS is usually preferred in early phases of the discovery phase when the exact base-pair sequence is not set. Given the hydrophilic and polyanionic properties of oligonucleotides, sample preparation prior to LC-MS is of importance. The advantage of LC-MS is its applicability to varying base-pair sequences, within a certain chemical class. However, the level of sensitivity can limit PK assessment, in particular for plasma exposure measurements where exposure might be more than thousand-fold lower compared to exposure in certain tissues (e.g., liver and kidney) [20–22]. While ELISA is generally more sensitive, it requires a synthesized and unique probe for each oligonucleotide sequence. Therefore, ELISA typically replaces LC-MS once the oligonucleotide, and its base-pair sequence, has been selected.

2.3 Pharmacokinetic Parameters

The key PK parameters, graphically presented in Fig. 1, are the following:

Maximum concentration (C_{max})—provides information of the maximum exposure level. This parameter tells if a sufficient drug level has been reached to anticipate a pharmacological action, and how this level relates to any future safety finding. The parameter T_{max} (time when concentration is at its maximum) is sometimes reported in conjunction with C_{max}.

Trough concentration (C_{trough})—provides information of the exposure level right before dosing, in a chronic study.

Area under the curve (AUC)—is a measure of the total drug plasma exposure level over time. To obtain an accurate value of AUC one needs to take continuous samples for at least 70–75% of the time the system is exposed to drug. One can then either report AUC up to last measured time point, $AUC_{0\text{-}t,last}$, or $AUC_{0\text{-}inf.}$ for which the remaining of the AUC is extrapolated based on the three previously measured time points (Fig. 1).

Volume of distribution (V_{ss})—is an indirect measure of the total extent of tissue distribution. This measure is derived from

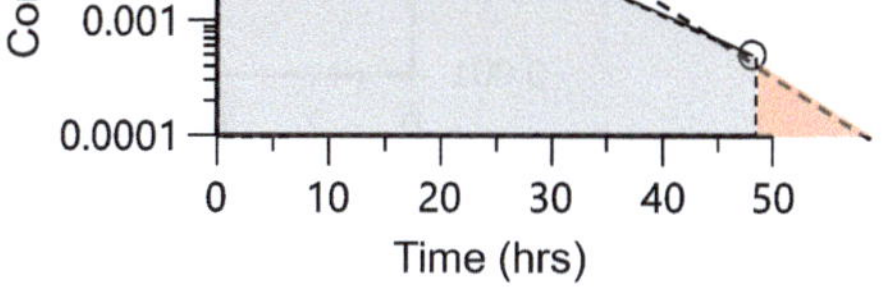

Fig. 1 Schematic illustration of the key PK parameters, C_{max} and half-life. AUC is the area under the plasma concentration curve (grey shaded area is the $AUC_{0\text{-}t,last}$ and the sum of the grey and red area is $AUC_{0\text{-}inf}$). Data were digitized from Yu et al. [23] where an antisense oligonucleotide (ISIS301012) was dosed with 5 mg/kg to mice

plasma/blood concentration of the drug and known amount of drug in the blood. It can be regarded as analogous to estimating the volume of a certain reservoir by mixing a certain amount of dye to it, ensure it is properly mixed, and then use the resultant concentration to estimate the volume (i.e., Volume = amount/concentration). Analogous to half-life, calculation of V_{ss} can be challenging since it requires that distribution equilibrium is reached between drug in tissues and in plasma. Immediately, after a single dose the maximum concentration can be measured to obtain an estimate of distribution but this is not V_{ss} since equilibrium has not been reached [24].

Half-life ($t_{1/2}$)—is the time it takes to half the concentration level. The parameter can be of value for assessing duration of pharmacological action. Since oligonucleotides have a multicompartmental kinetic plasma profile, one must distinguish between the initial half-life (time points 0.1–0.5 days and 0.5–3 days; Fig. 2)) or the terminal half-life (28–90 days; Fig. 2) [14, 23].

Half-life is a secondary PK parameter since it depends on both total clearance and V_{ss}. The relationship between half-life, clearance, and volume is as follows:

$$t_{1/2} = \log 2 \times \frac{V_{ss}}{\mathrm{Cl}} \quad (1)$$

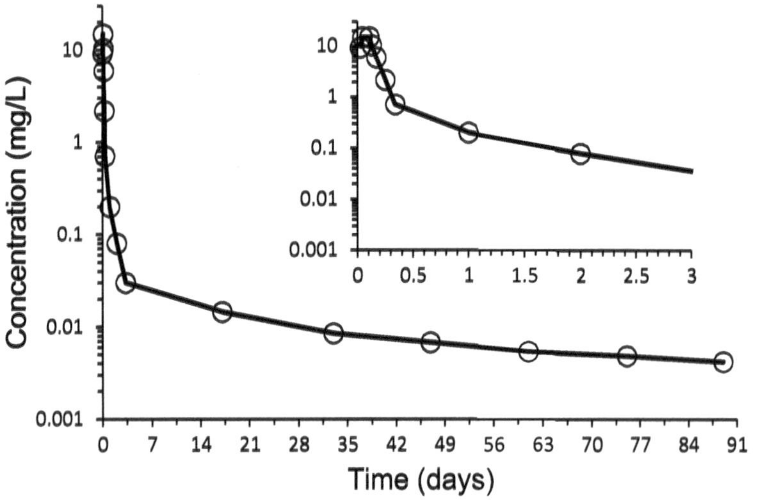

Fig. 2 The characteristic multicompartmental profile of an antisense oligonucleotide. The main graph corresponds to the full PK profile. The insert graph in the right corner corresponds to the PK profile during the first 3 days. The compound reaches the terminal half-life after approximately 28 days. Data were digitized and adapted from Yu et al. [23] where an antisense oligonucleotide (ISIS301012) was subcutaneously dosed (approximately 200 mg) to human

The above parameters can be obtained by noncompartmental analysis [25]. The parameters can also be estimated using mathematical modeling.

Tissue exposure—is a relevant measure when the target tissue is known. To date, liver (e.g., hepatocytes) is the most commonly targeted tissue by oligonucleotides. We note that total tissue exposure may not correlate with effective tissue exposure. Only the so-called productive tissue uptake gives rise to the desired PD effect [14]. The nonproductive uptake (e.g., uptake to the wrong cell-type in the tissue) does not cause the desired effect. In practice, the productive cell or tissue exposure cannot be directly measured, but indirectly assessed by measurement of downstream target-related variables such as the produced mRNA [25, 26]. For ASOs with drug target in the tissue, the terminal plasma half-life is considered to reflect tissue half-life. In such cases, the terminal plasma half-life can be determined and used as a surrogate measure for tissue half-life [14]. For siRNAs, mouse data indicate that the half-life of Ago2-loaded antisense siRNA reflects antisense half-life at target site [21].

Renal clearance—is largely dependent on fraction unbound in plasma. It is estimated from the amount of drug in urine up to at least 80% of the time for sampling of plasma AUC. The urine concentration is determined and multiplied with the total urine volume excretion. The renal clearance then is obtained as

$$\mathrm{Cl}\ (\mathrm{L/h}) = \frac{\text{Amount renally excreted (mg)}}{\mathrm{AUC}_{\mathrm{plasma}}\ (\mathrm{mg} \times \mathrm{h/L})} \tag{2}$$

Bioavailability—the fraction of the total drug that reaches the systemic circulation upon extravascular administration compared to intravenous administration.

2.4 Pharmacodynamic Parameters

For single- and double-stranded RNAs the level of mRNA, encoding the protein of interest, in the target tissue can be used as target-engagement biomarker. The reduction of mRNA can be quantified in preclinical in vivo studies by harvesting the tissue of interest and measuring the mRNA by real-time quantitative PCR. The effect on the corresponding protein in relevant tissue can also be quantified by ELISA or Western blot.

The key PD parameters, graphically presented in Fig. 3 based on data from Yu et al. [27], are as follows:

Baseline (E_0)—the basal level of mRNA or protein without treatment. Target engagement is often normalized to the mRNA or protein levels from control animals (treated with vehicle).

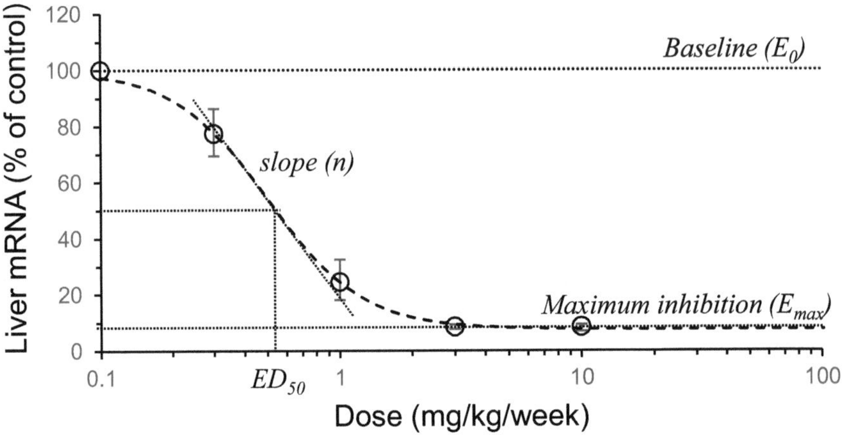

Fig. 3 Schematic illustration of the key PD parameters; E_{max}, E_0, ED_{50} and *n*. Data were digitized from Yu et al. [27] where a GalNAc-conjugated antisense oligonucleotide (ISIS 681257) was dosed subcutaneously for 6 weeks in human transgenic mice

Potency (EC_{50})—affinity of the drug to the target. Defined as the concentration of drug required for half-maximal reduction of mRNA or protein level.

Potency (ED_{50})—the dose of drug required for half-maximal reduction of mRNA or protein level (e.g., with unit mg/kg/week). The parameter is a conglomerate of underlying parameters, that is, clearance, half-life, and potency (e.g., EC_{50}).

Maximum inhibition (E_{max})—the maximum reduction of mRNA or protein. Expressed as fractional inhibition ($0 < E_{max} < 1$).

Sigmoidicity coefficient (n)—the steepness of the dose/concentration-response relationship.

PD half-life—the time it takes for the response to be reduced to half its initial value. The rate parameter determining the onset and duration of drug response for a given drug concentration.

The oligonucleotide dose–response data can often be described by an E_{max} function as:

$$E = E_0 - \frac{E_{max}\mathrm{Dose}^n}{\mathrm{ED}_{50}^n + \mathrm{Dose}^n} \quad (3)$$

or expressed as fractional inhibition ($0 < E_{max} < 1$) as

$$E = E_0\left(1 - \frac{E_{max}\mathrm{Dose}^n}{\mathrm{ED}_{50}^n + \mathrm{Dose}^n}\right) \quad (4)$$

Similarly, the relationship between the tissue or plasma trough concentrations and the mRNA or protein can be characterized by an E_{max} function:

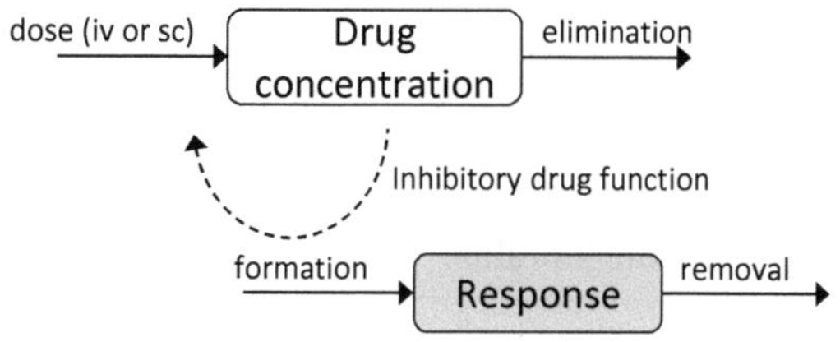

Fig. 4 The turnover model. The response has a continuous formation (e.g., constant rate of formation) and elimination (e.g., constant fraction of the response is cleared per unit of time). The drug is assumed to inhibit the production of the target (mRNA or protein) leading to reduced response levels

$$E = E_0 - \frac{E_{\max} C^n}{\mathrm{EC}_{50}^n + C^n} \quad \text{or} \quad E = E_0 \left(1 - \frac{E_{\max} C^n}{\mathrm{EC}_{50}^n + C^n}\right) \tag{5}$$

If both pharmacokinetic and pharmacodynamic data have been monitored over time one can build a PKPD model where the drug concentration drives the response. The turnover model (Fig. 4) is a common type of PKPD model used for oligonucleotide drugs. Here, the oligonucleotide is assumed to inhibit the production of the target (e.g., mRNA or protein) [28]. In drug discovery, the PKPD model used for human dose prediction may be based on a combination of PK data from higher species such as dog or monkey , and PD data from a human transgenic animal, commonly mouse. In cases where only response data have been monitored over time, a dose–response–time (DRT) model can be used to estimate both PK and PD rate parameters [7].

3 Tactics to Assess Pharmacokinetic and Pharmacodynamic Parameters

3.1 How to Design a Single-Dose Preclinical Pharmacokinetic Study?

To generate informative PK data of an oligonucleotide, one should first consider the drug's pharmacological mode of action. A single-stranded mRNA can be measured directly (*see* for example Geary et al. [29]). A double-stranded siRNA is delivered to the intracellular RNA endonuclease (Ago2) where the antisense strand elicits it pharmacological effect [2, 21, 30]. The intact drug causes a minor pharmacological effect. Therefore, the main interest is mostly put on the PK of the single-stranded oligonucleotide.

Plasma and tissue sample handling are dependent on the sample preparation and the analytical method to be used. One risk is drug degradation in the plasma or tissue-sample test tube. To avoid degradation, one should consult bioanalytical experts to ensure that samples are appropriately handled.

Table 1
Typical drug exposure levels in plasma, converted to concentration per unit administered dose

Type	Route of administration	Drug	C_{max}/dose ((mg/L)/(mg/kg))	C_{last}/dose ((mg/L)/(mg/kg))
Antisense oligonucleotide[a]	Subcutaneous	ISIS301012	0.5	0.0001 (48 h after dose)
siRNA, GalNac conjugated[b]	Intravenous	si-TTR2	4	0.02 (4 h after dose)
siRNA, GalNac conjugated[b]	Subcutaneous	si-TTR2	0.2	0.02 (4 h after dose)
Anti-microRNA[c]	Subcutaneous	RG-101	1	0.002 (average exposure over 168 h after dose)

For example, 10 mg/kg antisense oligonucleotide to mouse is predicted to give a C_{max} of 0.5 (mg/L)/(mg/kg) (as reported in the table) times the dose 10 mg/kg, which is equal to 5 mg/L
[a]Yu et al. [23]. Based on 5 mg/kg dose
[b]Nair et al. [21]. Based on 10 mg/kg dose for both intravenous and subcutaneous administration
[c]Neben et al. [31]. Based on 3 mg/kg dose

Typical drug-exposure levels in plasma that have been reported in the literature for ASOs, anti-miRs, and siRNAs in mice are summarized in Table 1. Exposure levels in rat are generally similar to, or a factor 2 greater, than those in mouse. Table data allow to estimate the range of drug exposure in plasma.

Prior to running more extensive PK studies, it is wise to carefully consider the purpose of such studies, and which PK parameters that are of greatest importance. We recommend a pilot PK study if prior information is sparse. Below is a general guidance on the information-content of each PK parameter and on how the sampling schedule should be designed for accurate determination of the parameters. For oligonucleotide drugs where the drug target is in tissue, the parameters below may also be determined in the tissue of interest.

To obtain an accurate value of C_{max}, frequent matrix sampling is required at time points where C_{max} is anticipated to occur. For a reliable value of $AUC_{0\text{-inf.}}$, the extrapolated curve should not be more than 20–25% of the $AUC_{0\text{-t, last}}$. Clearance (Cl) and administered dose determines the AUC according to the equation AUC = Bioavailability × Dose/Clearance. Bioavailability is commonly assumed to be 1 upon subcutaneous or intravenous administration of oligonucleotides. The correct term if estimating clearance from subcutaneous dosing only is $Cl_{subcutaneous}$.

The PK of oligonucleotides is often characterized by multi-compartment plasma kinetics with rapid (hours) distribution to tissue and slow (weeks) terminal half-life dependent on redistribution from tissue. For ASOs, the terminal plasma exposure half-life is commonly assumed to reflect tissue half-life. Due to the long tissue half-life, one can expect accumulation of drug in tissue for standard dosing intervals (like once weekly, or even for once monthly). Determination of tissue half-life is therefore of general interest to interpret safety aspects, and of specific interest if the target is situated in tissue. These aspects have several implications for the design of a single-dose preclinical PK study:

1. Select the sampling points to allow observation of plasma exposure during the terminal phase. For an ASO, sample densely over 48 h, and then in the order of once weekly for at least 4 weeks. For double-stranded RNAs, a shorter sampling period may be considered.
2. Choose a bioanalytic method that allows detection of low concentration levels. Sensitive methods such as ELISA can be required, while standard LC-MS methods will not always be sufficient.
3. Select a therapeutically relevant dose. Note that the choice of dose influences the chance of having drug concentrations above the lower level of quantification in the terminal samples. However, a super-therapeutic dose could result in concentrations in a nonlinear range not relevant for clinical administration.

The long terminal half-life may result in exposure levels that cannot be measurable. In such cases, only the initial distribution phase is monitored, resulting in an apparent short half-life in plasma that is not reflecting the terminal half-life. If this is suspected, the most straightforward way is to measure the tissue half-life by sampling tissue at two or more time-points. This approach may require a high single dose, as no tissue accumulation will occur. The approach is generally more powerful in a multiple-dosing study.

3.2 How to Design a Preclinical PKPD Study from a PK Perspective?

Based on information from a single-dose preclinical PK study one can design a repeated dosing PKPD study that reaches steady-state tissue exposure. For example, weekly dosing for 6 weeks, potentially with extra loading doses the first week to reach steady state rapidly.

Such a study gives a straightforward way to measure the tissue half-life. One alternative is to sample at two or more time-points during drug administration and infer the tissue half-life. For example, we want to determine the tissue half-life from once weekly dosing, and sample at day 7 (just before the second dose), and at an anticipated steady-state, 7 days after the last dose. Since we do not know the half-life we cannot guarantee to have a sample at steady state; in practice we sample after 4–8 weekly doses and assume steady-state conditions. The accumulation α, visualized in Fig. 5, is calculated as the fraction between exposure at steady state

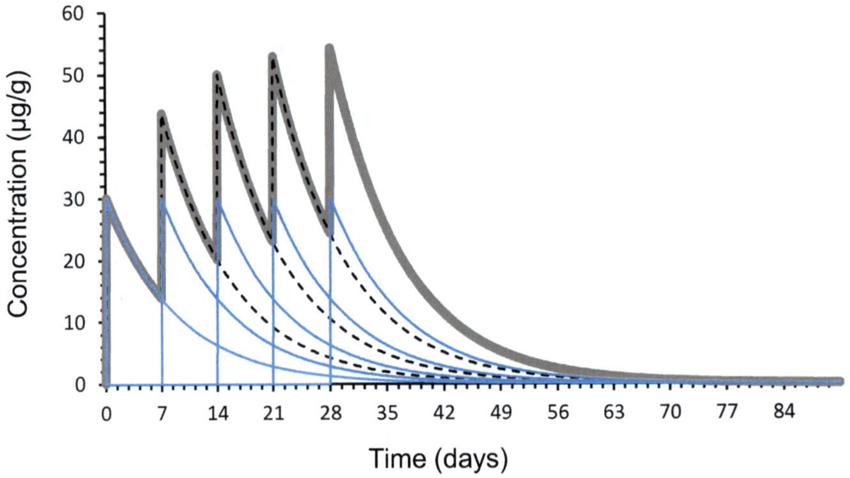

Fig. 5 Principle of using drug accumulation to estimate the half-life. The blue line corresponds to the PK profile after a single dose. The dashed line corresponds to accumulated drug per dosing occasion (sum of the concentration from the previous doses). The grey thick line is the actual observed concentration after repeated dosing. Simulations are based on a half-life of 6 days. The accumulation between day 7 and 28 is about twofold on the level of C_{through} (from 13 to 28 μg/g)

and after a single dose. The tissue half-life is then estimated from the equation

$$\alpha = \frac{1}{1 - e^{-\left(\frac{\log(2)}{t_{1/2}}\right) \times \tau}} \tag{6}$$

where τ represents the time between doses (in this case τ =7 days). Rearranging, we get

$$t_{1/2} = -\frac{\log(2) \times \tau}{\log\left(\frac{\alpha - 1}{\alpha}\right)} \tag{7}$$

Alternatively, one can sample during the washout phase. Be careful to observe at a therapeutically realistic exposure level. For instance, high-dose toxicological studies may not be appropriate due to nonlinearities in the kinetics.

If longitudinal target engagement biomarker data are available one can use dose-response-time modelling to infer the tissue half-life [7]. This alternative second approach requires a mathematical modelling analysis of the resulting data to extract the relevant parameters. Naturally, robustness increases if several approaches are combined.

3.3 How to Design a Preclinical PKPD Study from a PD Perspective?

To get a solid understanding of the dose or concentration that is needed to reduce the mRNA or protein to a certain level, a dose/concentration–response relationship can be established. The single- or double-stranded RNA can be weekly dosed (with potential

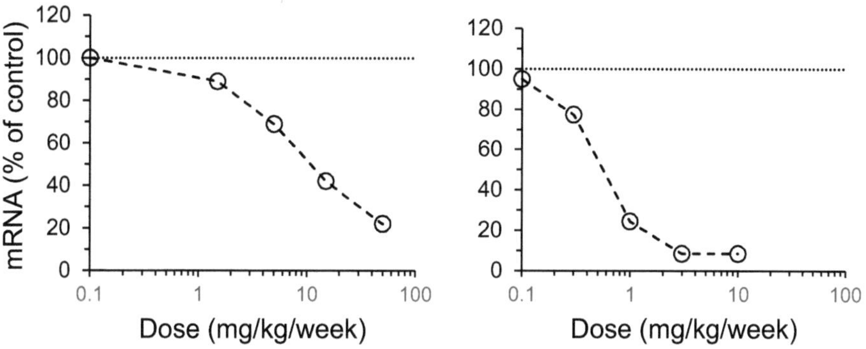

Fig. 6 Examples of dose-response data for two different study designs. In the design to the left the doses are sub-optimally spread and this design will give uncertain estimates of E_{max} and EC_{50}/ED_{50}. In the design to the right the selected doses are covering the full range of responses and will give more certain estimates of E_{max} and EC_{50}/ED_{50}. Data were digitized from Graham et al. 2013 [32] and Yu et al. 2006 [27]

loading doses the first week) in 3–5 dose levels for 4–8 weeks to approach pharmacokinetic steady state. The PD parameters can then be assessed by fitting an E_{max} function to the dose/concentration–response data. The doses should be spread to maximize the chance of determining the EC_{50}/ED_{50} and E_{max} (Fig. 6). Optimally, the lowest dose should have limited effect, the mid doses result in approximately 50% reduction, and the highest doses result in maximal reduction. If the mRNA or protein can be completely inhibited, one high dose resulting in full inhibition is enough to estimate E_{max}. If the fractional $E_{max} < 1$, two high doses both resulting in the same inhibition are needed to get a certain estimate of E_{max}. In Fig. 6, two different dose regimens are presented [27, 32]. The one to the left presents a sub-optimal range of doses where the maximum reduction of response cannot be assessed. The E_{max}, and subsequently the EC_{50}/ED_{50} parameters would be estimated with high uncertainty from these data. In contrast, the right graph shows data for doses that are optimally spread leading to more certain estimates of the E_{max} and EC_{50}/ED_{50} parameters.

We recommend running a pilot dose-response study with 2 or 3 dose levels in a few animals to get an understanding of what dose range to be used in the full dose-response study.

To obtain information about the onset and duration of the response (if the target situated in tissue and repeated sampling is not possible) the animals can be terminated at different time points after the last dose and preferably after different number of doses. A few animals can, for example, be terminated 48 h after a single dose and a few others a week after a single dose. The rest can be dosed for 4–8 weeks and then terminated, for example, 48 h, 1 week, 2 weeks, 3 weeks, and 4 weeks after the last dose. As mentioned previously, data can be analyzed using a dose–response–time model or a PKPD model to obtain the ED_{50}/EC_{50} and PK and PD half-lives.

If the site of action is situated in tissue, biomarkers in a surrogate tissue (e.g., plasma or urine) need to be identified, unless tissue biopsies are acceptable in the clinical studies. These biomarkers should be measurable in healthy volunteers and patients, and preferably be altered after a single dose. The relationship between biomarkers in a surrogate tissue and biomarkers in the target tissue should be established preclinically with respect to onset, intensity, and duration of the response. The relationship between the biomarker in different tissues is then assumed to be identical in animals and humans.

3.4 How to Design a Toxicology Study from a Pharmacokinetic Perspective?

All PK aspects described in the previous sections apply to the design of a toxicological study. A key difference is that higher dose levels will be used. In combination with repeated dosing, such high doses may result in very high exposure at steady-state. Therefore, the predicted steady-state exposure must be considered when designing the study. Naturally, one should consider one or several loading dose(s) to rapidly reach steady-state. In case loading doses are planned in early clinical studies, it can be relevant to use the same schedule in the toxicology study.

If the PK is linear, it is straightforward to predict the exposure in the toxicology study. However, in practice, the PK can be nonlinear as illustrated by nonhuman primate data for an ASO in Table 2. If linear kinetics applies over the dose range, the dose-adjusted parameters would be roughly constant. For the system in Table 2, plasma C_{max} is close to linear, while the plasma AUC and the liver exposure are clearly nonlinear. Note that dose-adjusted plasma AUC increases with dose, while dose-adjusted liver exposure decreases. A high-dose pharmacokinetic study, or literature data from previous studies of similar compounds, or a combination of those, help to inform about the level of nonlinearity to expect.

Table 2
Nonhuman primate PK of an ASO [33]

Dose (mg/kg/wk)	Plasma C_{max} (μg/mL)	Plasma C_{max}/dose	Plasma $AUC_{0-48\ h}$ (μg/mL × h)	Plasma $AUC_{0-48\ h}$/dose	Liver conc. (μg/g)	Liver conc./dose
1	0.960	0.960	2.89	2.89	126	126
3	4.03	1.34	12.2	4.07	243	81.0
12	23.5	1.96	130	10.8	519	43.2
40	62.2	1.56	553	13.8	1101	27.5

The ASO was administered once weekly, and average ($N = 4$–6) data sampled after 4 weeks are reported

A toxicology study often gives an opportunity to measure the terminal plasma half-life or tissue half-life in a higher specie like dog or monkey. This can be highly informative for the efficacy aspects of an oligonucleotide. As already described, one can either sample at two or more time-points during drug administration and infer the tissue half-life from drug accumulation or one can sample during the washout phase. As the low-dose group usually is closest to the anticipated therapeutic dose, that group may be most informative for the efficacy aspects of an oligonucleotide. Hence, one may want to sample more densely on that group if the number of tissue samples is limited. Naturally, the final study design is primarily based on toxicology considerations.

Finally, a toxicology study enables determination of metabolite PK in a higher specie. Key data would include the percentage of individual metabolites compared to the parent, and the half-lives of major metabolites.

3.5 What Aspects to Consider in Phase 1 Clinical Study Design?

When the oligonucleotide is administered repeatedly, accumulation is expected due to the long half-life. This implies that the maximum concentration after a single dose will be lower compared to the maximum concentration at steady state when the same dose has been given repeatedly according to:

$$\alpha = \frac{1}{1 - e^{-\left(\frac{\log(2)}{t_{\mathrm{half}}}\right) \times \tau}} = \frac{C_{\mathrm{max,\ steady\ state}}}{C_{\mathrm{max,\ single\ dose}}} \tag{8}$$

Rearranging, we get

$$C_{\mathrm{max,\ single\ dose}} = \frac{C_{\mathrm{max,\ steady\ state}}}{\alpha} \tag{9}$$

For safety reasons, the predicted tissue concentration range in the multiple ascending dose (MAD) study should be covered by corresponding range in the single ascending dose (SAD) study. If the drug is expected to be accumulated in tissues when dosed repeatedly ($\alpha > 1$), the single doses must be higher than the doses administered repeatedly. If the higher SAD doses are exceeding ~1000 mg they can be fractionated into 2–4 doses, separated in time by at least 24 h. Loading doses may be considered to reach steady state levels faster in the MAD study.

The PK and PD will not be at steady state after a single dose in the SAD study. The observed response will therefore depend on the PK and PD rate parameters. As described previously, the MAD study can be designed to reach a steady state. Here, the time to reach maximum response depends on the PK and PD rate parameters, while the maximum response per se does not.

For safety reasons sentinel dosing (start by dosing one subject + one placebo, dose the rest of the group after an appropriate time delay) is often used for each cohort in clinical Phase 1 studies. The multicompartment plasma kinetics of, for example, an ASO with rapid (hours) distribution to tissue and slow (weeks) terminal half-life results in a maximum drug concentration within ~48 h. The acute safety effects related to plasma exposure of the ASO can be expected to have occurred within ~72 h and the remaining subjects can therefore be dosed after this time delay.

As described in the previous sections of design of nonclinical studies, the terminal half-life can be assessed either by sampling during drug administration and by inferring the tissue half-life from drug accumulation, or by sampling during the washout phase. The half-life on an antisense oligonucleotide is roughly in the range of 10–40 days in humans which means that the washout period preferably should be at least two weeks [14, 29].

As described previously, biomarkers in a surrogate tissue such as plasma or urine may be used for targets situated in tissue. The relationship between drug-induced changes of the biomarker in different tissues should be established in animals. This relationship is then assumed to be applicable to humans.

3.6 How to Scale Pharmacokinetic Parameters from Animal to Human?

Scaling of PK is primarily done to predict a human dose, and to simulate the anticipated concentration-time course. Combined with scaled PD, one can predict the human PD response over time [28]. The PK of oligonucleotides appears to have disposition characteristics that are primarily governed by processes that are relatively conserved across species [1]. Intrinsically, this provides the possibility to scale animal PK to human, and data indicate that human PK is reasonable predictive from animal data for antisense oligonucleotides [22]. In the discovery phase, the predicted human PK of the majority of antisense oligonucleotides have been scaled from monkey. However, in principle, data from lower animal species can be used, potentially to the cost of lower accuracy [34]. To predict the human PK from animal data, one needs to scale clearance, and V_{ss} or half-life.

3.6.1 Scaling of AUC or Clearance

The magnitude of several body processes depends on the size of the organism [35]. For example, it has been shown that the metabolic rate of an organism depends on body weight (BW) as Metabolic rate $= a \times \text{BW}^b$, where a is a constant of appropriate unit, and b is approximately 0.75. Clearance is a rate parameter that is usually assumed to follow the same relationship. Based on empirical findings, this also holds for oligonucleotides. If the metabolic rate is converted to rate per kg body weight, we obtain converting factors (e.g., $\text{Cl}_{\text{animal, per kg}}/\text{Cl}_{\text{human, per kg}}$) which can be used to scale clearance, or AUC, from animal species to human. The ranges reported in Table 3 give a rough estimate of the uncertainty one can expect in the scaling of oligonucleotides. For antisense oligonucleotides, the PPB is slightly lower in mice compared to other species, which can result in a higher ratio between mice and human

Table 3
Theoretical ratio and observed range of clearance per kg body weight in relation to human body weight

Specie	Theoretical ratio	Observed ratio range for oligonucleotides (n)	Source
Mice, 0.025 kg	$Cl_{mice,0.025\ kg}/Cl_{human,70\ kg}$ ~7	3–16 ($n = 5$)	Yu et al. [34, 36] and Geary et al. [37]
Rat, 0.25 kg	$Cl_{rat,\ 0.25\ kg}/Cl_{human,70\ kg}$ ~4	1.5–5 ($n = 4$)	Yu et al. [36] and Geary et al. [37]
Monkey, 3 kg	$Cl_{Monkey,\ 3\ kg}/Cl_{human,70\ kg}$ ~2	0.8–2 ($n = 6$)	Yu et al. [34, 36] and Geary et al. [37]
Dog, 10 kg	$Cl_{dog,\ 10\ kg}/Cl_{human,70\ kg}$ ~1.5	2 ($n = 1$)	Geary et al. [37]

The numbers in the table can be used to predict clearance, or AUC, and its uncertainty range from nonclinical species

than theoretically anticipated [13]. If correcting for specie differences in PPB one obtains a ratio that is more in line with the anticipated theoretical value [23]. We note that the observed AUC scaling ratio from monkey to human tends to be less than the theoretical ratio of two [34]. As PK can be nonlinear for oligonucleotides (Table 2), a general recommendation is to scale PK based on animal doses that correspond to therapeutically relevant exposure.

3.6.2 Scaling of Volume of Distribution

For oligonucleotides, $t_{1/2}$ can be directly estimated from animal data, either using plasma or tissue. The parameter V_{ss} can then be derived from Cl and $t_{1/2}$ according to Eq. 1. There is limited literature information on the scalability of volume of distribution. For small molecules, V_{ss} scales approximately 1:1 on a per kg body weight basis. Geary et al. reported that for ISIS 104838, V_{ss} per kg body weight was similar in human, monkey and dog, but greater in rodents [37]. It is generally challenging to obtain an accurate estimate of V_{ss}, especially since oligonucleotides are metabolized in tissue.

3.6.3 Scaling of Pharmacokinetic Half-Life

No dedicated study has addressed scalability of the terminal PK half-life of oligonucleotides. An important factor to consider when assessing scalability of the terminal PK half-life is to truly obtain the terminal half-life.

For an antisense oligonucleotide (ISIS 301012), the terminal half-life was estimated in rat ($t_{1/2}$ ~ 4.7 days), monkey ($t_{1/2}$ ~ 16 days), and human ($t_{1/2}$ ~ 31 days). Hence, the half-lives in rat and monkey were approximately 15% and 50% of the human half-life. In this study, the authors mentioned that the terminal half-life in rat might have been underestimated [23]. Yu et al. compared liver and kidney terminal half-lives in monkey to plasma half-life in humans for five ASOs. The average monkey/human half-life ratio was ~1, and the range was 0.5 to 1.6 [38]. For one antisense oligonucleotide, the reported terminal half-lives in mouse and rat were 1.5–4 times shorter compared to monkey and human [13, 23].

For siRNA, there are also limited peer-reviewed published data. The terminal half-life is highly dependent on the chemical modification of the backbone. Based on dose-response time modelling (DRT) a crude estimate suggests that the liver half-life of one siRNA in mice was 1–2 weeks, whereas the corresponding estimated half-life in plasma was approximately 20 days [1, 7, 22]. Based on DRT modelling of PCSK9sc02, we have estimated that the effective half-life is approximately two to three times longer in human compared to monkey. We note that DRT modelling is an estimate of the biophase half-life. Additionally, the duration of action is slightly longer in human compared to NHP [1, 22]. In summary, based on current limited data the effective half-life in mice is 5–10 times shorter compared to monkey. The effective half-life for siRNA in humans is approximately 1–3 times that of monkey.

3.7 How to Scale PD Parameters from Animal to Human?

3.7.1 Potency and Pharmacodynamic Rate

Potency of oligonucleotide drugs in vivo is expressed in dose-units (i.e., a composite of PK and potency) or in concentration units. Commonly, in vivo dose/concentration–response data are generated for promising oligonucleotide drugs in the discovery phase. If preclinical concentration–response data are based on tissue exposure (e.g., liver tissue exposure), the tissue–plasma concentration ratio for the preclinical specie is used to convert predicted clinical plasma exposure to an anticipated human liver exposure. If preclinical concentration–response data have been generated, the scaling to human should take the following factors into account:

- Are the data sampled after a single dose or after repeated dosing? If data are sampled after repeated dosing, is the system at steady state (i.e., PK and PD steady state)? If not, can the steady state be estimated?
- What previous information is available about scaling effective concentration/dose for this cell type? If there are historical data for effective scaling from animals to human this information should be considered (e.g., liver/hepatocyte target). If only limited data are available for scaling efficacious concentrations for this particular tissue/cell, there will be intrinsic uncertainties in the scaling.
- Do you anticipate difference in affinity for the mRNA in the preclinical animal model compared to human?

- Yes—adjust for this difference in your scaling. If the difference is not known, generate in vitro data or transgenic animal data to find a correction factor.
- No—assume 1:1 scaling.

- Do you anticipate specie difference in PPB? This is relevant if potency is defined from plasma concentrations. For small-molecule drugs, one converts the plasma concentration to an unbound level and assume the unbound plasma potency scales 1:1.

Note that the effective concentration (e.g., EC_{50}) is an affinity parameter and not a rate parameter. This means, assuming that factors above have been considered, it can be scaled as 1:1.

The predicted PD rate parameters can either be based on literature data of this particular response or scaled from animal data. If scaled from animal data, the anticipated human PD response rate (ke) is modelled as $ke_{human} = ke_{animal} \times (BW_{animal}/BW_{human})^b$, where b is approximately 0.25. If response rate is defined as an half-life the equation would be $t_{1/2\ PD,\ human} = t_{1/2,\ PD,animal} \times (BW_{human}/BW_{animal})^b$, where, again, b is approximately 0.25 [35].

3.7.2 ED_{50} or Effective Dose

If potency (i.e., affinity of the drug to the target) can be assumed equal in preclinical species and in human, scaling of ED_{50} from animal to human is essentially a scaling of preclinical PK to human [1]. Below we provide scaling factors that can be useful to assess animal effective doses and how these would equate to a human dose. Here, they are defined as "ED_{50}," but the scaling factors can also be used for other types of "effective dose" measurements (e.g., daily dose required to reach 60% reduction of a circulating protein). Note that scaling factors are similar to clearance scaling factors (*see* Table 3).

$ED_{50,\ human} = ED_{50,\ mice}/3\text{–}10.$

$ED_{50,\ human} = ED_{50,\ rat}/3\text{–}8.$

$ED_{50,\ human} = ED_{50,\ NHP}/0.5\text{–}2.$

In addition to the aforementioned there also are some cautions and assumption that should be considered:

Duration of study: if the duration of the study is short (e.g., single dose), one cannot scale directly using the suggested factors. This is because the half-life is generally shorter in animals compared to human. However, if the study duration is sufficiently long (i.e., PKPD is near steady state) and assuming that the average drug tissue exposure drives the effect, the scaling factor can be used (*see* Figs. 5 and 7).

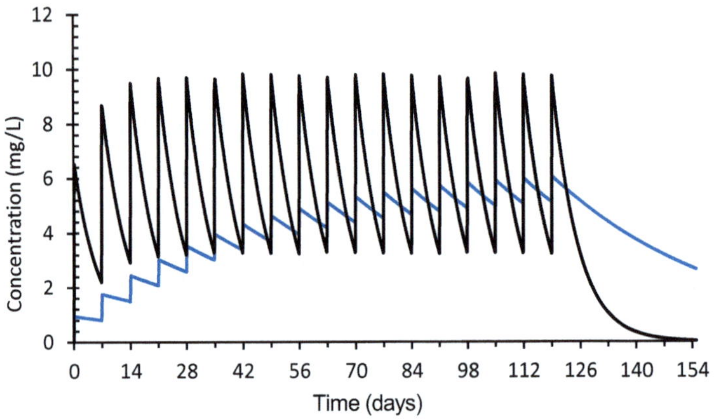

Fig. 7 Pharmacokinetic profiles for two species with different terminal half-life. The black line represents a hypothetical drug PK profile in tissue in mice. The half-life is 4 days and repeated dosing of 100 (arbitrary unit) every 7 days is applied. The blue line represents the PK of the same drug given to human. The half-life is scaled to ~30 days by adjusting clearance with a factor of 7, and the dose is 14 (scaled dose by a factor of 7) every seventh day. We notice that once steady-state has been reached (i.e., 90 days and onward) the average concentration is similar in mouse and human, although mouse reaches steady-state substantially earlier. Note the large difference in drug exposure after the first dose and the difference between C_{max} and $C_{through}$ at steady state

Biomarker used: in addition to difference in the PK profile, the type of biomarker used might also substantially influence the scaling. If a target-engagement biomarker is used (i.e., mRNA levels or circulating protein for the encoded mRNA) the scaling factor is more reliable than using a downstream biomarker (e.g., glucose levels or lipids).

4 Concluding Remarks

Based on a couple of general questions that relate to the PK and PD of oligonucleotides, we have addressed tactics and recommendations on the design and analysis of in vivo data. The chapter has focused on single-stranded oligonucleotides, as the literature is richer for this class of oligonucleotides compared to double-stranded RNAs.

Compared to PKPD of small-molecule compounds, oligonucleotides stand out in several respects. First, the PK is largely determined by the nucleotide backbone and sequence-independent within each class of oligonucleotides, something that opens for class-based rules of thumb for PK and scaling. Second, the terminal half-life of oligonucleotides is typically longer than for small-molecule drugs, affecting in vivo study design. Third, data on the target-engagement biomarker (i.e., the mRNA) are usually available. Fourth, oral bioavailability is very low for oligonucleotides, making oral administration infeasible, at least without permeability enhancers.

There are also similarities between PKPD of small-molecule compounds and oligonucleotides. The same mathematical framework can be used for both modalities. That includes noncompartmental analysis and standard compartment models for PK, and E_{max} models and turnover models for PD.

References

1. Andersson S, Antonsson M, Elebring M, Jansson-Lofmark R, Weidolf L (2018) Drug metabolism and pharmacokinetic strategies for oligonucleotide- and mRNA-based drug development. Drug Discov Today 23:1733. https://doi.org/10.1016/j.drudis.2018.05.030
2. Crooke ST, Witztum JL, Bennett CF, Baker BF (2018) RNA-targeted therapeutics. Cell Metab 27(4):714–739. https://doi.org/10.1016/j.cmet.2018.03.004
3. Valeur E, Gueret SM, Adihou H, Gopalakrishnan R, Lemurell M, Waldmann H, Grossmann TN, Plowright AT (2017) New modalities for challenging targets in drug discovery. Angew Chem Int Ed Engl 56(35):10294–10323. https://doi.org/10.1002/anie.201611914
4. Durham TB, Blanco MJ (2015) Target engagement in lead generation. Bioorg Med Chem Lett 25(5):998–1008. https://doi.org/10.1016/j.bmcl.2014.12.076
5. Morgan P, Brown DG, Lennard S, Anderton MJ, Barrett JC, Eriksson U, Fidock M, Hamren B, Johnson A, March RE, Matcham J, Mettetal J, Nicholls DJ, Platz S, Rees S, Snowden MA, Pangalos MN (2018) Impact of a five-dimensional framework on R&D productivity at AstraZeneca. Nat Rev Drug Discov 17(3):167–181. https://doi.org/10.1038/nrd.2017.244
6. Visser SA, Aurell M, Jones RD, Schuck VJ, Egnell AC, Peters SA, Brynne L, Yates JW, Jansson-Lofmark R, Tan B, Cooke M, Barry ST, Hughes A, Bredberg U (2013) Model-based drug discovery: implementation and impact. Drug Discov Today 18 (15-16):764–775. https://doi.org/10.1016/j.drudis.2013.05.012
7. Jansson-Lofmark R, Gennemark P (2018) Inferring half-lives at the effect site of oligonucleotide drugs. Nucleic Acid Ther 28:319–325. https://doi.org/10.1089/nat.2018.0739
8. Tillman LG, Geary RS, Hardee GE (2008) Oral delivery of antisense oligonucleotides in man. J Pharm Sci 97(1):225–236. https://doi.org/10.1002/jps.21084
9. Larson SD, Jackson LN, Chen LA, Rychahou PG, Evers BM (2007) Effectiveness of siRNA uptake in target tissues by various delivery methods. Surgery 142(2):262–269. https://doi.org/10.1016/j.surg.2007.03.011
10. Liang F, Lindgren G, Lin A, Thompson EA, Ols S, Rohss J, John S, Hassett K, Yuzhakov O, Bahl K, Brito LA, Salter H, Ciaramella G, Lore K (2017) Efficient targeting and activation of antigen-presenting cells in vivo after modified mRNA vaccine administration in rhesus macaques. Mol Ther 25(12):2635–2647. https://doi.org/10.1016/j.ymthe.2017.08.006
11. Svitkin YV, Cheng YM, Chakraborty T, Presnyak V, John M, Sonenberg N (2017) N1-methyl-pseudouridine in mRNA enhances translation through eIF2alpha-dependent and independent mechanisms by increasing ribosome density. Nucleic Acids Res 45 (10):6023–6036. https://doi.org/10.1093/nar/gkx135
12. Crooke ST (ed) (2001) Antisense drug technology: principles, strategies, and applications, 2nd edn. Marcel Dekker, New York, 948p
13. Watanabe TA, Geary RS, Levin AA (2006) Plasma protein binding of an antisense oligonucleotide targeting human ICAM-1 (ISIS 2302). Oligonucleotides 16(2):169–180. https://doi.org/10.1089/oli.2006.16.169
14. Geary RS, Norris D, Yu R, Bennett CF (2015) Pharmacokinetics, biodistribution and cell uptake of antisense oligonucleotides. Adv Drug Deliv Rev 87:46–51. https://doi.org/10.1016/j.addr.2015.01.008

15. Geary RS, Baker BF, Crooke ST (2015) Clinical and preclinical pharmacokinetics and pharmacodynamics of mipomersen (kynamro ((R))): a second-generation antisense oligonucleotide inhibitor of apolipoprotein B. Clin Pharmacokinet 54(2):133–146. https://doi.org/10.1007/s40262-014-0224-4
16. Baek MS, Yu RZ, Gaus H, Grundy JS, Geary RS (2010) In vitro metabolic stabilities and metabolism of 2′-O-(methoxyethyl) partially modified phosphorothioate antisense oligonucleotides in preincubated rat or human whole liver homogenates. Oligonucleotides 20 (6):309–316. https://doi.org/10.1089/oli.2010.0252
17. Kazmi F, Yerino P, McCoy C, Parkinson A, Buckley DB, Ogilvie BW (2018) An assessment of the in vitro inhibition of cytochrome P450 enzymes, UDP-glucuronosyltransferases, and transporters by phosphodiester- or phosphorothioate-linked oligonucleotides. Drug Metab Dispos 46(8):1066–1074. https://doi.org/10.1124/dmd.118.081729
18. Zou Y, Tiller P, Chen IW, Beverly M, Hochman J (2008) Metabolite identification of small interfering RNA duplex by high-resolution accurate mass spectrometry. Rapid Commun Mass Spectrom 22(12):1871–1881. https://doi.org/10.1002/rcm.3561
19. Wang L, Ji C (2016) Advances in quantitative bioanalysis of oligonucleotide biomarkers and therapeutics. Bioanalysis 8(2):143–155. https://doi.org/10.4155/bio.15.234
20. Hung G, Xiao X, Peralta R, Bhattacharjee G, Murray S, Norris D, Guo S, Monia BP (2013) Characterization of target mRNA reduction through in situ RNA hybridization in multiple organ systems following systemic antisense treatment in animals. Nucleic Acid Ther 23 (6):369–378. https://doi.org/10.1089/nat.2013.0443
21. Nair JK, Attarwala H, Sehgal A, Wang Q, Aluri K, Zhang X, Gao M, Liu J, Indrakanti R, Schofield S, Kretschmer P, Brown CR, Gupta S, Willoughby JLS, Boshar JA, Jadhav V, Charisse K, Zimmermann T, Fitzgerald K, Manoharan M, Rajeev KG, Akinc A, Hutabarat R, Maier MA (2017) Impact of enhanced metabolic stability on pharmacokinetics and pharmacodynamics of GalNAc-siRNA conjugates. Nucleic Acids Res 45(19):10969–10977. https://doi.org/10.1093/nar/gkx818
22. Gupta A (2015) Drug metabolism and pharmacokinetic (DMPK) properties of siRNA-GalNAc conjugates. DIA/FDA oligonucleotide based therapeutic conference, September 09–11, 2015. http://www.alnylam.com/web/assets/DIA_DMPK_09092015.pdf. Accessed 08 Aug 2018
23. Yu RZ, Kim TW, Hong A, Watanabe TA, Gaus HJ, Geary RS (2007) Cross-species pharmacokinetic comparison from mouse to man of a second-generation antisense oligonucleotide, ISIS 301012, targeting human apolipoprotein B-100. Drug Metab Dispos 35(3):460–468. https://doi.org/10.1124/dmd.106.012401
24. Rowland M, Tozer TN (1995) Clinical pharmacokinetics: concepts and applications. Lippincott Williams & Wilkins, Baltimore
25. Graham MJ, Crooke ST, Monteith DK, Cooper SR, Lemonidis KM, Stecker KK, Martin MJ, Crooke RM (1998) In vivo distribution and metabolism of a phosphorothioate oligonucleotide within rat liver after intravenous administration. J Pharmacol Exp Ther 286 (1):447–458
26. Donner AJ, Wancewicz EV, Murray HM, Greenlee S, Post N, Bell M, Lima WF, Swayze EE, Seth PP (2017) Co-administration of an excipient oligonucleotide helps delineate pathways of productive and nonproductive uptake of phosphorothioate antisense oligonucleotides in the liver. Nucleic Acid Ther 27 (4):209–220. https://doi.org/10.1089/nat.2017.0662
27. Yu RZ, Graham MJ, Post N, Riney S, Zanardi T, Hall S, Burkey J, Shemesh CS, Prakash TP, Seth PP, Swayze EE, Geary RS, Wang Y, Henry S (2016) Disposition and pharmacology of a GalNAc3-conjugated ASO targeting human lipoprotein (a) in mice. Mol Ther Nucleic Acids 5:e317. https://doi.org/10.1038/mtna.2016.26
28. Callies S, Andre V, Patel B, Waters D, Francis P, Burgess M, Lahn M (2011) Integrated analysis of preclinical data to support the design of the first in man study of LY2181308, a second generation antisense oligonucleotide. Br J Clin Pharmacol 71(3):416–428. https://doi.org/10.1111/j.1365-2125.2010.03836.x
29. Geary RS (2009) Antisense oligonucleotide pharmacokinetics and metabolism. Expert Opin Drug Metab Toxicol 5(4):381–391. https://doi.org/10.1517/17425250902877680
30. Park J, Park J, Pei Y, Xu J, Yeo Y (2016) Pharmacokinetics and biodistribution of recently-developed siRNA nanomedicines. Adv Drug Deliv Rev 104:93–109. https://doi.org/10.1016/j.addr.2015.12.004
31. Steven Neben KL, Jia Tay, Nelson Chau, Yoshio Morikawa, Balkrishnan Bhat, Neil Gibson (2015) RG-101, A novel GalNac-conjugate inhibitor of microRNA-122, demonstrates significant viral load reduction

and reduces liver steatosis in human hepatocyte chimeric mice infected with genotype 1A or hard-to-treat genotype 3A hepatitis C virus (HCV). EASL 50th congress of hepatology. http://ir.regulusrx.com/static-files/bebec48e-c06f-4289-bf25-723ba3f856af. Accessed 13 Aug 2018.

32. Graham MJ, Lee RG, Bell TA 3rd, Fu W, Mullick AE, Alexander VJ, Singleton W, Viney N, Geary R, Su J, Baker BF, Burkey J, Crooke ST, Crooke RM (2013) Antisense oligonucleotide inhibition of apolipoprotein C-III reduces plasma triglycerides in rodents, nonhuman primates, and humans. Circ Res 112 (11):1479–1490. https://doi.org/10.1161/CIRCRESAHA.111.300367

33. Yu RZ, Gunawan R, Post N, Zanardi T, Hall S, Burkey J, Kim TW, Graham MJ, Prakash TP, Seth PP, Swayze EE, Geary RS, Henry SP, Wang Y (2016) Disposition and pharmacokinetics of a GalNAc3-conjugated antisense oligonucleotide targeting human lipoprotein (a) in monkeys. Nucleic Acid Ther 26 (6):372–380. https://doi.org/10.1089/nat.2016.0623

34. Yu RZ, Grundy JS, Henry SP, Kim TW, Norris DA, Burkey J, Wang Y, Vick A, Geary RS (2015) Predictive dose-based estimation of systemic exposure multiples in mouse and monkey relative to human for antisense oligonucleotides with 2′-o-(2-methoxyethyl) modifications. Mol Ther Nucleic Acids 4: e218. https://doi.org/10.1038/mtna.2014.69

35. Gabrielsson J, Weiner D (2012) Non-compartmental analysis. Methods Mol Biol 929:377–389. https://doi.org/10.1007/978-1-62703-050-2_16

36. Yu RZ, Lemonidis KM, Graham MJ, Matson JE, Crooke RM, Tribble DL, Wedel MK, Levin AA, Geary RS (2009) Cross-species comparison of in vivo PK/PD relationships for second-generation antisense oligonucleotides targeting apolipoprotein B-100. Biochem Pharmacol 77(5):910–919. https://doi.org/10.1016/j.bcp.2008.11.005

37. Geary RS, Yu RZ, Watanabe T, Henry SP, Hardee GE, Chappell A, Matson J, Sasmor H, Cummins L, Levin AA (2003) Pharmacokinetics of a tumor necrosis factor-alpha phosphorothioate 2′-O-(2-methoxyethyl) modified antisense oligonucleotide: comparison across species. Drug Metab Dispos 31 (11):1419–1428. https://doi.org/10.1124/dmd.31.11.1419

38. Rosie Z, Yu PK and PD (2014) Properties of antisense oligonucleotides: bridging nonclinical to clinical. AAPS NBC 19–21 May 2014, San Diego, California https://cms.psav.com/efb7b65/public/download_uploaded_media/pdf/64

Index

Olof Gissberg et al. (eds.), *Oligonucleotide-Based Therapies: Methods and Protocols*, Methods in Molecular Biology, vol. 2036, https://doi.org/10.1007/978-1-4939-9670-4, © Springer Science+Business Media, LLC, part of Springer Nature 2019

E

F

G

H

I

L

M

N

O

U

V

W

Z

MIX
Papier aus verantwortungsvollen Quellen
Paper from responsible sources
FSC® C105338

If you have any concerns about our products,
you can contact us on
ProductSafety@springernature.com

In case Publisher is established outside the EU,
the EU authorized representative is:
Springer Nature Customer Service Center GmbH
Europaplatz 3, 69115 Heidelberg, Germany

Printed by Libri Plureos GmbH
in Hamburg, Germany